Treatment Guidelines for Medicine and Primary Care

2008 Edition

New Treatment Guidelines

Paul D. Chan, MD
Margaret T. Johnson, MD

Current Clinical Strategies Publishing

www.ccspublishing.com/ccs

Current Clinical Strategies Publishing
PO Box 1753
Blue Jay, CA 92317
Phone: 800-331-8227 or 909-744-8070
Fax: 800-965-9420
E-mail: info@ccspublishing.com
www.ccspublishing.com/ccs

Printed in USA

ISBN 978-1-934323-12-0

Table of Contents

Cardiovascular Disorders

Acute Coronary Syndromes (ST-Segment Elevation MI, Non-ST-Segment Elevation MI, and Unstable Angina)

Acute myocardial infarction (AMI) and unstable angina are part of a spectrum known as the acute coronary syndromes (ACS), which have in common a ruptured atheromatous plaque. Plaque rupture results in platelet activation, adhesion, and aggregation, leading to partial or total occlusion of the artery.

These syndromes include ST-segment elevation MI, non-ST-segment elevation MI, and unstable angina. The ECG presentation of ACS includes ST-segment elevation infarction, ST-segment depression (including non–Q-wave MI and unstable angina), and nondiagnostic ST-segment and T-wave abnormalities. Patients with ST-segment elevation MI require immediate reperfusion, mechanically or pharmacologically. The clinical presentation of myocardial ischemia is most often acute chest pain or discomfort.

I. **Characteristics of chest pain and associated symptoms**
   A. **Ischemic chest pain** can be characterized by the the OPQRST mnemonic. Symptoms associated with the highest relative risk of myocardial infarction (MI) include radiation to an upper extremity, particularly when there is radiation to both arms, and pain associated with diaphoresis or with nausea and vomiting. The patient should be asked if current pain is reminiscent of prior MI.
      1. **Onset.** Ischemic pain is typically gradual in onset, although the intensity of the discomfort may wax and wane.
      2. **Provocation and palliation.** Ischemic pain is generally provoked by an activity. Ischemic pain does not change with respiration or position. It may or may not respond to nitroglycerin.
      3. **Quality.** Ischemic pain is often characterized more as a discomfort than pain, and it may be difficult to describe. The patient may describe the pain as squeezing, tightness, pressure, constriction, crushing, strangling, burning, heartburn, fullness in the chest, band-like sensation, knot in the center of the chest, lump in throat, ache, heavy weight on chest. It is usually not described as sharp, fleeting, knife-like, stabbing, or pins and needles-like. The patient may place his clenched fist in the center of the chest, which is known as the "Levine sign."
      4. **Radiation.** Ischemic pain often radiates to other parts of the body including the upper abdomen (epigastrium), shoulders, arms (upper and forearm), wrist, fingers, neck and throat, lower jaw and teeth (but not upper jaw), and not infrequently to the back (specifically the interscapular region). Pain radiating to the upper extremities is highly suggestive of ischemic pain.
      5. **Site.** Ischemic pain is not felt in one specific spot, but rather it is a diffuse discomfort that may be difficult to localize. The patient often indicates the entire chest, rather than localizing it to a specific area by pointing a single finger.
      6. **Time course.** Angina is usually brief (two to five minutes) and is relieved by rest or with nitroglycerin. In comparison, patients with an acute coronary syndrome (ACS) may have chest pain at rest, and the duration is variable but generally lasts longer than 30 minutes. Classic anginal pain lasting more than 20 minutes is particularly suggestive of an ACS.

7. **Associated symptoms.** Ischemic pain is often associated with is shortness of breath, which may reflect pulmonary congestion. Other symptoms may include belching, nausea, indigestion, vomiting, diaphoresis, dizziness, lightheadedness, clamminess, and fatigue. Elderly women and diabetics are more likely to present with such "atypical" symptoms in lieu of classic chest pain.

B. **Characteristics of nonischemic chest discomfort:**
   1. Pleuritic pain, sharp or knife-like pain related to respiratory movements or cough.
   2. Primary or sole location in the mid or lower abdominal region.
   3. Any discomfort localized with one finger.
   4. Any discomfort reproduced by movement or palpation.
   5. Constant pain lasting for days.
   6. Fleeting pains lasting for a few seconds or less.
   7. Pain radiating into the lower extremities or above the mandible.

C. Some patients with ACS present with atypical types of chest pain. Acute ischemia is diagnosed in 22 percent of patients who present with sharp or stabbing pain and 13 percent who presented with pleuritic-type pain.

D. **Atypical symptoms.** Some patients with acute coronary syndrome (ACS) present with atypical symptoms rather than chest pain. One-third have no chest pain on presentation to the hospital. These patients often present with symptoms such as dyspnea alone, nausea and/or vomiting, palpitations, syncope, or cardiac arrest. They are more likely to be older, diabetic, and women.

E. **Additional history and exam**
   1. **Historical features increasing likelihood of ACS**
      a. Patients with a prior history of coronary heart disease (CHD) have a significantly increased risk of recurrent ischemic events.
      b. A prior history of other vascular disease is associated with a risk of cardiac ischemic events comparable to that seen with a prior history of CHD.
      c. Risk factors for CHD, including especially age, sex, diabetes, hypertension, hyperlipidemia, and cigarette smoking.
      d. Recent cocaine use.
   2. **Focused physical exam**
      a. Responsiveness, airway, breathing and circulation.
      b. Evidence of systemic hypoperfusion (hypotension; tachycardia; impaired cognition; cool, clammy, pale, ashen skin). Cardiogenic shock complicating acute MI requires aggressive evaluation and management.
      c. Ventricular arrhythmias. Sustained ventricular tachyarrhythmias in the periinfarction period must be treated immediately because of their deleterious effect on cardiac output, possible exacerbation of myocardial ischemia, and the risk of deterioration into VF.
      d. Evidence of heart failure (jugular venous distention, rales, S3 gallop, hypotension, tachycardia).
      e. A screening neurologic examination should be performed to assess for focal lesions or cognitive deficits that might preclude safe use of thrombolytic therapy.

Differential diagnosis of severe or prolonged chest pain

Myocardial infarction
Unstable angina
Aortic dissection
Gastrointestinal disease (esophagitis, esophageal spasm, peptic ulcer disease, biliary colic, pancreatitis)
Pericarditis
Chest-wall pain (musculoskeletal or neurologic)
Pulmonary disease (pulmonary embolism, pneumonia, pleurisy, pneumothorax)
Psychogenic hyperventilation syndrome

---

      f. Exam findings increasing likelihood of MI. Findings on physical examination associated with significantly increased risk of myocardial infarction are hypotension (systolic blood pressure <80) and signs of pump failure (ie, new or worsening pulmonary crackles, new S3, new or worsening MR murmur).

II. Immediate management

A. During the initial assessment phase, the following steps should be accomplished for any patient with significant risk of ACS:

  1. Airway, breathing, and circulation assessed
  2. 12-lead ECG obtained
  3. Resuscitation equipment brought nearby
  4. Cardiac monitor attached
  5. Oxygen given
  6. IV access and blood work obtained
  7. Aspirin 162 to 325 mg given
  8. Nitrates and morphine given (unless contraindicated)

B. Twelve-lead ECG should be obtained in all patients with possible coronary ischemia. The 12-lead ECG provides the basis for initial diagnosis and management. The initial ECG is often not diagnostic in patients with ACS. The ECG should be repeated at 5 to 10 minute intervals, if the initial ECG is not diagnostic but the patient remains symptomatic and there is a high clinical suspicion for MI.

C. Cardiac monitoring should be initiated with emergency resuscitation equipment (including a defibrillator and airway equipment) nearby.

D. Supplemental oxygen should be initiated to maintain oxygen saturation above 90 percent.

E. Intravenous access should be established, with blood drawn for initial laboratory work, including cardiac biomarkers.

F. Aspirin should be given to all patients at a dose of 162 to 325 mg to chew and swallow, unless there is a compelling contraindication (eg, history of anaphylactic reaction) or it has been taken prior to presentation.

G. Sublingual nitroglycerin should be administered at a dose of 0.4 mg every five minutes for a total of three doses, after which an assessment is made about the need for intravenous nitroglycerin. Before this is done, all men should be questioned about the use of sildenafil (Viagra), vardenafil (Levitra), or tadalafil (Cialis); nitrates are contraindicated if these drugs have been used in the last 24 hours (36 hours with tadalafil) because of the risk of severe hypotension.

  1. Extreme care should also be taken before giving nitrates in the setting of an inferior myocardial infarction with possible involvement of the right ventricle. Nitrate use can cause severe hypotension in this setting.

H. Intravenous morphine sulfate at an initial dose of 2 to 4 mg, with increments of 2 to 8 mg, repeated at 5 to 15 minute intervals, should be given for the relief of chest pain and anxiety.

III. **ECG-based management of the Four major ischemic syndromes**
   A. ST elevation (Q wave) MI is manifested by Q waves that are usually preceded by hyperacute T waves and ST elevations, and followed by T wave inversions. Clinically significant ST segment elevation is considered to be present if it is greater than 1 mm (0.1 mV) in at least two anatomically contiguous leads.
   B. Non-ST elevation (Non-Q wave) MI is manifested by ST depressions or T-wave inversions without Q waves.
   C. Noninfarction subendocardial ischemia (classic angina), manifested by transient ST segment depressions.
   D. Noninfarction transmural ischemia (Prinzmetal's variant angina) is manifested by transient ST segment elevations or paradoxical T wave normalization.
   E. **Localization of ischemia.** The anatomic location of a transmural infarct is determined by which ECG leads show ST elevation and/or increased T wave positivity:
      1. Acute transmural anterior wall ischemia - one or more of the precordial leads (V1-V6)
      2. Anteroseptal ischemia - leads V1 to V3
      3. Apical or lateral ischemia - leads aVL and I, and leads V4 to V6
      4. Inferior wall ischemia - leads II, III, and aVF
      5. Right ventricular ischemia - right-sided precordial leads
   F. The right-sided leads V4R, V5R, and V6R should be obtained if there is evidence of inferior wall ischemia, demonstrated by ST elevation in leads II, III, and aVF. The posterior leads V7, V8, and V9 may also be helpful if there is evidence of posterior wall ischemia, as suggested by prominent R waves and ST depressions in leads V1 and V2.
   G. **Serial ECGs.** The initial ECG is often not diagnostic in patients with ACS. Therefore, if the initial ECG is not diagnostic, but the patient remains symp-tomatic and there is a high clinical suspicion for MI, it is recommended that the ECG be repeated at 5 to 10 minute intervals.
   H. **LBBB or pacing.** Both LBBB, which is present in 7 percent of patients with an acute MI, and pacing can interfere with the electrocardiographic diagnosis of coronary infarction. Careful evaluation of the ECG may show some evidence of ACS in patients with these abnormalities. The clinical history and cardiac enzymes are of primary importance in diagnosing an ACS in this setting.
   I. **ST elevation.** Regardless of the presence or absence of Q waves, an ST elevation MI (STEMI) is diagnosed in the following circumstances:
      1. ST segment elevation ≥1 mm is present in two or more anatomically contiguous leads.
      2. The elevations are considered to represent ischemia and not pericarditis or left ventricular aneurysm.
   J. The patient should also be presumed to have an acute STEMI if the ECG shows a left bundle branch block that is not known to be old and the clinical suspicion for an ACS is high.
   K. **Reperfusion therapy.** A patient with an acute STEMI should undergo reperfusion therapy with either primary percutaneous intervention (PCI) or thrombolysis, if less than 12 hours has elapsed from the onset of symptoms. Benefit from thrombolysis is significantly greater when given within four hours of the onset of symptoms. Primary PCI is preferred to thrombolysis when readily available.
   L. **Antiplatelet therapy** is indicated in all patients with STEMI, regardless of whether they undergo reperfusion therapy, unless an absolute contraindication exists.
      1. Aspirin is the preferred antiplatelet agent and should be given in a dose of 162 to 325 mg to chew and swallow as soon as possible to any patient with

STEMI.

2. Clopidogrel (Plavix) is recommended in all patients treated with primary PCI and stenting. A 600 mg loading dose should begin in these patients, and primary PCI should be done within 90 minutes. Benefit from the use of clopidogrel in addition to aspirin has also been demonstrated in patients under 75 years of age undergoing thrombolysis. Patients over 75 years of age generally receive 75 mg because of the increased risk of hemorrhage.

3. Clopidogrel (300 mg loading dose followed by 75 mg once daily) is given to patients who are managed without reperfusion therapy in this setting based upon the benefit demonstrated in nonrevascularized patients with non-ST elevation syndromes.

4. Clopidogrel can also be given in the rare case where aspirin is contraindicated.

M. **Glycoprotein IIb/IIIa inhibitors**. Treatment with abciximab should be started as early as possible prior to PCI, with or without stent, in patients with STEMI.

N. **Beta blockers** should be administered to all patients with ST elevation MI without contraindications. Early intravenous use of a cardioselective agent, such as metoprolol or atenolol, is recommended:

1. Intravenous metoprolol can be given in 5 mg increments by slow intravenous administration (5 mg over one to two minutes), repeated every five minutes for a total initial dose of 15 mg. Patients who tolerate this regimen should then receive oral therapy beginning 15 minutes after the last intravenous dose (25 to 50 mg every six hours for 48 hours) followed by a maintenance dose of 100 mg twice daily.

2. Intravenous atenolol can be given in a 5 mg dose, followed by another 5 mg, five minutes later. Patients who tolerate this regimen should then receive oral therapy beginning one to two hours after the last intravenous dose (50 to 100 mg/day).

3. Esmolol (Brevibloc) (50 mcg/kg per min increasing to a maximum of 200 to 300 mcg/kg per min) can be used if an ultrashort acting beta blocker is required.

O. **Intravenous nitroglycerin** can be given for treatment of persistent pain, congestive heart failure, or hypertension, provided there are no contraindications (eg, use of drugs for erectile dysfunction or right ventricular infarction). The goal of therapy is a 10 percent reduction in the systolic blood pressure or a 30 percent reduction in hypertensive patients.

Therapy for Non-ST Segment Myocardial Infarction and Unstable Angina	
Treatment	**Recommendations**
Antiplatelet agent	Aspirin, 325 mg (chewable)
Nitrates	Sublingual nitroglycerin (Nitrostat), one tablet every 5 min for total of three tablets initially, followed by IV form (Nitro-Bid IV, Tridil) if needed
Beta-blocker	• IV therapy recommended for prompt response, followed by oral therapy. • Metoprolol (Lopressor), 5 mg IV every 5 min for three doses • Atenolol (Tenormin) 5 mg IV q5min x 2 doses • Esmolol (Brevibloc), initial IV dose of 50 micrograms/kg/min and adjust up to 200-300 micrograms/kg/min

Treatment	Recommendations
Heparin	80 U/kg IVP, followed by 15 U/kg/hr. Goal: aPTT 50-70 sec
Enoxaparin (Lovenox)	1 mg/kg IV, followed by 1 mg/kg subcutaneously bid
Glycoprotein IIb/IIIa inhibitors	Eptifibatide (Integrilin) or tirofiban (Aggrastat) for patients with high-risk features in whom an early invasive approach is planned
Adenosine diphosphate receptor-inhibitor	Consider clopidogrel (Plavix) therapy, 300 mg x 1, then 75 mg qd.
Cardiac catheterization	Consideration of early invasive approach in patients at intermediate to high risk and those in whom conservative management has failed

P. Potassium. The ACC/AHA guidelines recommend maintaining the serum potassium concentration above 4.0 meq/L in an acute MI. Maintaining a serum magnesium concentration above 2.0 meq/L is recommended.

Q. Unfractionated heparin (UFH) is given to patients with with STEMI undergoing percutaneous or surgical revascularization, and to patients undergoing thrombolysis with selective fibrinolytic agents. Low molecular weight heparin (LMWH) is an alternative to UFH in patients receiving thrombolysis provided they are younger than 75 years of age and have no renal dysfunction.

Treatment Recommendations for ST-Segment Myocardial Infarction

Supportive Care for Chest Pain
- All patients should receive supplemental oxygen, 2 L/min by nasal canula, for a minimum of three hours
- Two large-bore IVs should be placed

Aspirin:	
Inclusion	Clinical symptoms or suspicion of AMI
Exclusion	Aspirin allergy, active GI bleeding
Recommendation	Chew and swallow one dose of160-325 mg, then orally qd

Thrombolytics:	
Inclusion	All patients with ischemic pain and ST-segment elevation ($\geq$1 mm in $\geq$2 contiguous leads) within 6 hours of onset of persistent pain, age <75 years. All patients with a new bundle branch block and history suggesting acute MI.
Exclusion	Active internal bleeding; history of cerebrovascular accident; recent intracranial or intraspinal surgery or trauma; intracranial neoplasm, arteriovenous malformation, or aneurysm; known bleeding diathesis; severe uncontrolled hypertension
Recommendation	**Reteplase (Retavase)** 10 U IVP over 2 min x 2. Give second dose of 10 U 30 min after first dose **OR** **Tenecteplase (TNKase):** <60 kg: 30 mg IVP; 60-69 kg: 35 mg IVP; 70-79 kg: 40 mg IVP; 80-89 kg: 45 mg IVP; $\geq$90 kg: 50 mg IVP **OR** **t-PA (Alteplase, Activase)** 15 mg IV over 2 minutes, then 0.75 mg/kg (max 50 mg) IV over 30 min, followed by 0.5 mg/kg (max 35 mg) IV over 30 min.

Heparin:	
Inclusion	**Administer concurrently with thrombolysis**
Exclusion	Active internal or CNS bleeding
Recommendation	Heparin 60 U/kg (max 4000 U) IVP, followed by 12 U/kg/hr (max 1000 U/h) continuous IV infusion x 48 hours. Maintain aPTT 50-70 seconds

Beta-Blockade:	
Inclusion	All patients with the diagnosis of AMI. Begin within 12 hours of diagnosis of AMI
Exclusion	Severe COPD, hypotension, bradycardia, AV block, pulmonary edema, cardiogenic shock
Recommendation	Metoprolol (Lopressor), 5 mg IV push every 5 minutes for three doses; followed by 25 mg PO bid. Titrate up to 100 mg PO bid **OR** Atenolol (Tenormin), 5 mg IV, repeated in 5 minutes, followed by 50-100 mg PO qd.

Nitrates:	
Inclusion	All patients with ischemic-type chest pain
Exclusion	Hypotension; caution in right ventricular infarction
Recommendation	0.4 mg NTG initially q 5 minutes, up to 3 doses or nitroglycerine aerosol, 1 spray sublingually every 5 minutes. IV infusion of NTG at 10-20 mcg/min, titrating upward by 5-10 mcg/min q 5-10 minutes (max 3 mcg/kg/min). Slow or stop infusion if systolic BP <90 mm Hg

ACE-Inhibitors or Angiotensin Receptor Blockers:	
Inclusion	All patients with the diagnosis of AMI. Initiate treatment within 24 hours after AMI
Exclusion	Bilateral renal artery stenosis, angioedema caused by previous treatment
Recommendation	Lisinopril (Prinivil) 2.5-5 mg qd, titrate to 10-20 mg qd. Maintain systolic BP >100 mmHg or Valsartan (Diovan) 40 mg bid, titrate to 160 mg bid

IV. **Non-ST elevation.** Patients with coronary ischemia but who do not manifest ST elevations on ECG are considered to have unstable angina (UA) or a non-ST elevation myocardial infarction (NSTEMI). UA and NSTEMI comprise part of the spectrum of ACS.

  A. Angina is considered unstable if it presents in any of the following three ways:
  1. Rest angina, generally lasting longer than 20 minutes
  2. New onset angina that markedly limits physical activity
  3. Increasing angina that is more frequent, lasts longer, or occurs with less exertion than previous angina

  B. NSTEMI is distinguished from UA by the presence of elevated serum biomarkers. ST segment elevations and Q waves are absent in both UA and NSTEMI. Unstable angina and NSTEMI are frequently indistinguishable initially because an elevation in serum biomarkers is usually not detectable for four to six hours after an MI, and at least 12 hours are required to detect elevations in all patients.

  C. **Risk stratification**
  1. The TIMI investigators developed a 7-point risk stratification tool that predicted the risk of death, reinfarction, or urgent revascularization at 14 days after presentation. This scoring system includes the following elements:
     a. Age >65.
     b. Three or more cardiac risk factors.
     c. Aspirin use in the preceding seven days.
     d. Two or more anginal events in the preceding 24 hours.
     e. ST-segment deviation on presenting ECG.
     f. Increased cardiac biomarkers.
     g. Prior coronary artery stenosis >50 percent.
  2. Patients are considered to be high risk if they have a TIMI risk score of 5 or greater (one point is given for each element) and low risk if the score is 2 or below.
  3. Additional factors associated with death and reinfarction at 30 days after presentation include:
     a. Bradycardia or tachycardia
     b. Hypotension
     c. Signs of heart failure (new or worsening rales, MR murmur, S3 gallop)
     d. Sustained ventricular tachycardia

  D. **Reperfusion.** Thrombolytic therapy should not be administered to patients with UA or NSTEMI unless subsequent ECG monitoring documents ST segment elevations that persist. An aggressive approach to reperfusion using PCI is best suited for patients with a TIMI risk score >5 or possibly other high-risk features.

  E. **Antiplatelet therapy** is a cornerstone of treatment in UA and NSTEMI.
  1. Aspirin is the preferred antiplatelet agent and should be given to all patients with suspected ACS.
  2. Clopidogrel (300-600 mg) is indicted in patients undergoing PCI. A class IIa

recommendation was given to their use in patients with high-risk features in whom PCI is not planned.

F. **Beta-blocker, nitroglycerin, morphine.** The use of these agents in NSTEMI is similar to that in STEMI.

G. **Electrolyte repletion.** Low electrolytes, particularly potassium and magnesium, which are associated with an increased risk of ventricular fibrillation in the setting of ACS, should be replaced.

H. **Heparin.** The ACC/AHA guidelines recommend the use of enoxaparin in preference to unfractionated heparin in patients with UA/NSTEMI, provided there is no evidence of renal failure and CABG is not planned within 24 hours.

I. **Disposition of NSTEMI**

1. **High-risk patients** have a high-risk ACS if ST segment depression (≥ 0.05 mV [0.5 mm]) is present in two or more contiguous leads and/or the TIMI risk score is ≥ 5. This patient is admitted to an intensive care unit, coronary care unit, or monitored cardiac unit depending upon the persistence of symptoms and evidence of hemodynamic compromise. Those with persistent pain or hemodynamic compromise generally undergo urgent angiography and revascularization. Others with resolution of symptoms and stable hemodynamics are typically referred for early elective angiography and revascularization if appropriate.

   a. If there is no ST segment elevation or depression or new LBBB, regardless of the presence or absence of Q waves, the patient with definite or probable ACS should still be admitted to a monitored care unit for further evaluation. Those patients manifesting high-risk features either on presentation or during their emergency room course should be considered for early PCI.

2. **Moderate-risk patient.** Patients who have no ECG changes and are at moderate risk for ACS can be admitted to a chest pain observation unit, if available, for further evaluation because a small percentage (2 to 4 percent) will have an ACS.

3. **Low-risk patient.** Patients with no ECG changes, a TIMI risk score below 3, and no other concerning features in their presentation can be considered for early provocative testing or possible discharge with outpatient follow-up. Patients at very low risk in whom there is clear objective evidence for a non-ischemic cause of their chest pain can be discharged with outpatient follow-up.

V. **Cardiac biomarkers (enzymes).** Serial serum biomarkers (also called cardiac enzymes) of acute myocardial damage, such as troponin T and I, creatine kinase (CK)-MB, and myoglobin, are essential for confirming the diagnosis of infarction. The most commonly used are troponin T or I and CK-MB, which can be measured by rapid bedside assay.

A. **Sensitivity and specificity.** An elevation in the serum concentration of one or more of the above markers is seen in virtually all patients with an acute MI. However, the sensitivity of these tests is relatively low until four to six hours after symptom onset. Thus, a negative test in this time period does not exclude infarction. Furthermore, some patients do not show a biomarker elevation for as long as 12 hours.

B. Therefore, in patients who have an acute STEMI, reperfusion therapy should not await the results of cardiac biomarkers. In patients without diagnostic ST segment elevation, serial biomarker testing is performed after four or more hours if the initial values are indeterminate, the ECG remains nondiagnostic, and clinical suspicion remains high.

Common Markers for Acute Myocardial Infarction			
Marker	Initial Elevation After MI	Mean Time to Peak Elevations	Time to Return to Baseline
Myoglobin	1-4 h	6-7 h	18-24 h
CTnI	3-12 h	10-24 h	3-10 d
CTnT	3-12 h	12-48 h	5-14 d
CKMB	4-12 h	10-24 h	48-72 h
CKMBiso	2-6 h	12 h	38 h

CTnI, CTnT = troponins of cardiac myofibrils; CPK-MB, MM = tissue isoforms of creatine kinase.

   C. Unstable angina. Patients with cardiac biomarker elevations and unstable angina are considered to have an NSTEMI and should be treated appropriately.

References, see page 372.

Stable Angina Pectoris

Stable angina pectoris is responsible for 11 percent of chest pain episodes; unstable angina or myocardial infarction occur in only 1.5 percent. Musculoskeletal chest pain accounts for 36 percent of all diagnoses (of which costochondritis accounted for 13 percent) followed by reflux esophagitis (13 percent).

I. **Assessment and management of chest pain in the office**
   A. Myocardial infarction, pulmonary embolus, aortic dissection, or tension pneumothorax may cause chest pain and sudden death. Any patient with a recent onset of chest pain who may be potentially unstable should be transported immediately to an emergency department in an ambulance equipped with a defibrillator. Stabilization includes supplemental oxygen, intravenous access, and placement of a cardiac monitor. A 12-lead electrocardiogram and a blood sample for cardiac enzymes should be obtained.
   B. Patients who with possible myocardial infarction should chew a 325 mg aspirin tablet.
   C. Sublingual nitroglycerin should be given unless the patient has relatively low blood pressure or has recently taken a phosphodiesterase inhibitor such as sildenafil (Viagra).
II. **Clinical evaluation**
   A. **Quality of the pain.** The patient with myocardial ischemia may describe the pain as squeezing, tightness, pressure, constriction, strangling, burning, heart burn, fullness in the chest, a band-like sensation, knot in the center of the chest, lump in the throat, ache, weight on chest, and toothache. In some cases, the patient may place his fist in the center of the chest ("Levine sign").
   B. **Region or location of pain.** Ischemic pain is a diffuse discomfort that may be difficult to localize. Pain that localizes to a small area on the chest is more likely of chest wall or pleural origin.

C. **Radiation.** The pain of myocardial ischemia may radiate to the neck, throat, lower jaw, teeth, upper extremity, or shoulder. Chest pain radiation increases the probability of myocardial infarction. Pain radiating to either arm is indicative of coronary ischemia.

D. **Acute cholecystitis** can present with right shoulder pain and right upper quadrant pain. Chest pain that radiates between the scapulae suggests aortic dissection.

E. **Temporal elements**
   1. The pain with a pneumothorax or an aortic dissection or acute pulmonary embolism typically has an abrupt onset.
   2. Ischemic pain usually has gradual onset with an increasing intensity over time.
   3. "Functional" or nontraumatic musculoskeletal chest pain has a vague onset.

F. **Duration of pain**
   1. Chest discomfort that lasts only for seconds or pain that is constant over weeks is not due to ischemia. A span of years without progression makes it more likely that the origin of pain is functional. The pain from myocardial ischemia generally lasts for a few minutes.
   2. Myocardial ischemia is more likely to occur in the morning, correlating with an increase in sympathetic tone.

G. **Provocative factors**
   1. Discomfort that reliably occurs with eating is suggestive of upper gastrointestinal disease.
   2. Chest discomfort provoked by exertion is a classic symptom of angina.
   3. Other factors that may provoke ischemic pain include cold, emotional stress, meals, or sexual intercourse.
   4. Pain made worse by swallowing is usually of esophageal origin.
   5. Body position or movement, as well as deep breathing, may exacerbate chest pain of musculoskeletal origin..
   6. Pleuritic chest pain is worsened by respiration. Causes of pleuritic chest pain include pulmonary embolism, pneumothorax, viral or idiopathic pleurisy, pneumonia, and pleuropericarditis.

H. **Palliation**
   1. Pain that is palliated by antacids or food is likely of gastroesophageal origin.
   2. Pain that responds to sublingual nitroglycerin usually has a cardiac etiology or to be due to esophageal spasm. Pain relief with nitroglycerin not helpful in distinguishing cardiac from noncardiac chest pain.
   3. Pain that abates with cessation of activity suggests an ischemic origin.
   4. **Pericarditis pain** improves with sitting up and leaning forward.

I. **Severity** of pain is not a useful predictor of CHD. One-third of myocardial infarctions may go unnoticed by the patient.

J. **Associated symptoms**
   1. **Belching**, a bad taste in the mouth, and difficult or painful swallowing are suggestive of esophageal disease, although belching and indigestion also may be seen with myocardial ischemia.
   2. **Vomiting** may occur with myocardial ischemia (particularly transmural myocardial infarction) or with peptic ulcer disease, cholecystitis, and pancreatitis.
   3. **Diaphoresis** is more frequently associated with myocardial infarction than esophageal disease.
   4. **Exertional dyspnea** is common when chest pain is due to myocardial ischemia or a pulmonary disorders.
   5. **Cough** may be caused by congestive heart failure, pulmonary embolus, neoplasm, or pneumonia.

K. **Syncope.** The patient with myocardial ischemia may describe presyncope.

Syncope should raise a concern for aortic dissection, pulmonary embolus, a ruptured abdominal aortic aneurysm, or critical aortic stenosis.

L. Palpitations. Patients with ischemia can feel palpitations resulting from ventricular ectopy. Atrial fibrillation is associated with chronic CHD.

M. Risk factors
1. **Hyperlipidemia, left ventricular hypertrophy, or a family history of premature CHD** increase the risk for myocardial ischemia.
2. **Hypertension** is a risk factor for both CHD and aortic dissection.
3. **Cigarette smoking** is a nonspecific risk factor for CHD, thromboembolism, aortic dissection, pneumothorax, and pneumonia
4. **Cocaine** use may be suggestive of myocardial infarction.
5. **Viral infection** may precede pericarditis or myocarditis. Other risk factors for pericarditis include chest trauma, autoimmune disease, recent myocardial infarction or cardiac surgery, and the use of procainamide, hydralazine, or isoniazid.

N. Age. Among patients older than age 40, chest pain resulting from CHD or an acute coronary syndrome (unstable angina or myocardial infarction) becomes increasingly common.
1. Men older than age 60 are most likely to suffer aortic dissection, while young men are at highest risk for primary spontaneous pneumothorax. Young adults of both sexes are diagnosed with viral pleurisy more often than are older patients.
2. A past history of CHD, symptomatic gastroesophageal reflux, peptic ulcer disease, gallstones, panic disorder, bronchospasm, or cancer is very helpful. Diabetics often have nonclassic presentation of CHD.

O. Physical examination
1. **General appearance of the patient** suggests the severity and the seriousness of the symptoms.
2. **Vital signs** can provide clues to the clinical significance of the pain.
3. **Palpation of the chest wall** may evoke pain. Hyperesthesia, particularly when associated with a rash, is often caused by herpes zoster.
4. **Cardiac examination** should include auscultation and palpation in a sitting and supine position to establish the presence of a pericardial rub or signs of acute aortic insufficiency or aortic stenosis. Ischemia may result in a mitral insufficiency murmur or an S4 or S3 gallop.
5. Asymmetric breath sounds and wheezes, crackles or evidence of consolidation should be assessed.
6. Abdomenal examination should assess the right upper quadrant, epigastrium, and the abdominal aorta.

P. Ancillary studies
1. **Normal electrocardiogram.** A normal ECG markedly reduces the probability that chest pain is due to acute myocardial infarction, but it does not exclude a serious cardiac etiology (particularly unstable angina). 1 to 4 percent of patients with normal ECGs will have an acute infarction. A normal ECG in a patient with the recent onset of chest pain suggests stable angina. Aortic dissection should be considered in patients with ongoing pain and a normal ECG.
2. **Abnormal electrocardiogram.** ST segment elevation, ST segment depression or new Q waves are indications of acute myocardial infarction or unstable angina.
3. **Chest radiograph** may assist in the diagnosis of chest pain if a cardiac, pulmonary, or neoplastic etiology is being considered. Aortic dissection, pneumothorax, and pneumomediastinum may be diagnosed.
4. **Exercise stress testing** is indicated for patients with suspected ischemic heart disease who do not have an unstable coronary syndrome (eg, acute

myocardial infarction or unstable angina).

5. **Transthoracic echocardiography** can identify regional wall motion abnormalities within seconds of acute coronary artery occlusion. TTE is also appropriate to assist in the identification of pericarditis with effusion, aortic dissection, and possibly pulmonary embolism.

6. **Myocardial perfusion imaging (MPI)** is a sensitive test for detecting acute myocardial infarction, particularly if the chest pain is ongoing at the time of the study. It can be used to assist in emergency department triage of patients with chest pain. The specificity of acute rest MPI is limited in patients with a previous myocardial infarction.

III. **Medical therapy of stable angina pectoris**

A. Nitrates are a first-line therapy for the treatment of acute anginal symptoms. The primary antiischemic effect of nitrates is to decrease myocardial oxygen demand by producing systemic vasodilation more than coronary vasodilation.

B. **Sublingual nitroglycerin** is the therapy of choice for acute anginal episodes and prophylactically for activities known to elicit angina. The onset of action is within several minutes and the duration of action is 40 minutes. The initial dose is 0.3 mg; one-half the dose (0.15 mg) can be used if the patient becomes hypotensive.

C. **The patient should contact EMS** if chest pain is unimproved or worsening five minutes after one nitroglycerin dose has been taken.

D. **Chronic nitrate therapy** in the form of an oral or transdermal preparation (isosorbide dinitrate, isosorbide mononitrate, or transdermal nitroglycerin) can prevent or reduce the frequency of recurrent anginal episodes and improve exercise tolerance. However, tolerance to long-acting nitrates can develop and has limited their use as first-line therapy. A 12 to 14 hour nitrate-free interval must be observed in order to avoid tolerance. As a result, chronic nitrate therapy is reserved for second-line antianginal therapy.

1. **Dosing for isosorbide dinitrate** begins with a dose of 10 mg at 8 AM, 1 PM, and 6 PM, which results in a 14 hour nitrate dose-free interval. The dose is increased to 40 mg three times daily as needed. Alternatively, isosorbide dinitrate can be taken twice daily at 8 AM and 4 PM.

   a. The extended release preparation of isosorbide mononitrate, which is administered once per day, may be preferable to improve compliance. The starting dose is 30 mg once daily and can be titrated to 120 mg once daily as needed. This preparation is particularly useful in patients who have effort-induced angina. However, since the effect lasts only about 12 hours, some patients may develop nocturnal or rebound angina. Such patients require twice daily dosing or additional antianginal therapy.

   b. Transdermal nitroglycerin patch is a convenient way to administer nitroglycerin. The patient must remove the patch for 12 to 14 hours. Since most patients have angina with activity, the patch should be applied at 8 AM and removed at 8 PM. The occasional patient with significant nocturnal angina can be treated with a patch-on period from 8 PM to 8 AM. Initial dose is 0.2 mg per hour; the dose can be increased to 0.8 mg per hour as needed.

   c. Side effects associated with nitrate use are headache, lightheadedness, and flushing which are due to the vasodilatation. These symptoms tend to improve with time.

Dosages of Nitroglycerine Preparations				
Preparation	Route of administration	Onset of action, minutes	Duration of action	Dose
Nitroglycerin	Sublingual tablet	2-5	15-30 min	0.15-0.9 mg
	Sublingual spray	2-5	15-30 min	0.4 mg
	Ointment	2-5	Up to 7 hours	2 percent, 15x15 cm
	Transdermal	30	8-14 hours	0.2-0.8 mg/hour q12h
	Oral sustained release	30	4-8 hours	2.5-13 mg
	Intravenous	2-5	During infusion, tolerance in 7-8 hours	5-200 ug/min
Isosorbide dinitrate	Sublingual	2-5	Up to 60 min	2.5-15 mg
	Oral	30	Up to 8 hours	5-80 mg BID or TID
	Spray	2-5	2-3 min	1.25 mg/day
	Chewable	2-5	2-2.25 hours	5 mg
	Oral slow release	30	Up to 8 hours	40 mg QD or BID
	Intravenous	2-5	During infusion, tolerance in 7-8 hours	1.25-5 mg/hour
Isosorbide mononitrate, extended release	Oral	30	12-24 hours	20-40 mg BID 60-240 mg/day
Isosorbide mononitrate, extended release	Oral	30-60	12 hours	30-120 mg once daily

E. **Beta blockers** relieve anginal symptoms by competitively inhibiting sympathetic stimulation of the heart, reducing both heart rate and contractility.
   1. **Choice of agent.** Lower doses of the cardioselective beta blockers (atenolol and metoprolol) have the advantage of blocking beta-1-receptor mediated stimulation of the heart with lesser inhibition of the peripheral vasodilation and bronchodilation induced by the beta-2 receptors.
      a. Long-acting cardioselective agents (atenolol or metoprolol) are preferred for stable angina. There are no advantages of a nonselective agent, other than the low cost of propranolol, and there are disadvantages in obstructive lung disease, asthma, peripheral vascular disease, diabetes, and depression.
      b. **Atenolol (Tenormin)** starting dose is 25 mg once daily which can be increased as tolerated to a maximum of 200 mg once a day until the resting heart rate is 50 to 60 beats/min and does not exceed 100 beats/min with ordinary activity.
      c. **Metoprolol (Lopressor)** starting dose is 25 mg BID, which can be increased to 200 mg BID as tolerated. An extended release form of

metoprolol, given once per day, can be substituted once an effective dose has been established.

d. Beta blockers are well tolerated and extremely effective in reducing anginal episodes and improving exercise tolerance. Beta blockers are the only antianginal drugs proven to prevent reinfarction and to improve survival after an MI.

2. **Achieving adequate beta blockade.** Reasonable goals when titrating the dose include:
   a. Resting heart rate between 50 and 60 beats/min. The target heart rate for some patients with more severe angina can be <50 beats/min, as long as the bradycardia is asymptomatic and heart block does not develop.

3. Patients with resting bradycardia prior to therapy can be treated with a calcium channel blocker (such as diltiazem or nifedipine), nitrates, or a drug with intrinsic sympathomimetic activity if a beta blocker is necessary.

4. **Beta-blocker side effects.** Bradycardia, conduction disturbances, bronchoconstriction, worsening of symptoms of peripheral vascular disease, fatigue, central nervous system side effects, and impotence. As a result, beta blockers should be used with caution in patients with obstructive airways disease or peripheral vascular disease and, initially at very low doses in patients with heart failure.

5. Beta blockers should not be used in patients with vasospastic or variant (Prinzmetal) angina. In such patients, they are ineffective and may increase the tendency to induce coronary vasospasm from unopposed alpha-receptor activity.

Adverse Effects of Beta-blockers

Bradycardia, decreased contractility, AV node conduction delay
Bronchoconstriction can be induced by nonselective agents and high doses of cardioselective agents.
Worsening of symptoms of peripheral vascular disease or Raynaud's phenomenon.
Fatigue may be due to the reduction in cardiac output or to direct effects on the central nervous system.
Central side effects include depression, nightmares, insomnia, and hallucinations.
Impotence is often a problem.

Beta-blockers

Class	Drug name	Starting dose	Maximal dose
Cardioselective	Atenolol (Tenormin)	25 mg QD	100 mg QD
Cardioselective	Metoprolol (Lopressor)	25 mg BID	100 mg BID
	Metoprolol extended release (Toprol XL)	50 mg qd	200 mg qd
Nonselective	Nadolol (Corgard)	25 mg QD	240 mg QD

Class	Drug name	Starting dose	Maximal dose
Nonselective	Propranolol (Inderal)	40 mg BID	120 mg BID
Intrinsic sympathomimetic	Pindolol (Visken)	5 mg BID	30 mg BID
Alpha blocker	Labetalol (Normo-dyne)	100 mg BID	600 mg BID

F. **Calcium channel blockers** prevent calcium entry into vascular smooth muscle cells and myocytes, which leads to coronary and peripheral vasodilatation, decreased atrioventricular (AV) conduction, and reduced contractility. In patients with angina, these effects result in decreased coronary vascular resistance and increased coronary blood flow. Calcium blockers also decrease myocardial oxygen demand by reducing systemic vascular resistance and arterial pressure and a negative inotropic effect.
1. **Choice of agent**
   a. Verapamil is a negative inotrope that also slows sinus rate and decreases AV conduction (negative chronotrope). It is a much less potent vasodilator than the dihydropyridines.
   b. The dihydropyridines (eg, nifedipine, nicardipine, felodipine, amlodipine) have a greater selectivity for vascular smooth muscle than for the myocardium. They are potent vasodilators with less effect on contractility and AV conduction.
   c. Diltiazem (Cardizem) is a modest negative inotropic and chronotropic agent and vasodilator and has intermediate effects between the dihydropyridines and verapamil.
   d. If a calcium channel blocker is used, long-acting diltiazem or verapamil or a second generation dihydropyridine (amlodipine or felodipine) should be selected. Short-acting dihydropyridines, especially nifedipine, should be avoided unless used in conjunction with a beta blocker in the management of CHD because of evidence of an increase in mortality after an MI and an increase in acute MI in hypertensive patients.
   e. **When to use.** All of the calcium channel blockers reduce anginal symptoms and increase exercise tolerance and exercise time before the onset of angina or ischemia. They should be used in combination with beta blockers when initial treatment with beta blockers is not successful. They may be a substitute for a beta blocker when beta blockers are contraindicated or cause side effects. Calcium channel blockers (eg, diltiazem at a dose of 240 to 360 mg per day) are effective in patients with vasospastic or variant (Prinzmetal) angina; they are the preferred agents in this setting.
   f. **Side effects** include symptomatic bradycardia, heart block, worsening heart failure, constipation, flushing, headache, dizziness, and pedal edema.
G. **General measures.** Treatment of any underlying medical conditions that might aggravate myocardial ischemia, such as hypertension, fever, tachyarrhythmias (eg, atrial fibrillation), thyrotoxicosis, anemia or polycythemia, hypoxemia, or valvular heart disease should be undertaken. Asymptomatic low grade arrhythmias are not treated routinely.
H. **Aspirin** should be given unless contraindicated (81 to 325 mg/day). Patients who have a gastrointestinal bleed on low dose aspirin should be treated with

aspirin (81 mg/day) plus a proton pump inhibitor. Clopidogrel (Plavix)is an alternative in patients who are allergic to aspirin.

I. Risk factor reduction includes treatment of hypertension, cessation of smoking, lipid lowering with a regimen that includes statin therapy, weight reduction, and glycemic control in diabetics.

J. Measurement of left ventricular systolic function. Most patients with chronic stable angina do not need measurement of LV systolic function. Measurement of LV systolic function is recommended in patients with the following:

1. History of prior MI, pathologic Q waves, or symptoms or signs of heart failure.
2. A systolic murmur suggesting mitral regurgitation.
3. Complex ventricular arrhythmias.

K. Exercise testing. A stress test should be performed in patients with stable angina to evaluate the efficacy of the antiischemic program and for prognostic information.

1. A standard exercise ECG is preferred as the initial test in patients with a normal resting ECG who are able to exercise and are not taking digoxin.
2. Exercise testing can identify a subset of high-risk patients who have an annual mortality of more than 3 per cent. In comparison, low-risk patients, with an annual mortality below one per cent, are able to exercise into stage 3 of a Bruce protocol with a normal ECG.
3. Low- and intermediate-risk patients are generally treated medically, while high-risk patients or those with angina refractory to medical therapy undergo coronary angiography and revascularization with either PCI or CABG.

L. Coronary angiography and revascularization. There are two primary indications for coronary angiography followed by revascularization of appropriate lesions:

1. Angina that significantly interferes with a patient's lifestyle despite maximal tolerable medical therapy.
2. Patients with high-risk criteria and selected patients with intermediate-risk criteria on noninvasive testing, regardless of anginal severity.
3. Revascularization is performed in appropriate patients in whom angiography reveals anatomy for which revascularization has a proven benefit.
4. The choice between PCI and CABG is based upon anatomy and other factors such as left ventricular function and the presence or absence of diabetes. PCI is increasingly performed for most lesions because of the availability of drug-eluting stents.

References, see page 372.

Heart Failure

Heart failure (HF) has a mortality rate of 50 percent at two years and 60 to 70 percent at three years. Heart failure can result from any structural or functional cardiac disorder that impairs the ability of the ventricle to fill with or eject blood.

I. New York Heart Association (NYHA) classification of heart failure severity:

Class I - symptoms of HF only at activity levels that would limit normal individuals

Class II - symptoms of HF with ordinary exertion

Class III - symptoms of HF with less than ordinary exertion

Class IV - symptoms of HF at rest

Stages of heart failure:

Stage A. High risk for HF, without structural heart disease or symptoms

Stage B. Heart disease with asymptomatic left ventricular dysfunction

Stage C. Prior or current symptoms of HF

Stage D. Advanced heart disease and severely symptomatic or refractory HF
II. Etiology
   A. **Systolic dysfunction** is most commonly caused by coronary heart disease, idiopathic dilated cardiomyopathy, hypertension, and valvular disease.
   B. **Diastolic dysfunction** can be caused by hypertension, ischemic heart disease, hypertrophic obstructive cardiomyopathy, and restrictive cardiomyopathy.
III. Clinical evaluation of heart failure
   A. **History.** There are two major classes of symptoms in HF: those due to excess fluid accumulation (dyspnea, edema, hepatic congestion, and ascites) and those due to a reduction in cardiac output (fatigue, weakness). Fluid retention in HF is initiated by the fall in cardiac output.
   B. **The acuity of HF is suggested by the presenting symptoms:**
   1. **Acute and subacute presentations** (days to weeks) are characterized by shortness of breath, at rest and/or with exertion. Also common are orthopnea, paroxysmal nocturnal dyspnea, and, with right HF, right upper quadrant discomfort due to hepatic congestion. Atrial and/or ventricular tachyarrhythmias may cause palpitations and lightheadedness.
   2. **Chronic presentations** (months) differ in that fatigue, anorexia, bowel distension, and peripheral edema may be more pronounced than dyspnea.
   3. The absence of dyspnea on exertion makes the diagnosis of HF unlikely, while a history of myocardial infarction and a displaced apical impulse, or S3 on physical examination, strongly suggest the diagnosis.
   C. **Clues to the cause of heart failure**
   1. **Exertional angina** usually indicates ischemic heart disease.
   2. **Flu-like illness** before acute HF suggests viral myocarditis.
   3. **Hypertension or alcohol** use suggests hypertensive or alcoholic cardiomyopathy.
   4. **Amyloidosis** should be excluded in patients who also have a history of heavy proteinuria.
   5. **Primary valvular dysfunction** should be considered in a patient with a history of murmurs.
   6. **Antiarrhythmic agents** may provoke HF. Antiarrhythmics include disopyramide and flecainide; calcium channel blockers, particularly verapamil; beta blockers. Nonsteroidal antiinflammatory drugs (NSAIDs) may provoke HF.
   7. **Acute pulmonary edema** occurring during, or shortly after, infusion of blood products suggests transfusional volume overload.

Factors Associated with Worsening Heart Failure
Cardiovascular factors
Superimposed ischemia or infarction Hypertension Primary valvular disease Worsening secondary mitral regurgitation Atrial fibrillation Excessive tachycardia Pulmonary embolism

Systemic factors
Inappropriate medications Superimposed infection Anemia Uncontrolled diabetes Thyroid dysfunction Electrolyte disorders Pregnancy

Patient-related factors
Medication noncompliance Dietary indiscretion Alcohol consumption Substance abuse

IV. Physical examination

A. **Heart sounds.** An S3 gallop indicates left atrial pressures exceeding 20 mmHg.

B. **Decreased cardiac output.** Decreased tissue perfusion, results in shunting of the cardiac output to vital organs, leading to sinus tachycardia, diaphoresis, and peripheral vasoconstriction (cool, pale or cyanotic extremities).

C. **Manifestations of volume overload in HF** include pulmonary congestion, peripheral edema, and elevated jugular venous pressure.

D. **Rales** are often absent even though the pulmonary capillary pressure is still elevated.

E. **Peripheral edema** is manifested by swelling of the legs, ascites, hepatomegaly, and splenomegaly. Manual compression of the right upper quadrant may elevate the central venous pressure (hepatojugular reflux).

F. **Elevated jugular venous pressure** is usually present if peripheral edema is due to HF. Jugular venous pressure can be estimated with the patient sitting at 45° either from the height above the left atrium of venous pulsations in the internal jugular vein.

G. **Ventricular chamber size** can be estimated by precordial palpation. An apical impulse that is laterally displaced past the midclavicular line is usually indicative of left ventricular enlargement. Left ventricular dysfunction can also lead to sustained apical impulse which may be accompanied by a parasternal heave.

H. **Blood tests for patients with signs or symptoms of heart failure:**
1. **Complete blood count** since anemia can exacerbate preexisting HF.
2. **Serum electrolytes and creatinine**
3. **Liver function tests**, which may be affected by hepatic congestion.
4. **Fasting blood glucose** to detect underlying diabetes mellitus.

I. If it is determined that dilated cardiomyopathy is responsible for HF and the cause is not apparent, several other blood tests may be warranted:
1. **Thyroid function tests**, particularly in patients over the age of 65 or in patients with atrial fibrillation. Thyrotoxicosis is associated with atrial fibrillation, and hypothyroidism may present as HF.
2. **Iron studies** (ferritin and TIBC) to screen for hereditary hemochromatosis (HH).

J. **Other studies that may be undertaken:**
1. ANA and other serologic tests for lupus

    2. Viral serologies and antimyosin antibody if myocarditis is suspected

    3. Evaluation for pheochromocytoma

    4. Thiamine, carnitine, and selenium levels

    5. Genetic testing and counseling (in patients suspected of familial cardiomyopathy

K. Plasma brain natriuretic peptide

    1. In chronic HF, atrial myocytes secrete increased amounts of atrial natriuretic peptide (ANP) and ventricular myocytes secrete ANP and brain natriuretic peptide (BNP) in response to the high atrial and ventricular filling pressures. Both hormones are increased in patients with left ventricular dysfunction.

    2. Rapid bedside measurement of plasma BNP is useful for distinguishing between HF and a pulmonary cause of dyspnea.

    3. Plasma concentrations of BNP are markedly higher in patients with HF. Intermediate values were found in the patients with baseline left ventricular dysfunction without an acute exacerbation (346 pg/mL).

    4. A value >100 pg/mL has a sensitivity, specificity, and predictive accuracy of 90, 76, and 83 percent, respectively. A low BNP concentrations has a high negative predictive value, and is useful in ruling out HF.

    5. **Plasma N-pro-BNP.** The active BNP hormone is cleaved from prohormone, pro-BNP. The N-terminal fragment, N-pro-BNP, is also released into the circulation. In normal subjects, the plasma concentrations of BNP and N-pro-BNP are similar (10 pmol/L). However, in LV dysfunction, plasma N-pro-BNP concentrations are four-fold higher than BNP concentrations.

    6. An elevated plasma BNP suggests the diagnosis of HF, while a low plasma BNP may be particularly valuable in ruling out HF.

L. Chest x-ray is useful to differentiate HF from primary pulmonary disease.

    1. Findings suggestive of HF include cardiomegaly (cardiac-to-thoracic width ratio above 50 percent), cephalization of the pulmonary vessels, Kerley B-lines, and pleural effusions.

    2. The presence of pulmonary vascular congestion and cardiomegaly on chest x-ray support the diagnosis of HF.

M. Electrocardiogram detects arrhythmias such as asymptomatic ventricular premature beats, runs of nonsustained ventricular tachycardia, or atrial fibrillation, which may be the cause of HF.

    1. Dilated cardiomyopathy is frequently associated with first degree AV block, left bundle branch block, left anterior fascicular block, or a nonspecific intraventricular conduction abnormality. Potential findings on ECG include:

        a. Signs of ischemic heart disease.

        b. Left ventricular hypertrophy due to hypertension.

        c. Low limb lead voltage on the surface ECG with a pseudo-infarction pattern (loss of precordial R wave progression in leads V1-V6) suggest an infiltrative process such as amyloidosis.

        d. Low limb lead voltage with precordial criteria for left ventricular hypertrophy is most suggestive of idiopathic dilated cardiomyopathy. A widened QRS complex and/or a left bundle branch block pattern is also consistent with this diagnosis.

        e. Most patients with HF due to systolic dysfunction have a significant abnormality on ECG. A normal ECG makes systolic dysfunction extremely unlikely.

N. Echocardiography should be performed in all patients with new onset HF and can provide information about ventricular size and function. The following findings can be detected:

1. Regional wall motion abnormalities are compatible with coronary heart disease.
2. Pericardial thickening in constrictive pericarditis.
3. Mitral or aortic valve disease, as well as interatrial and interventricular shunts.
4. Abnormal myocardial texture in infiltrative cardiomyopathies.
5. Right ventricular size and function in right HF.
6. Estimation of pulmonary artery wedge pressure.
7. Right atrial and pulmonary artery pressures can be used to assess left ventricular filling pressures.
8. Cardiac output can be measured.
9. Echocardiography, especially with the use of dobutamine, is also useful in predicting recovery of cardiac function.
10. Echocardiography should be performed in all patients with new onset HF. Echocardiography has a high sensitivity and specificity for the diagnosis of myocardial dysfunction, and may determinethe etiology of HF.

O. **Detection of coronary heart disease**
   1. Heart failure resulting from coronary disease is usually irreversible due to myocardial infarction and ventricular remodeling. However, revascularization may be of benefit in the appreciable number of patients with hibernating myocardium.
   2. Exercise testing should be part of the initial evaluation of any patient with HF.
   3. With severe heart failure, measurement of the maximal oxygen uptake (VO_2max) provides an objective estimate of the severity of the myocardial dysfunction. VO_2max is one of the best indices of prognosis in patients with symptomatic HF and can aid in the determination of the necessity and timing of cardiac transplantation.
   4. **Coronary arteriography**
      a. **Recommendations for coronary arteriography**: Coronary arteriography should be performed in patients with angina and in patients with known or suspected coronary artery disease who do not have angina.
      b. Patients with unexplained HF should be evaluated for coronary heart disease. If the exercise test is normal and HF is unexplained, cardiac catheterization should be strongly considered.

Laboratory Workup for Suspected Heart Failure

Blood urea nitrogen	Thyroid-stimulating hormone
Cardiac enzymes (CK-MB, troponin)	Urinalysis
Complete blood cell count	Echocardiogram
Creatinine	Electrocardiography
Electrolytes	Atrial natriuretic peptide (ANP)
Liver function tests	Brain natriuretic peptide (BNP)
Magnesium	

V. **Treatment of heart failure due to systolic dysfunction**
   A. **Treatment of the underlying cardiac disease**
      1. **Hypertension** is the primary cause of HF in many patients. Angiotensin converting enzyme (ACE) inhibitors, beta blockers, and angiotensin II receptor blockers (ARBs) are the preferred antihypertensive agents be-

cause they improve survival in HF. Beta blockers can also provide anginal relief in ischemic heart disease and rate control in with atrial fibrillation.

2. **Renovascular disease.** Testing for renovascular disease is indicated if there is severe or refractory hypertension, a sudden rise in blood pressure, or repeated episodes of flash pulmonary edema.

3. **Ischemic heart disease.** Coronary atherosclerosis is the most common cause of cardiomyopathy, comprising 50 to 75 percent of patients with HF.

   a. All patients with documented ischemic heart disease should be treated medically for relief of angina and with risk factor reduction, such as control of serum lipids.

   b. Myocardial revascularization with angioplasty or bypass surgery may improve exercise capacity and prognosis in patients with hibernating myocardium. Revascularization should also be considered for repeated episodes of acute left ventricular dysfunction and flash pulmonary edema.

4. **Valvular disease** is the primary cause of HF 10 to 12 percent.

5. **Other causes of heart failure:** Alcohol abuse, cocaine abuse, obstructive sleep apnea, nutritional deficiencies, myocarditis, hemochromatosis, sarcoidosis, thyroid disease, and rheumatologic disorders such as systemic lupus erythematosus.

B. **Pharmacologic therapy of heart failure**

1. **Improvement in symptoms** can be achieved by digoxin, diuretics, beta blockers, ACE inhibitors, and angiotensin II receptor blockers (ARBs).

2. **Prolongation of survival** has been documented with ACE inhibitors, beta blockers, ARBs, hydralazine/nitrates, and spironolactone and eplerenone.

3. **Order of therapy:**

   a. **Loop diuretics** are used first for fluid control in overt HF. The goal is relief of dyspnea and peripheral edema.

   b. **ACE inhibitors**, or if not tolerated, angiotensin II receptor blockers (ARBs) are initiated during or after the optimization of diuretic therapy. These drugs are usually started at low doses and then titrated.

   c. **Beta blockers** are initiated after the patient is stable on ACE inhibitors, beginning at low doses with titration to goals.

   d. **Digoxin** is initiated in patients who continue to have symptoms of HF despite the above regimen; and, in atrial fibrillation, digoxin may be used for rate control.

   e. An ARB, aldosterone antagonist, or, particularly in black patients, the combination of hydralazine and a nitrate may be added in patients who are persistently symptomatic.

C. **ACE inhibitors and beta blockers.** Begin with a low dose of an ACE inhibitor (eg, lisinopril 5 mg/day), increase to a moderate dose (eg, lisinopril 15 to 20 mg/day) at one to two week intervals, and then begin a beta blocker, gradually increasing toward the target dose or the highest tolerated dose. When the beta blocker titration is completed, the ACE inhibitor titration is completed.

1. All patients with asymptomatic or symptomatic left ventricular dysfunction should be started on an ACE inhibitor. Beginning therapy with low doses (eg, 2.5 mg of enalapril (Vasotec) twice daily, 6.25 mg of captopril (Capotin) three times daily, or 5 mg of lisinopril (Prinivil) once daily) will reduce the likelihood of hypotension and azotemia.

2. If initial therapy is tolerated, the dose is then gradually increased at one to two week intervals to a target dose of 20 mg twice daily of enalapril, 50 mg three times daily of captopril, or up to 40 mg/day of lisinopril or quinapril. Plasma potassium and creatinine should be assessed one to two weeks after starting or changing a dose and periodically.

3. An ARB should be administered in patients who cannot tolerate ACE inhibitors. An ARB should be added to HF therapy in patients who are still symptomatic on ACE inhibitors and beta blockers or are hypertensive. In patients with renal dysfunction or hyperkalemia, the addition of an ARB must be done with caution. An ARB should not be added to an ACE inhibitor in the immediate post-MI setting.

D. Beta blockers. Carvedilol, metoprolol, and bisoprolol, improve survival in patients with New York Heart Association (NYHA) class II to III HF and probably in class IV HF. Beta blockers with intrinsic sympathomimetic activity (such as pindolol and acebutolol) should be avoided.

1. Carvedilol (Coreg), metoprolol (Toprol-XL), or bisoprolol (Ziac) is recommended for all patients with symptomatic HF, unless contraindicated. Relative contraindications to beta blocker therapy in patients with HF include:
   a. Heart rate <60 bpm
   b. Symptomatic hypotension
   c. Signs of peripheral hypoperfusion
   d. PR interval >0.24 sec
   e. Second- or third-degree atrioventricular block
   f. Severe chronic obstructive pulmonary disease
   g. Asthma

2. **Choice of agent.** Metoprolol has a high degree of specificity for the beta-1 adrenergic receptor, while carvedilol blocks beta-1, beta-2, and alpha-1 adrenergic receptors. Patients with low blood pressure may tolerate metoprolol better than carvedilol. Those with high blood pressure may have a greater lowering of blood pressure with carvedilol.

3. **Initiation of therapy.** Prior to initiation of therapy, the patient should have no fluid retention and should not have required recent intravenous inotropic therapy. Therapy should be begun at very low doses and the dose doubled every two weeks until the target dose is reached or symptoms become limiting. Initial and target doses are:
   a. **Carvedilol (Coreg),** 3.125 mg BID initially and 25 to 50 mg BID ultimately (the higher dose being used in subjects over 85 kg)
   b. **Extended-release metoprolol (Toprol-XL),** 12.5 mg daily in patients with NYHA class III or IV or 25 mg daily in patients with NYHA II, and ultimately 200 mg/day. If patients receive short acting metoprolol for cost reasons, the dosage is 6.25 mg BID initially and 50 to 100 mg BID ultimately.
   c. **Bisoprolol (Ziac),** 1.25 mg QD initially and 5 to 10 mg QD ultimately.

E. The patient should weigh himself daily and call the physician if there has been a 1 to 1.5 kg weight gain. Weight gain may be treated with diuretics.

F. Digoxin is given to patients with HF and systolic dysfunction to control symptoms and, in atrial fibrillation, to control the ventricular rate. Digoxin therapy is associated with a significant reduction in hospitalization for HF but no benefit in overall mortality.

1. Digoxin should be started in patients with left ventricular systolic dysfunction (left ventricular ejection fraction [LVEF] <40 percent) who continue to have NYHA functional class II, III, and IV symptoms despite therapy including an ACE inhibitor, beta blocker, and a diuretic. The usual daily dose is 0.125 mg or less, based upon renal function. The serum digoxin concentration should be maintained between 0.5 and 0.8 ng/mL.

G. Diuretics

1. A loop diuretic should be given to control pulmonary and/or peripheral edema. The most commonly used loop diuretic for the treatment of HF is

furosemide, but some patients respond better to bumetanide or torsemide because of superior absorption.

   2. The usual starting dose is 20 to 40 mg of furosemide. In patients who are volume overloaded, a reasonable goal is weight reduction of 1.0 kg/day.
H. **Aldosterone antagonists.** Spironolactone and eplerenone, which compete with aldosterone for the mineralocorticoid receptor, prolong survival in selected patients with HF.

   1. Treatment should begin with spironolactone (Aldactone, 25 to 50 mg/day), and switched to eplerenone (Inspra, 25 and after four weeks 50 mg/day) if endocrine side effects occur.
   2. Serum potassium and creatinine should be checked one to two weeks after starting spironolactone or eplerenone and periodically thereafter. Patients with poor renal function are at risk for hyperkalemia.

Treatment Classification of Patients with Heart Failure Caused by Left Ventricular Systolic Dysfunction

Symptoms	Pharmacology
Asymptomatic	ACE inhibitor or angiotensin-receptor blocker Beta blocker
Symptomatic	ACE inhibitor or angiotensin-receptor blocker Beta blocker Diuretic If symptoms persist: digoxin (Lanoxin)
Symptomatic with recent history of dyspnea at rest	Diuretic ACE inhibitor or angiotensin-receptor blocker Spironolactone (Aldactone) Beta blocker Digoxin
Symptomatic with dyspnea at rest	Diuretic ACE inhibitor or angiotensin-receptor blocker Spironolactone (Aldactone) Digoxin

Dosages of Primary Drugs Used in the Treatment of Heart Failure

Drug	Starting Dosage	Target Dosage
Drugs that decrease mortality and improve symptoms		
ACE inhibitors		
Captopril (Capoten)	6.25 mg three times daily (one-half tablet)	12.5 to 50 mg three times daily
Enalapril (Vasotec)	2.5 mg twice daily	10 mg twice daily
Lisinopril (Zestril)	5 mg daily	10 to 20 mg daily
Ramipril (Altace)	1.25 mg twice daily	5 mg twice daily
Trandolapril (Mavik)	1 mg daily	4 mg daily
Angiotensin-Receptor Blockers (ARBs)		
Candesartan (Atacand)	4 mg bid	16 mg bid

Drug	Starting Dosage	Target Dosage
Irbesartan (Avapro)	75 mg qd	300 mg qd
Losartan (Cozaar)	12.5 mg bid	50 mg bid
Valsartan (Diovan)	40 mg bid	160 mg bid
Telmisartan (Micardis)	20 mg qd	80 mg qd
Aldosterone antagonists		
Spironolactone (Aldactone)	25 mg daily	25 mg daily
Eplerenone (Inspra)	25 mg daily	25 mg daily
Beta blockers		
Bisoprolol (Zebeta)	1.25 mg daily (one-fourth tablet)	10 mg daily
Carvedilol (Coreg)	3.125 mg twice daily	25 to 50 mg twice daily
Metoprolol tartrate (Lopressor)	12.5 mg twice daily (one-fourth tablet)	50 to 75 mg twice daily
Metoprolol succinate (Toprol-XL)	12.5 mg daily (one-half tablet)	200 mg daily
Drugs that treat symptoms		
Thiazide diuretics		
Hydrochlorothiazide (Esidrex)	25 mg daily	25 to 100 mg daily
Metolazone (Zaroxolyn)	2.5 mg daily	2.5 to 10 mg daily
Loop diuretics		
Bumetanide (Bumex)	1 mg daily	1 to 10 mg once to three times daily
Ethacrynic acid (Edecrin)	25 mg daily	25 to 200 mg once or twice daily
Furosemide (Lasix)	40mg daily	40 to 400 mg once to three times daily
Torsemide (Demadex)	20 mg daily	20 to 200 mg once or twice daily
Inotrope		
Digoxin (Lanoxin)	0.125 mg daily	0.125 to 0.375 mg daily

VI. Lifestyle modification
   A. Cessation of smoking.
   B. Restriction of alcohol consumption.
   C. Salt restriction to 2 to 3 g (or less) of sodium per day to minimize fluid accumulation.
   D. Daily weight monitoring to detect fluid accumulation before it becomes symptomatic.
   E. Weight reduction in obese subjects with a goal of being within 10 percent of ideal body weight.
   F. A cardiac rehabilitation program for all stable patients.

References, see page 372.

Atrial Fibrillation

Atrial fibrillation (AF) is more prevalent in men and with increasing age. AF can have adverse consequences related to a reduction in cardiac output and to atrial thrombus formation that can lead to systemic embolization.

I. Classification

A. Atrial fibrillation occurs in the normal heart and in the presence of organic heart disease. Classification of Atrial fibrillation:

1. **Paroxysmal (ie, self-terminating) AF** in which the episodes of AF generally last less than seven days (usually less than 24 hours) and may be recurrent.

2. **Persistent AF** fails to self-terminate and lasts for longer than seven days. Persistent AF may also be paroxysmal if it recurs after reversion. AF is considered recurrent when the patient experiences two or more episodes.

3. **Permanent AF** is considered to be present if the arrhythmia lasts for more than one year and cardioversion either has not been attempted or has failed.

4. **"Lone" AF** describes paroxysmal, persistent, or permanent AF in individuals without structural heart disease.

B. If the AF is secondary to cardiac surgery, pericarditis, myocardial infarction (MI), hyperthyroidism, pulmonary embolism, pulmonary disease, or other reversible causes, therapy is directed toward the underlying disease as well as the AF.

II. Clinical evaluation

A. **History and physical examination.** Associated symptoms with AF should be sought; the clinical type or "pattern" should be defined; the onset or date of discovery of the AF; the frequency and duration of AF episodes; any precipitating causes and modes of termination of AF; the response to drug therapy; and the presence of heart disease or potentially reversible causes (eg, hyperthyroidism).

B. The frequency and duration of AF episodes are determined from the history. Symptoms include palpitations, weakness, dizziness, and dyspnea. However, among patients with paroxysmal AF, up to 90% of episodes are not recognized by the patient.

C. **Electrocardiogram** is used to verify the presence of AF; identify left ventricular hypertrophy, pre-excitation, bundle branch block, or prior MI; define P-wave duration and morphology.

D. **Chest x-ray** is useful in assessing the lungs, vasculature, and cardiac outline.

E. **Transthoracic echocardiography** is required to evaluate the size of the right and left atria and the size and function of the right and left ventricles; to detect possible valvular heart disease, left ventricular hypertrophy, and pericardial disease; and to assess peak right ventricular pressure. It may also identify a left atrial thrombus, although the sensitivity is low. Transesophageal echocardiography is much more sensitive for atrial thrombi and can be used to determine the need for three to four weeks of anticoagulation prior to cardioversion.

F. **Assessment for hyperthyroidism.** A low-serum thyroid-stimulating hormone (TSH) value is found in 5.4% of patients with AF; only 1% have clinical hyperthyroidism. Measurement of serum TSH and free T4 is indicated in all patients with a first episode of AF, when the ventricular response to AF is difficult to control, or when AF recurs unexpectedly after cardioversion. Patients with low TSH values (<0.5 mU/L) and normal serum free T4 probably have subclinical hyperthyroidism.

G. Additional testing

1. **Exercise testing** is often used to assess the adequacy of rate control in permanent AF, to reproduce exercise-induced AF, and to evaluate for ischemic heart disease.
2. **Holter monitoring** or event recorders are used to identify the arrhythmia if it is intermittent and not captured on routine electrocardiography.
3. **Electrophysiologic studies** may be required with wide QRS complex tachycardia or a possible predisposing arrhythmia, such as atrial flutter or a paroxysmal supraventricular tachycardia.

III. General treatment issues

Risk-based Approach to Antithrombotic Therapy in Atrial Fibrillation	
Patient features	**Antithrombotic therapy**
Age <60 years No heart disease (line AF)	Aspirin (325 mg per day) or no therapy
Age <60 years Hear disease by no risk factors*	Aspirin (325 mg per day)
Age ≥60 years No risk factors*	Aspirin (325 mg per day)
Age ≥60 years With diabetes mellitus or CAD	Oral anticoagulation (INR 2 to 3) Addition of aspirin, 81 to 162 mg/day is optional
Age ≥75 years, especially women	Oral anticoagulation (INR ≈ 2.0)
Heart failure (HF) LVEF ≤0.35 Thyrotoxicosis Hypertension	Oral anticoagulation (INR 2 to 3)
Rheumatic heart disease (mitral stenosis) Prosthetic heart valves Prior thromboembolism Persistent atrial thrombus on TEE	Oral anticoagulation (INR 2.5 to 3.5 or higher may be apropriate)

*Risk factors for thromboembolism include heart failure, left ventricular ejection fraction (LVEF) less than 0.35, and hypertension.

A. Rate control with chronic anticoagulation is recommended for the majority of patients with AF.
B. Beta-blockers (eg, atenolol or metoprolol), diltiazem, and verapamil are recommended for rate control at both rest and exercise; digoxin is not effective during exercise and should be used in patients with heart failure or as a second-line agent.
C. Anticoagulation should be achieved with adjusted-dose warfarin unless the patient is considered at low embolic risk or has a contraindication. Aspirin may be used in such patients.

    D. When rhythm control is chosen, both DC and pharmacologic cardioversion are appropriate options. To prevent dislodgment of pre-existing thrombi, warfarin therapy should be given for three to four weeks prior to cardioversion unless transesophageal echocardiography demonstrates no left atrial thrombi. Anticoagulation is continued for at least one month after cardioversion to prevent de novo thrombus formation.

    E. After cardioversion, antiarrhythmic drugs to maintain sinus rhythm are not recommended, since the risks outweigh the benefits, except for patients with persistent symptoms during rate control that interfere with the patient's quality of life. Recommended drugs are amiodarone, disopyramide, propafenone, and sotalol.

IV. Rhythm control

    A. Reversion to NSR. Patients with AF of more than 48 hours duration or unknown duration may have atrial thrombi that can embolize. In such patients, cardioversion should be delayed until the patient has been anticoagulated at appropriate levels for three to four weeks or transesophageal echocardiography has excluded atrial thrombi.

        1. DC cardioversion is indicated in patients who are hemodynamically unstable. In stable patients in whom spontaneous reversion due to correction of an underlying disease is not likely, either DC or pharmacologic cardioversion can be performed. Electrical cardioversion is usually preferred because of greater efficacy and a low risk of proarrhythmia. The overall success rate of electrical cardioversion for AF is 75 to 93 percent and is related inversely both to the duration of AF and to left atrial size.

        2. Antiarrhythmic drugs will convert 30 to 60 percent of patients.

        3. Rate control with an atrioventricular (AV) nodal blocker (beta-blocker, diltiazem, or verapamil), or (if the patient has heart failure or hypotension) digoxin should be attained before instituting a class IA drug.

    B. Maintenance of NSR. Only 20 to 30 percent of patients who are successfully cardioverted maintain NSR for more than one year without chronic antiarrhythmic therapy. This is more likely to occur in patients with AF for less than one year, no enlargement of the left atrium (ie, <4.0 cm), and a reversible cause of AF such as hyperthyroidism, pericarditis, pulmonary embolism, or cardiac surgery.

        1. Prophylactic antiarrhythmic drug therapy is indicated only in patients who have a moderate-to-high risk for recurrence.

        2. Evidence of efficacy is best for amiodarone, propafenone, disopyramide, sotalol, flecainide, and quinidine. Flecainide may be preferred in patients with no or minimal heart disease, while amiodarone is preferred in patients with a reduced left ventricular (LV) ejection fraction or heart failure and sotalol in patients with coronary heart disease. Concurrent administration of an AV nodal blocker is indicated in patients who have demonstrated a moderate-to-rapid ventricular response to AF.

        3. Amiodarone is significantly more effective for maintenance of sinus rhythm than other antiarrhythmic drugs. Amiodarone should be used as first-line therapy in patients without heart failure.

V. Rate control in chronic AF. Rapid ventricular rate in patients with AF should be prevented because of hemodynamic instability and/or symptoms.

    A. Rate control in AF is usually achieved by slowing AV nodal conduction with a beta-blocker, diltiazem, verapamil, or, in patients with heart failure or hypotension, digoxin. Amiodarone is also effective in patients who are not cardioverted to NSR.

    B. Heart rate control include:

        1. Rest heart rate <80 beats/min.

2. 24-hour Holter average $\leq$100 beats/min and no heart rate >110% of the age-predicted maximum.
3. Heart rate $\leq$110 beats/min in six minute walk.

C. **Nonpharmacologic approaches.** The medical approaches to either rate or rhythm control described above are not always effective.

1. **Rhythm control.** Alternative methods to maintain NSR in patients who are refractory to conventional therapy include surgery, radiofrequency catheter ablation, and pacemakers.

2. **Rate control.** Radio-frequency AV nodal-His bundle ablation with permanent pacemaker placement or AV nodal conduction modification are nonpharmacologic therapies for achieving rate control in patients who do not respond to pharmacologic therapy.

Intravenous Agents for Heart Rate Control in Atrial Fibrillation

Drug	Loading Dose	Onset	Maintenance Dose	Major Side Effects
Diltiazem	0.25 mg/kg IV over 2 min	2–7 min	5–15 mg per hour infusion	Hypotension, heart block, HF
Esmolol	0.5 mg/kg over 1 min	1 min	0.05–0.2 mg/kg/min	Hypotension, heart block, bradycardia, asthma, HF
Metoprolol	2.5–5 mg IV bolus over 2 min up to 3 doses	5 min	5 mg IV q6h	Hypotension, heart block, bradycardia, asthma, HF
Verapamil	0.075–0.15 mg/kg IV over 2 min	3–5 min	5-10 mg IV q6h	Hypotension, heart block, HF
Digoxin	0.25 mg IV q2h, up to 1.5 mg	2 h	0.125–0.25 mg daily	Digitalis toxicity, heart block, bradycardia

Oral Agents for Heart Rate Control

Drug	Loading Dose	Usual Maintenance Dose	Major Side Effects
Digoxin	0.25 mg PO q2h up to 1.5 mg	0.125–0.375 mg daily	Digitalis toxicity, heart block, bradycardia
Diltiazem Extended Release	NA	120–360 mg daily	Hypotension, heart block, HF
Metoprolol	NA	25–100 mg BID	Hypotension, heart block, bradycardia, asthma, HF

Drug	Loading Dose	Usual Mainte-nance Dose	Major Side Effects
Propranolol Extended Release	NA	80–240 mg daily	Hypotension, heart block, bradycardia, asthma, HF
Verapamil Extended Release	NA	120–360 mg daily	Hypotension, heart block, HF, digoxin interaction
Amiodarone	800 mg daily for 1 wk 600 mg daily for 1 wk 400 mg daily for 4–6 wk	200 mg daily	Pulmonary toxicity, skin dis-coloration, hypo or hyper-thyroidism, corneal deposits, optic neuropathy, warfarin interaction, proarrhythmia (QT prolongation)

VI. Prevention of systemic embolization

A. Anticoagulation during restoration of NSR

1. **AF for more than 48 hours or unknown duration.** Outpatients without a contraindication to warfarin who have been in AF for more than 48 hours should receive three to four weeks of warfarin prior to and after cardiover-sion. This approach is also recommended for patients with AF who have valvular disease, evidence of left ventricular dysfunction, recent thromboembolism, or when AF is of unknown duration, as in an asymptom-atic patient.

   a. The recommended target INR is 2.5 (range 2.0 to 3.0). The INR should be ≥ 2.0 in the weeks before cardioversion.

   b. An alternative approach that eliminates the need for prolonged anticoagulation prior to cardioversion is the use of transesophageal echocardiography-guided cardioversion.

   c. Thus, the long-term recommendations for patients who have been cardioverted to NSR but are at high risk for thromboembolism are similar to those in patients with chronic AF, even though the patients are in sinus rhythm.

2. **Atrial fibrillation for less than 48 hours.** A different approach with respect to anticoagulation can be used in low-risk patients (no mitral valve disease, severe left ventricular dysfunction, or history of recent thromboembolism) in whom there is reasonable certainty that AF has been present for less than 48 hours. Such patients have a low risk of clinical thromboembolism if converted early (0.8%), even without a screening TEE.

3. Long-term anticoagulation prior to cardioversion is not recommended in such patients, but heparin use is recommended at presentation and during the pericardioversion period.

Antithrombotic Therapy in Cardioversion for Atrial Fibrillation	
Timing of cardioversion	**Anticoagulation**
Early cardioversion in patients with atrial fibrillation for less than 48 hours	Heparin during cardioversion period to achieve PTT of 50-70 seconds. Heparin 70 U/kg load, 15 U/kg/hr drip.

Timing of cardioversion	Anticoagulation
Early cardioversion in patients with atrial fibrillation for more than 48 hours or an unknown duration, but with documented absence of atrial thrombi	Heparin during cardioversion period to achieve PTT of 50-70 seconds. Warfarin (Coumadin) for 4 weeks after cardioversion to achieve target INR of 2.0 to 3.0.
Elective cardioversion in patients with atrial fibrillation for more than 48 hours or an unknown duration	Warfarin for 3 weeks before and 4 weeks after cardioversion to achieve target INR of of 2.0 to 3.0.

4. Current practice is to administer aspirin for a first episode of AF that converts spontaneously and warfarin for at least four weeks to all other patients.
5. Aspirin should not be considered in patients with AF of less than 48 hours duration if there is associated rheumatic mitral valve disease, severe left ventricular dysfunction, or recent thromboembolism. Such patients should be treated the same as patients with AF of longer duration: one month of oral anticoagulation with warfarin or shorter-term anticoagulation with screening TEE prior to elective electrical or pharmacologic cardioversion followed by prolonged warfarin therapy after cardioversion.

B. Anticoagulation in chronic AF

1. The incidence of stroke associated with AF is 3 to 5 percent per year in the absence of anticoagulation; compared with the general population, AF significantly increases the risk of stroke (relative risk 2.4 in men and 3.0 in women).
2. The incidence of stroke is relatively low in patients with AF who are under age 65 and have no risk factors. The prevalence of stroke associated with AF increases strikingly with age and with other risk factors including diabetes, hypertension, previous stroke as clinical risk factors, and left ventricular dysfunction.
3. **Choice of antiembolism therapy**
   a. Patients with a CHADS2 score of 0 are at low risk of embolization (0.5% per year) and can be managed with aspirin.
   b. Patients with a CHADS2 score ≥ 3 are at high risk (5.3 to 6.9 percent per year) and should, in the absence of a contraindication, be treated with warfarin.
   c. Patients with a CHADS2 score of 1 or 2 are at intermediate risk of embolization (1.5 to 2.5 percent per year). In this group, the choice between warfarin therapy and aspirin will depend upon many factors, including patient preference.
4. An INR between 2.0 and 3.0 is recommended for most patients with AF who receive warfarin therapy. A higher goal (INR between 2.5 and 3.5) is reasonable for patients at particularly high risk for embolization (eg, prior thromboembolism, rheumatic heart disease, prosthetic heart valves). An exception to the latter recommendation occurs in patients over the age of 75 who are at increased risk for major bleeding. A target INR of 1.8 to 2.5 is recommended for this age group.

C. Anticoagulation in paroxysmal AF.
The stroke risk appears to be equivalent in paroxysmal and chronic AF. The factors governing the choice between warfarin and aspirin therapy and the intensity of warfarin therapy are similar to patients with chronic AF.

VII. Presentation and management of recent onset AF

A. Indications for hospitalization

    1. For the treatment of an associated medical problem, which is often the reason for the arrhythmia.

    2. For elderly patients who are more safely treated for AF in hospital.

    3. For patients with underlying heart disease who have hemodynamic consequences from the AF or who are at risk for a complication resulting from therapy of the arrhythmia.

B. Search for an underlying cause, such as heart failure (HF), pulmonary problems, hypertension, or hyperthyroidism.

C. Serum should be obtained for measurement of thyroid stimulating hormone (TSH) and free T4. This should be done even if there are no symptoms suggestive of hyperthyroidism, since the risk of AF is increased up to threefold in patients with subclinical hyperthyroidism. The latter disorder is characterized by low serum TSH (<0.5 mU/L) and normal serum free T4.

D. If AF appears to have been precipitated by a reversible medical problem, cardioversion should be postponed until the condition has been successfully treated, which will often lead to spontaneous reversion. If this treatment is to be initiated as an outpatient, anticoagulation with warfarin should be begun with cardioversion performed, if necessary, after three to four weeks of adequate anticoagulation. If the patient is to be admitted to the hospital for treatment of the underlying disease, it is prudent to begin heparin therapy and then institute oral warfarin. Cardioversion is again performed after anticoagulation if the patient does not revert to NSR. In either case, three to four weeks of anticoagulation is not necessary if TEE shows no left atrial thrombus.

E. Indications for urgent cardioversion

    1. Active ischemia.

    2. Significant hypotension, to which poor LV systolic function, diastolic dysfunction, or associated mitral or aortic valve disease may contribute.

    3. Severe manifestations of HF.

    4. The presence of a pre-excitation syndrome, which may lead to an extremely rapid ventricular rate.

    5. In a patient who has truly urgent indications for cardioversion, the need for restoration of NSR takes precedence over the need for protection from thromboembolic risk. If feasible, the patient should still be heparinized for the cardioversion procedure.

F. Initial rate control with mild-to-moderate symptoms Initial treatment directed at slowing the ventricular rate will usually result in improvement of the associated symptoms. This can be achieved with beta-blockers, calcium channel blockers (verapamil and diltiazem), or digoxin.

    1. Digoxin is the preferred drug only in patients with AF due to HF. Digoxin can also be used in patients who cannot take or who respond inadequately to beta-blockers or calcium channel blockers. The effect of digoxin is additive to both of these drugs.

    2. A beta-blocker, diltiazem, or verapamil is the preferred drug in the absence of HF. Beta-blockers are particularly useful when the ventricular response increases to inappropriately high rates during exercise, after an acute MI, and when exercise-induced angina pectoris is also present. A calcium channel blocker is preferred in patients with chronic lung disease.

G. Elective cardioversion. In some patients, antiarrhythmic drugs are administered prior to cardioversion to increase the chance of successful reversion and to prevent recurrence. Patients who are successfully cardioverted generally require antiarrhythmic drugs to increase the likelihood of maintaining sinus rhythm.

H. **Immediate cardioversion.** There is a low risk of systemic embolization if the duration of the arrhythmia is 48 hours or less and there are no associated cardiac abnormalities (mitral valve disease or LV enlargement). In such patients, electrical or pharmacologic cardioversion can be attempted after systemic heparinization. Aspirin should be administered for a first episode of AF that converts spontaneously and warfarin for at least four weeks to all other patients.

I. **Delayed cardioversion.** It is preferable to anticoagulate with warfarin for three to four weeks before attempted cardioversion to allow any left atrial thrombi to resolve if:
   1. The duration of AF is more than 48 hours or of unknown duration.
   2. There is associated mitral valve disease or cardiomyopathy or HF.
   3. The patient has a prior history of a thromboembolic event.
   4. During this time, rate control should be maintained with an oral AV nodal blocker. The recommended target INR is 2.5 (range 2.0 to 3.0). The INR should be consistently ≥2.0 in the weeks before cardioversion.

J. **Trans-esophageal echocardiogram** immediately prior to elective cardioversion should be considered for those patients at increased risk for left atrial thrombi (eg, rheumatic mitral valve disease, recent thromboembolism, severe LV systolic dysfunction). Among patients with AF of recent onset (but more than 48 hours) who are not being anticoagulated, an alternative approach to three to four weeks of warfarin therapy before cardioversion is TEE-based screening with cardioversion performed if no thrombi are seen.

References, see page 372.

Hypertension

The prevalence of hypertension (systolic >140 and/or diastolic >90 mm Hg) is 32 percent in the non-Hispanic black population and 23 percent in the non-Hispanic white and Mexican-American populations.

I. **Definitions.** The following definitions have been suggested by the seventh report of the Joint National Committee (JNC 7). Based upon the average of two or more readings at each of two or more visits after an initial screen, the following classification is used.
   A. The prehypertension category recognizes that the correlation between the risk of adverse outcomes (including stroke and death) and blood pressure level is a continuous variable in which there is an increased incidence of poor outcomes as the blood pressure rises, even within the previously delineated "normal" range.

II. **Etiology/risk factors**
   A. **Essential hypertension** has been associated with a number of risk factors:
      1. Hypertension is about twice as common in subjects who have one or two hypertensive parents.
      2. Increased salt intake is a necessary but not a sufficient cause for hypertension.
      3. There is a clear association between excess alcohol intake and hypertension.
      4. Obesity and weight gain appears to be a main determinant of the rise in blood pressure (BP).
   B. **Secondary hypertension**
      1. **Primary renal disease.** Hypertension is a frequent finding in renal disease, particularly with glomerular or vascular disorders.
      2. **Oral contraceptives** can induce hypertension.

3. **Pheochromocytoma.** About one-half of patients with pheochromocytoma have paroxysmal hypertension, most of the rest have what appears to be essential hypertension.

Classification and Management of Blood Pressure for Adults Aged 18 Years or Older					
				Initial drug therapy	
BP classification	Systolic BP	Diastolic BP	Lifestyle Modification	Without compelling indication	With compelling indications
Normal	<120 and	<60	Encourage		
Prehypertension	120-139 or	80-89	Yes	No antihypertensive drug indicated	Drug(s) for the compelling indications
Stage 1 hypertension	140-159 or	90-99	Yes	Thiazide-type diuretics for most, may consider ACE inhibitor, ARB, beta blocker, CCB, or combination	Drug(s) for the compelling indications Other antihypertensive drugs (diuretics, ACE inhibitor, ARB, beta blocker, CCB) as needed
Stage 2 hypertension	$\geq$160 or	$\geq$100	Yes	2-drug combination for most (usually thiazide-type diuretic and ACE inhibitor or ARB or beta blocker, CCB)	Drug(s) for the compelling indications Other antihypertensive drugs (diuretics, ACE inhibitor, ARB, beta blocker, CCB) as needed

4. **Primary hyperaldosteronism.** The presence of primary mineralocorticoid excess, primarily aldosterone, should be suspected in any patient with the triad of hypertension, unexplained hypokalemia and metabolic alkalosis. Some patients have a normal plasma potassium concentration.
5. **Cushing's syndrome.** Moderate diastolic hypertension is a major cause of morbidity and death in patients with Cushing's syndrome.
6. **Other endocrine disorders.** Hypertension may be induced by hypothyroidism, hyperthyroidism, and hyperparathyroidism.
7. **Sleep apnea syndrome.** Disordered breathing during sleep is an independent risk factor for awake systemic hypertension.
8. **Coarctation of the aorta** is one of the major causes of hypertension in young children.

III. **Complications of hypertension**
   A. Hypertension is the major risk factor for premature cardiovascular disease, being more common than cigarette smoking, dyslipidemia, and diabetes, the other major risk factors.
   B. Hypertension increases the risk of heart failure.

C. Left ventricular hypertrophy is a common problem in patients with hypertension, and is associated with an enhanced incidence of heart failure, ventricular arrhythmias, death following myocardial infarction, and sudden cardiac death.

D. Hypertension is the most common and most important risk factor for stroke.

E. Hypertension is the most important risk factor for intracerebral hemorrhage.

F. Hypertension is a risk factor for chronic renal insufficiency.

IV. Diagnosis

A. Blood pressure should be measured at each office visit for patients over the age of 21.

B. In the absence of end-organ damage, the diagnosis of mild hypertension should not be made until the blood pressure has been measured on at least three to six visits, spaced over a period of weeks to months.

C. **White-coat hypertension and ambulatory monitoring.** 20 to 25 percent of patients with mild office hypertension (diastolic pressure 90 to 104 mm Hg) have "white-coat" or isolated office hypertension in that their blood pressure is repeatedly normal when measured at home, at work, or by ambulatory blood pressure monitoring. Ambulatory monitoring can be used to confirm the presence of white-coat hypertension.

V. Evaluation

A. **History.** The history should search for the presence of precipitating or aggravating factors, the natural course of the blood pressure, the extent of target organ damage, and the presence of other risk factors for cardiovascular disease.

B. **Physical examination** should evaluate for signs of end-organ damage (such as retinopathy) and for evidence of a cause of secondary hypertension.

C. **Laboratory testing**

1. Hematocrit, urinalysis, and routine blood chemistries (glucose, creatinine, electrolytes).

2. Fasting (9 to 12 hours) lipid profile (total and HDL-cholesterol, triglycerides).

3. Electrocardiogram.

History in the Patient with Hypertension

Duration of hypertension 　Last known normal blood pressure 　Course of the blood pressure **Prior treatment of hypertension** 　Drugs: doses, side effects **Intake of agents that may cause hypertension** 　Estrogens, sympathomimetics, adrenal 　steroids, excessive sodium **Family history** 　Hypertension 　Premature cardiovascular disease or 　death 　Familial diseases: pheochromocytoma, 　renal disease, diabetes, gout **Symptoms of secondary cause** 　Muscle weakness 　Spells of tachycardia, sweating, tremor 　Thinning of the skin 　Flank pain	**Symptoms of target organ damage** 　Headaches 　Transient weakness or blindness 　Loss of visual acuity 　Chest pain 　Dyspnea 　Claudication **Other risk factors** 　Smoking 　Diabetes 　Dyslipidemias 　Physical inactivity **Dietary history** 　Sodium 　Alcohol 　Saturated fats

---

Physical Examination in the Patient with Hypertension

Accurate measurement of blood pressure
General appearance: distribution of body fat, skin lesions, muscle strength, alertness
Funduscope
Neck: palpation and auscultation of carotids, thyroid
Heart: size, rhythm, sounds Lungs: rhonchi, rales
Abdomen: renal masses, bruits over aorta or renal arteries, femoral pulses
Extremities: peripheral pulses, edema
Neurologic assessment

D. Testing for renovascular hypertension. Renovascular hypertension is the most common correctable cause of secondary hypertension. It occurs in less than one percent of patients with mild hypertension. In comparison, between 10 and 45 percent of white patients with severe or malignant hypertension have renal artery stenosis.

  1. Signs suggesting renovascular hypertension or other cause of secondary hypertension:

     a. Severe or refractory hypertension, including retinal hemorrhages or papilledema; bilateral renovascular disease may be present in patients who also have a plasma creatinine above 1.5 mg/dL (132 µmol/L).

     b. An acute rise in blood pressure over a previously stable baseline.

     c. Age of onset before puberty or above 50.

     d. An acute elevation in the plasma creatinine concentration that is either unexplained or occurs after the institution of an angiotensin converting enzyme inhibitor or angiotensin II receptor blocker (in the absence of an excessive reduction in blood pressure).

     e. Moderate-to-severe hypertension in a patient with diffuse atherosclerosis or an incidentally discovered asymmetry in renal disease. A unilateral small kidney ($\leq$9 cm) has a 75 percent correlation with the presence of large vessel occlusive disease.

     f. A systolic-diastolic abdominal bruit that lateralizes to one side.

     g. Negative family history for hypertension.

     h. Moderate-to-severe hypertension in patients with recurrent episodes of acute (flash) pulmonary edema or otherwise unexplained congestive heart failure.

  2. Spiral CT scanning or 3D time-of-flight MR angiography are minimally invasive diagnostic methods. Duplex Doppler ultrasonography may be useful both for diagnosis and for predicting the outcome of therapy.

E. Testing for other causes of secondary hypertension

  1. The presence of primary renal disease is suggested by an elevated plasma creatinine concentration and/or an abnormal urinalysis.

  2. **Pheochromocytoma** should be suspected if there are paroxysmal elevations in blood pressure, particularly if associated with the triad of headache (usually pounding), palpitations, and sweating.

  3. **Plasma renin activity** is usually performed only in patients with possible low-renin forms of hypertension, such as primary hyperaldosteronism. Otherwise unexplained hypokalemia is the primary clinical clue to the latter disorder in which the plasma aldosterone to plasma renin activity ratio is a screening test.

  4. **Cushing's syndrome** (including that due to corticosteroid administration) is usually suggested by cushingoid facies, central obesity, ecchymoses, and muscle weakness.

5. **Sleep apnea syndrome** should be suspected in obese individuals who snore loudly while asleep, awake with headache, and fall asleep inappropriately during the day.
6. **Coarctation of the aorta** is characterized by decreased or lagging peripheral pulses and a vascular bruit over the back.
7. Hypertension may be induced by both hypothyroidism and primary hyperparathyroidism, suspected because of hypercalcemia.

Evaluation of Secondary Hypertension	
Renovascular Hypertension	Captopril test: Plasma renin level before and 1 hr after captopril 25 mg. A greater than 150% increase in renin is positive Captopril renography: Renal scan before and after 25 mg MRI angiography Arteriography (DSA)
Hyperaldosteronism	Serum potassium Serum aldosterone and plasma renin activity CT scan of adrenals
Pheochromocytoma	24 hr urine catecholamines CT scan Nuclear MIBG scan
Cushing's Syndrome	Plasma cortisol Dexamethasone suppression test
Hyperparathyroidism	Serum calcium Serum parathyroid hormone

VI. Treatment of essential hypertension
A. **Benefits of blood pressure control.** Antihypertensive therapy is associated with 35 to 40 percent reduction in stroke incidence; 20 to 25 percent in myocardial infarction; and more than 50 percent in heart failure. Optimal control to below 130/80 mm Hg could prevent 37 and 56 percent of coronary heart disease events.
B. All patients should undergo lifestyle modification. A patient should not be labeled as having hypertension unless the blood pressure is persistently elevated after three to six visits over a several-month period.

Lifestyle Modifications in the Management of Hypertension		
Modification	**Recommendation**	**Approximate systolic BP reduction, range**[*]
Weight reduction	Maintain normal body weight (BMI), 18.5 to 24.9 kg/m^2	5 to 20 mm Hg per 10-kg weight loss
DASH eating plan	Consume a diet rich in fruits, vegetables, and low-fat dairy products, with a reduced content of saturated and total fat	8 to 14 mm Hg

Modification	Recommendation	Approximate systolic BP reduction, range*
Dietary sodium reduction	Reduce dietary sodium intake to no more than 100 meq/day (2.4 sodium or 6 g sodium chloride)	2 to 8 mm Hg
Physical activity	Regular aerobic physical activity, such as brisk walking (at least 30 minutes per day, most days of the week)	4 to 9 mm Hg
Moderate consumption of alcohol consumption	Limit consumption to no more than 2 drinks per day in most men and no more than 1 drink per day in women	2 to 4 mm Hg

- **C.** Antihypertensive medications should be begun if the systolic pressure is persistently $\geq$140 mm Hg and/or the diastolic pressure is persistently $\geq$90 mm Hg in the office and at home despite attempted nonpharmacologic therapy. Starting with two drugs may be considered in patients with a baseline blood pressure more than 20/10 mm Hg above goal.
- **D.** In patients with diabetes or chronic renal failure, antihypertensive therapy is indicated when the systolic pressure is persistently above 130 mm Hg and/or the diastolic pressure is above 80 mm Hg.
- **E.** Patients with office hypertension, normal values at home, and no evidence of end-organ damage should undergo ambulatory blood pressure monitoring.
- **F. Lifestyle modifications**
  - **1.** Treatment of hypertension generally begins with nonpharmacologic therapy, including dietary sodium restriction, weight reduction in the obese, avoidance of excess alcohol, and regular aerobic exercise.
  - **2.** A low-sodium diet will usually lower high blood pressure and may prevent the onset of hypertension. The overall impact of moderate sodium reduction is a fall in blood pressure of 4.8/2.5 mm Hg. Dietary intake should be reduced to 2.3 g of sodium or 6 g of salt.
  - **3.** Weight loss in obese individuals can lead to a significant fall in blood pressure.
  - **4. Goal blood pressure**
    - **a.** The goal of antihypertensive therapy in patients with uncomplicated combined systolic and diastolic hypertension is a blood pressure of below 140/90 mm Hg.
    - **b.** For individuals over age 65 with isolated systolic hypertension (eg, a diastolic blood pressure below 90 mm Hg), caution is needed not to inadvertently lower the diastolic blood pressure to below 65 mm Hg to attain a goal systolic pressure <140 mm Hg, since this level of diastolic pressure has been associated with an increased risk of stroke.
    - **c.** A goal blood pressure of less than 130/80 mm Hg is recommended in patients with diabetes mellitus; and patients with slowly progressive chronic renal failure, particularly those excreting more than 1 g of protein per day.

VII. Drug therapy in essential hypertension

A. Each of the antihypertensive agents is roughly equally effective, producing a good antihypertensive response in 30 to 50 percent of cases.

B. A thiazide diuretic is recommended as initial drug therapy in most patients. African American patients generally responding better to monotherapy with a thiazide diuretic or calcium channel blocker and relatively poorly to an ACE inhibitor or beta-blocker.

C. Initial therapy

1. The seventh Joint National Committee (JNC 7) report recommends initiating therapy in uncomplicated hypertensives with a thiazide diuretic (eg, 12.5 to 25 mg of hydrochlorothiazide or chlorthalidone). This regimen is associated with a low rate of metabolic complications, such as hypokalemia, glucose intolerance, and hyperuricemia.

2. If low-dose thiazide monotherapy fails to attain goal blood pressure in uncomplicated hypertensives, an ACE inhibitor/ARB, beta-blocker, or calcium channel blocker can be sequentially added or substituted. Most often an ACE inhibitor/ARB, which acts synergistically with a diuretic, is used.

Considerations for Individualizing Antihypertensive Therapy	
Indication	**Antihypertensive drugs**
Compelling indications (major improvement in outcome independent of blood pressure)	
Systolic heart failure	ACE inhibitor or ARB, beta blocker, diuretic, aldosterone antagonist
Post-myocardial infarction	beta blocker, ACE inhibitor, aldosterone antagonist
Proteinuric chronic renal failure	ACE inhibitor and/or ARB
High coronary disease risk	Diuretic, perhaps ACE inhibitor
Diabetes mellitus (no proteinuria)	Diuretic, perhaps ACE inhibitor
Angina pectoris	Beta blocker, calcium channel blocker
Atrial fibrillation rate control	Beta blocker, nondihydropyridine calcium channel blocker
Atrial flutter rate control	Beta blocker, nondihydropyridine calcium channel blocker
Likely to have a favorable effect on symptoms in comorbid conditions	
Essential tremor	Beta blocker (noncardioselective)
Hyperthyroidism	Beta blocker
Migraine	Beta blocker, calcium channel blocker

Indication	Antihypertensive drugs
Osteoporosis	Thiazide diuretic
Raynaud's syndrome	Dihydropyridine calcium channel blocker

Contraindications to Specific Antihypertensive Agents	
Indication	**Antihypertensive drugs**
Bronchospastic disease	Beta blocker
Pregnancy	ACE inhibitor, ARB (includes women likely to become pregnant)
Second or third degree heart block	Beta blocker, nondihydropyridine calcium channel blocker
May have adverse effect on comorbid conditions	
Depression	Beta blocker, central alpha agonist
Gout	Diuretic
Hyperkalemia	Aldosterone antagonist, ACE inhibitor, ARB
Hyponatremia	Thiazide diuretic
Renovascular disease	ACE inhibitor or ARB

D. Diuretics

1. A low-dose thiazide diuretic provides better cardioprotection than an ACE inhibitor or a calcium channel blocker in patients with risk factors for coronary artery disease, including left ventricular hypertrophy, type 2 diabetes, previous myocardial infarction or stroke, current cigarette smoking habits, hyperlipidemia, or atherosclerotic cardiovascular disease.
2. Diuretics should also be given for fluid control in patients with heart failure or nephrotic syndrome; these settings usually require loop diuretics. In addition, an aldosterone antagonist is indicated in patients with advanced HF who have relatively preserved renal function and for the treatment of hypokalemia.

Thiazide Diuretics	
Drug	**Usual dose**
Hydrochlorothiazide (HCTZ, Hydrodiuril)	12.5-25 mg qd
Chlorthalidone (Hygroton)	12.5-25 mg qd
Chlorothiazide (Diuril)	125-500 mg qd
Indapamide (Lozol)	1.25 mg qd

Drug	Usual dose
Metolazone (Zaroxolyn)	1.25-5 mg qd

E. ACE inhibitors provide survival benefits in heart failure and myocardial infarction (particularly ST elevation) and renal benefits in proteinuric chronic renal failure. Thus, an ACE inhibitor should be used in heart failure, prior myocardial infarction, asymptomatic left ventricular dysfunction, type 1 diabetics with nephropathy, and nondiabetic proteinuric chronic renal failure. The use of ACE inhibitors in these settings is independent of the need for BP control.

Angiotensin-converting enzyme inhibitors		
Drug	**Usual doses**	**Maximum dose**
Benazepril (Lotensin)	10-40 mg qd or divided bid	80 mg/d
Captopril (Capoten)	50 mg bid-qid	450 mg/d
Enalapril (Vasotec, Vasotec IV)	10-40 mg qd or divided bid	40 mg/d
Fosinopril (Monopril)	20-40 mg qd or divided bid	80 mg/d
Lisinopril (Prinivil, Zestril)	20-40 mg qd	40 mg/d
Moexipril (Univasc)	15-30 mg qd	30 mg/d
Quinapril (Accupril)	20-80 mg qd or divided bid	80 mg/d
Ramipril (Altace)	5-20 mg qd or divided bid	20 mg/d
Trandolapril (Mavik)	1-4 mg qd	8 mg/d
Perindopril (Aceon)	4-8 mg qd-bid	8 mg/d

F. ARBs. The indications for and efficacy of ARBs are the same as those with ACE inhibitors. An ARB is particularly indicated in patients who do not tolerate ACE inhibitors (mostly because of cough).

Angiotensin II Receptor Blockers		
Drug	**Usual dose**	**Maximum dose**
Losartan (Cozaar)	50 mg qd	100 mg/d
Candesartan (Atacand)	4-8 mg qd	16 mg/d
Eprosartan (Teveten)	400-800 mg qd	800 mg/d
Irbesartan (Avapro)	150-300 mg qd	300 mg/d
Telmisartan (Micardis)	40-80 mg qd	80 mg/d

Drug	Usual dose	Maximum dose
Valsartan (Diovan)	80 mg qd	320 mg/d

G. Beta-blockers. A beta-blocker without intrinsic sympathomimetic activity should be given after an acute myocardial infarction and to stable patients with heart failure or asymptomatic left ventricular dysfunction (beginning with very low doses). The use of beta-blockers in these settings is in addition to the recommendations for ACE inhibitors in these disorders. Beta-blockers are also given for rate control in atrial fibrillation and for angina.

Beta-blockers		
Drug	Usual dose	Maximum dose
Acebutolol (Sectral)	200-800 mg/d (qd or bid)	1.2 g/d (bid)
Atenolol (Tenormin)	50-100 mg qd	100 mg qd
Betaxolol (Kerlone)	10 mg qd	20 mg qd
Bisoprolol (Zebeta)	5 mg qd	20 mg qd
Carteolol (Cartrol)	2.5 mg qd	10 mg qd
Carvedilol (Coreg)	6.26-25 mg bid	100 mg/d
Labetalol (Normodyne, Trandate)	100-600 mg bid	1200 mg/d
Metoprolol (Toprol XL)	100-200 mg qd	400 mg qd
Metoprolol (Lopressor)	100-200 mg/d (qd or bid)	450 mg/d (qd or bid)
Nadolol (Corgard)	40 mg qd	320 mg/d
Penbutolol (Levatol)	20 mg qd	NA
Pindolol (Visken)	5 mg bid	60 mg/d
Propranolol (Inderal, Inderal LA)	120-160 mg qd (LA 640 mg/d)	
Timolol (Blocadren)	10-20 mg bid	60 mg/d (bid)

H. Calcium channel blockers. Like beta-blockers, they can be given for rate control in patients with atrial fibrillation or for control of angina. Calcium channel blockers may be preferred in obstructive airways disease.

Calcium channel blockers	
Drug	Dosage
Diltiazem extended-release (Cardizem SR)	120-360 mg in 2 doses

Drug	Dosage
Diltiazem CD (Cardizem CD)	120-360 mg in 1 dose
Diltiazem XR (Dilacor XR)	120-480 mg in 1 dose
Verapamil (Calan)	120-480 mg in 2 or 3 doses
Verapamil extended-release (Calan SR)	120-480 mg in 1 or 2 doses
Verapamil HS (Covera-HS)	180-480 mg in 1 dose
Dihydropyridines	
Amlodipine (Norvasc)	2.5-10 mg in 1 dose
Felodipine (Plendil)	2.5-10 mg in 1 dose
Isradipine (DynaCirc)	5-10 mg in 2 doses
Isradipine extended-release (DynaCirc CR)	5-10 mg in 1 dose
Nicardipine (Cardene)	60-120 mg in 3 doses
Nicardipine extended-release (Cardene SR)	60-120 mg in 2 doses
Nifedipine extended-release (Adalat CC, Procardia XL)	30-90 mg in 1 dose
Nisoldipine (Sular)	10-60 mg in 1 dose

I. **Combination therapy**
   1. If two drugs are required, use of a low dose of a thiazide diuretic as one of the drugs increases the response rate to all other agents. By minimizing volume expansion, diuretics increase the antihypertensive effect of all other antihypertensive drugs.
   2. The combination of a thiazide diuretic with a beta-blocker, an ACE inhibitor, or an ARB has a synergistic effect, controlling the BP in up to 85 percent of patients.
   3. **Fixed-dose combination.** A wide variety of (low) dose combination preparations are available, including low doses of a diuretic with a beta-blocker, ACE inhibitor, or ARB. Combination preparations include:
      a. Sustained-release verapamil (180 mg) - trandolapril (2 mg).
      b. Atenolol (100 mg) - chlorthalidone (25 mg).
      c. Lisinopril (20 mg) - hydrochlorothiazide (12.5 mg).
      d. The three combinations were equally effective, normalizing the blood pressure or lowering the diastolic pressure by more than 10 mm Hg in 69 to 76 percent of patients. All are well tolerated.

Combination Agents for Hypertension

Drug	Initial dose	Comments
Beta-Blocker/Diuretic		
Atenolol/chlorthalidone (Tenoretic)	50 mg/25 mg, 1 tab qd	Additive vasodilation
Bisoprolol/HCTZ (Ziac)	2.5 mg/6.25 mg, 1 tab qd	
Metoprolol/HCTZ (Lopressor HCTZ)	100 mg/25 mg, 1 tab qd	
Nadolol/HCTZ (Corzide)	40 mg/5 mg, 1 tab qd	
Propranolol/HCTZ (Inderide LA)	80 mg/50 mg, 1 tab qd	
Timolol/HCTZ (Timolide)	10 mg/25 mg, 1 tab qd	
ACE inhibitor/Diuretic		
Benazepril/HCTZ (Lotensin HCT)	5 mg/6.25 mg, 1 tab qd	ACE inhibitor conserves potassium and magnesium; combination beneficial for CHF patients with HTN
Captopril/HCTZ (Capozide)	25 mg/15 mg, 1 tab qd	
Enalapril/HCTZ (Vaseretic)	5 mg/12.5 mg, 1 tab qd	
Lisinopril/HCTZ (Zestoretic, Prinzide)	10 mg/12.5 mg, 1 tab qd	
Moexipril/HCTZ (Uniretic)	7.5 mg/12.5 mg, 1 tab qd	
ACE inhibitor/Calcium-channel blocker		
Benazepril/amlodipine (Lotrel)	2.5 mg/10 mg, 1 tab qd	
Enalapril/felodipine (Lexxel)	5 mg/5 mg, 1 tab qd	
Enalapril/diltiazem (Teczem)	5 mg/180 mg, 1 tab qd	
Trandolapril/verapamil (Tarka)	2 mg/180 mg, 1 tab qd	
Angiotensin II receptor blocker/Diuretic		
Losartan/HCTZ (Hyzaar)	50 mg/12.5 mg, 1 tab qd	
Valsartan/HCTZ (Diovan HCT)	80 mg/12.5 mg, 1 tab qd	
Alpha-1-Blocker/Diuretic		
Prazosin/polythiazide (Minizide)	1 mg/0.5 mg, 1 cap bid	Synergistic vasodilation
K$^+$-sparing diuretic/Thiazide		

Drug	Initial dose	Comments
Amiloride/HCTZ (Moduretic)	5 mg/50 mg, 1 tab qd	Electrolyte-sparing effect
Triamterene/HCTZ (Dyazide, Maxzide)	37.5 mg/25 mg, 1/2 tab qd	

References, see page 372.

Hypertensive Urgencies

Hypertensive urgency is defined as severe hypertension without symptoms. Severe hypertension is defined as systolic blood pressure 180 mmHg and/or diastolic blood pressure 120 mmHg. When hypertension of this degree is asymptomatic with no acute signs of end-organ damage it is designated hypertensive urgency. Severe hypertension can occur when patients are noncompliant with antihypertensive regimens and following ingestion of large quantities of sodium.

I. **Treatment.** Blood pressure should be confirmed with a repeat measurement.
   A. **Blood pressure reduction goals.** Cerebral or myocardial ischemia or infarction can be induced by aggressive antihypertensive therapy. In the absence of signs of acute end-organ damage, the goal of management is to reduce the blood pressure to 160/100 mmHg over several hours to days.
   B. **Management of previously treated hypertension:**
      1. Increase the dose of existing antihypertensive medications, or add another agent.
      2. Restart medications in non-adherent patients.
      3. Add a diuretic, and reinforcement of dietary sodium restriction, in patients who have worsening hypertension due to high sodium intake.
   C. **Management of previously untreated hypertension:**
      1. **Initial blood pressure reduction** should take place over several hours. Give oral furosemide (if the patient is not volume depleted) at a dose of 20 mg; or a small dose of oral clonidine (0.2 mg); or a small dose of oral captopril (6.25 or 12.5 mg). Following administration of one of these agents, the patient is observed for a few hours, to observe a reduction in blood pressure of 20 to 30 mmHg. Thereafter, a longer acting agent is prescribed and the patient is sent home to follow-up within a few days.
      2. **Blood pressure reduction over one to two days.** A calcium channel blocker, beta blocker or angiotensin converting enzyme (ACE) inhibitor or receptor blocker can be started. Examples are nifedipine (Procardia XL) 30 mg once or twice daily, metoprolol (Lopressor) 50 mg twice daily, or enalapril (Vasotec) 5 mg once or twice daily (patients with normal kidney function usually require twice daily dosing).
      3. **Choice of agent** should take into consideration the type of antihypertensive agent that is most appropriate in the long term.
         a. **Hydrochlorothiazide** 12.5 to 25 mg; initial therapy for many patients without other medical problems.
         b. **Enalapril (Vasotec)** 10-40 mg qd or divided bid; use for patients with systolic heart failure.
         c. **Metoprolol (Lopressor)** 50 mg twice daily; use for post-myocardial infarction.
         d. **Nifedipine extended-release (Procardia XL)** 30-90 mg qd; calcium channel blockers are preferred over ACE inhibitors and beta blockers in blacks.

4. Over subsequent weeks and months, the dose and selection of medications should be adjusted as needed to achieve desired goals (eg, <140/90 or <130/80 mmHg) with longer acting agents.

Considerations for Individualizing Antihypertensive Therapy	
Indication	Antihypertensive drugs
Compelling indications (major improvement in outcome independent of blood pressure)	
Systolic heart failure	ACE inhibitor or ARB, beta blocker, diuretic, aldosterone antagonist
Post-myocardial infarction	beta blocker, ACE inhibitor, aldosterone antagonist
Proteinuric chronic renal failure	ACE inhibitor and/or ARB
High coronary disease risk	Diuretic, perhaps ACE inhibitor
Diabetes mellitus (no proteinuria)	Diuretic, perhaps ACE inhibitor
Angina pectoris	Beta blocker, calcium channel blocker
Atrial fibrillation rate control	Beta blocker, nondihydropyridine calcium channel blocker
Atrial flutter rate control	Beta blocker, nondihydropyridine calcium channel blocker
Likely to have a favorable effect on symptoms in comorbid conditions	
Essential tremor	Beta blocker (noncardioselective)
Hyperthyroidism	Beta blocker
Migraine	Beta blocker, calcium channel blocker
Osteoporosis	Thiazide diuretic
Raynaud's syndrome	Dihydropyridine calcium channel blocker

Hypertensive Emergencies

Hypertensive emergency is defined as severe hypertension associated with acute end-organ damage, such as hypertensive encephalopathy, subarachnoid or intracerebral hemorrhage, acute pulmonary edema, or aortic dissection. Severe hypertension is defined as systolic blood pressure 180 mmHg and/or diastolic blood pressure 120 mmHg. Immediate but careful reduction in blood pressure is indicated for hypertensive emergency. Excessive hypotension caused by drug treatment is dangerous and could result in stroke, myocardial infarction or blindness.

I. Antihypertensive drugs

A. Nitroprusside, an arteriolar and venous dilator, is given as an intravenous infusion. Initial dose: 0.25 to 0.5 µg/kg per min; maximum dose: 8 to 10 µg/kg per min.

B. Nitroglycerin, a venous and arteriolar dilator, is given as an intravenous infusion. Initial dose: 5 µg/min; maximum dose: 100 µg/min.

C. Labetalol (Trandate), an alpha- and ß-adrenergic blocker, is given as an intravenous bolus or infusion. Bolus: 20 mg initially, followed by 20 to 80 mg every 10 minutes to a total dose of 300 mg. Infusion: 0.5 to 2 mg/min.

D. Nicardipine (Cardene), a calcium channel blocker, given as an intravenous infusion. Initial dose: 5 mg/h; maximum dose: 15 mg/h.

E. Fenoldopam (Corlopam), a peripheral dopamine-1 receptor agonist, is given as an intravenous infusion. Initial dose: 0.1 µg/kg per min; the dose is titrated at 15 min intervals, depending upon the blood pressure response.

F. Hydralazine, an arteriolar dilator, is given as an intravenous bolus. Initial dose: 10 mg given every 20 to 30 minutes; maximum dose: 20 mg.

G. Propranolol (Inderol) a ß-adrenergic blocker, is given as an intravenous infusion and then followed by oral therapy. Dose: 1 to 10 mg load, followed by 3 mg/h.

H. Phentolamine, an a-adrenergic blocker, is given as an intravenous bolus. Dose: 5 to 10 mg every 5 to 15 minutes.

I. Enalaprilat (Vasotec IV) an angiotensin converting enzyme inhibitor, is given as an intravenous bolus. Dose: 1.25 mg every six hours.

II. Choice of agent for hypertensive emergencies

A. Nitroprusside is the most rapid-acting and potent parenteral antihypertensive agent. It acts within seconds and has a duration of action of only 2 to 5 minutes. Hypotension can be easily reversed by temporarily discontinuing the infusion. The major limitation is the development of cyanide toxicity with high doses, for a prolonged period (>24 to 48 hours), or with underlying renal insufficiency.

B. Alternatives to nitroprusside include intravenous labetalol, nicardipine, and fenoldopam. These agents are better than nitroprusside because hypotension is uncommon with these drugs and cyanide toxicity does not occur.

C. Intravenous fenoldopam, a dopamine agonist that acts at the vasodilator DA1 receptors, is as effective and almost as short-acting as nitroprusside. It has the advantages of increasing renal blood flow and sodium excretion, of not causing accumulation of cyanide, and of not requiring shielding from light.

Parenteral drugs for treatment of hypertensive emergencies					
Drug	Dose	Onset	Duration	Adverse effects	Indications
Vasodilators					
Nitroprusside	0.25-10 µg/kg/min as IV infusion	Immediate	1-2 min	Nausea, vomiting, muscle twitching, sweating, thiocynate and cyanide intoxication	Most hypertensive emergencies; caution with high intracranial pressure or azotemia

Drug	Dose	Onset	Duration	Adverse effects	Indications
Nicardipine (Cardene)	5-15 mg/h IV	5-10 min	15-30 min, may exceed 4 h	Tachycardia, headache, flushing, local phlebitis	Most hypertensive emergencies except acute heart failure; caution with coronary ischemia
Fenoldopam (Corlopam)	0.1-0.3 µg/kg per min IV infusion	<5 min	30 min	Tachycardia, headache, nausea, flushing	Most hypertensive emergencies; caution with glaucoma
Nitroglycerin	5-100 µg/min as IV infusion	2-5 min	5-10 min	Headache, vomiting, methemoglobinemia, tolerance with prolonged use	Coronary ischemia
Enalaprilat (Vasotec IV)	1.25-5 mg every 6 h IV	15-30 min	6-12 h	Precipitous fall in pressure in high-renin states; variable response	Left ventricular failure; avoid in acute myocardial infarction
Hydralazine	10-20 mg IV	10-20 min IV	1-4 h IV	Tachycardia, flushing, headache, vomiting, angina	Eclampsia
	10-40 mg IM	20-30 min IM	4-6 h IM		
Andrenergic inhibitors					
Labetalol (Trandate)	20-80 mg IV bolus every 10 min	5-10 min	3-6 h	Vomiting, scalp tingling, bronchoconstriction, dizziness, nausea, heart block, orthostatic hypotension	Most hypertensive emergencies except acute heart failure
	0.5-2.0 mg/min IV infusion				
Esmolol (Brevibloc)	250-500 µg/kg/min by infusion; may repeat bolus after 5 min or increase infusion to 300 µg/min	1-2 min	10-30 min	Hypotension, nausea, asthma, first-degree heart block, HF	Aortic dissection, perioperative

Drug	Dose	Onset	Dura-tion	Adverse ef-fects	Indications
Phentolamine	5-15 mg IV bolus	1-2 min	10-30 min	Tachycardia, flushing, head-ache	Catecholamine excess

III. **Treatment of specific hypertensive emergencies**
   A. **Ischemic stroke or subarachnoid or intracerebral hemorrhage.** The benefit of reducing the BP in these disorders must be weighed against possible worsening of cerebral ischemia caused by the thrombotic lesion or by cerebral vasospasm. These cerebrovascular events manifest as an abrupt onset of focal neurologic findings. Hypertensive encephalopathy, however, manifests as gradual insidious onset of headache, nausea, vomiting, and confusion.
   B. **Acute pulmonary edema.** Hypertension in patients with acute left ventricular failure due to systolic dysfunction should be treated with vasodilators. Nitroprusside or nitroglycerin with a loop diuretic is the regimen of choice. Drugs that decrease cardiac contractility (labetalol, other beta blockers) should be avoided.
   C. **Angina pectoris or acute myocardial infarction.** Acute coronary insufficiency frequently increases the systemic blood pressure. Intravenous parenteral vasodilators, such as nitroprusside and nitroglycerin, are effective and reduce mortality in patients with acute myocardial infarction with hypertension. Labetalol is also effective in this setting. Drugs that increase cardiac work (hydralazine) are contraindicated.
   D. **Aortic dissection.** The initial aim of medical therapy is to decrease the systolic pressure to 100-120 mmHg and reduce cardiac contractility. These goals are achieved by the combination of nitroprusside and an intravenous beta blocker, such as propranolol or labetalol. Nitroprusside should not be given without a beta blocker.
   E. **Withdrawal of antihypertensive therapy.** Abrupt discontinuation of a short-acting sympathetic blocker (such as clonidine or propranolol) can lead to severe hypertension and coronary ischemia. Control of the BP can be achieved in this setting by readministration of the discontinued drug and, if necessary, phentolamine, nitroprusside, or labetalol.
   F. **Acute increase in sympathetic activity.** Increased adrenergic activity can lead to severe hypertension.
      1. Pheochromocytoma.
      2. Autonomic dysfunction, as in the Guillain-Barré syndrome or post-spinal cord injury.
      3. Sympathomimetic drugs, such as, cocaine, amphetamines, phencyclidine, or the combination of an MAO (monoamine oxidase) inhibitor and tyramine-containing foods (fermented cheeses, smoked or aged meats, Chianti, champagne, and avocados).
      4. Control of the hypertension in these disorders can be achieved with phentolamine, labetalol, or nitroprusside. Administration of a ß-blocker alone is contraindicated, since inhibition of ß-receptor-induced vasodilation results in unopposed alpha-adrenergic vasoconstriction and a further rise in BP.
   G. **Malignant hypertension** is marked hypertension with retinal hemorrhages, exudates, or papilledema. Malignant hypertension is usually associated with a diastolic pressure above 120 mmHg.
      1. Malignant hypertension most often occurs in patients with long-standing uncontrolled hypertension, many of whom have discontinued antihypertensive therapy.

H. **Hypertensive encephalopathy** refers to cerebral edema caused by severe and sudden rises in blood pressure.
   1. Hypertensive encephalopathy can be seen at diastolic pressures as low as 100 mmHg in previously normotensive patients with acute hypertension due to preeclampsia or acute glomerulonephritis.
   2. Hypertensive encephalopathy is characterized by the gradual onset of headache, nausea, and vomiting, followed by restlessness, confusion, seizures, and coma.
   3. These neurologic symptoms differ from the abrupt onset of focal neurologic symptoms seen with a stroke or hemorrhage. However, an MRI scan should be obtained to exclude stroke or hemorrhage.

IV. **Goal of therapy**
   A. The initial aim of treatment in hypertensive crises is to rapidly lower the diastolic pressure to about 100 to 105 mmHg within two to six hours, with the maximum initial fall in BP not exceeding 25 percent of the presenting value.
   B. More aggressive hypotensive therapy may reduce the blood pressure below the autoregulatory range, possibly leading to ischemic events (such as stroke or coronary disease).
   C. Once the BP is controlled, the patient should be switched to oral therapy, with the diastolic pressure being gradually reduced to 85 to 90 mmHg over two to three months.

Hypertensive Emergencies
Accelerated-malignant hypertension with papilloedema
Cerebrovascular Hypertensive encephalopathy Atherothrombotic brain infarction with severe hypertension Intracerebral hemorrhage Subarachnoid hemorrhage
Cardiac Acute aortic dissection Acute left ventricular failure Acute or impending myocardial infarction After coronary bypass surgery
Renal Acute glomerulonephritis Renal crises from collagen vascular diseases Severe hypertension after kidney transplantation
Excessive circulating catecholamines Pheochromocytoma crisis Food or drug interactions with monoamine-oxidase inhibitors Sympathomimetic drug use (cocaine) Rebound hypertension after sudden cessation of antihypertensive drugs
Eclampsia
Surgical Severe hypertension in patients requiring immediate surgery Postoperative hypertension Postoperative bleeding from vascular suture lines

| Severe body burns |
| Severe epistaxis |

References, see page 372.

Syncope

Syncope is defined as the abrupt and transient loss of consciousness associated with loss of postural tone, followed by a rapid and complete recovery. Although syncope can be a premonitory sign of many diseases and can resemble a cardiac arrest, it usually has a benign and self-limited cause. Syncope can be a warning sign of impending cardiac arrest in patients with organic heart disease.

I. Causes of syncope
A. Cardiac cause, most often a bradyarrhythmia or tachyarrhythmia — 23 percent
B. Neurally mediated cause — 58 percent
C. Neurologic or psychiatric cause — 1 percent
D. Unexplained syncope — 18 percent
E. Syncope and cardiac arrest are different entities that must be distinguished from each other. Patients in whom cardiopulmonary resuscitation or electric or pharmacologic cardioversion have been required should be designated a cardiac arrest and not syncope. Patients with cardiac syncope have a very high incidence of subsequent cardiac arrest (24 percent).
F. The evaluation of the patient with syncope is the same as that for presyncope, which is the prodromal symptom of fainting.

II. History
A. **Number of episodes.** Benign causes of syncope usually present with a single syncopal episode or with multiple episodes spread out over many years. A serious underlying disorder is likely when multiple episodes of syncope occur over a short period of time.
B. **Associated symptoms.** Dyspnea is indicative of an acute pulmonary embolism; angina indicates an underlying cardiac cause; a history of focal neurologic abnormalities implies a neurologic origin; nausea, vomiting, diaphoresis, and pallor after an episode suggest high vagal tone; and urination and defecation suggest a seizure.
C. **Prodrome.** Neurocardiogenic syncope (ie, vasovagal syncope) is usually associated with a prodrome of nausea, warmth, pallor, lightheadedness, and/or diaphoresis."Auras" occur before seizures.
D. **Position.** Neurocardiogenic syncope commonly occurs when the patient is erect, not usually when supine. Syncope resulting from orthostatic hypotension is frequently associated with the change from a supine to erect posture. Syncope that occurs when the patient is supine suggests an arrhythmia.
E. **Warning.** Sudden loss of consciousness without warning is most likely to result from an arrhythmia (bradycardia or tachycardia).
F. **Preceding events.** Coughing, eating, drinking cold liquid, urinating, and defecating can all cause syncope; these causes are designated situational syncope.
G. **Duration of symptoms.** Prolonged loss of consciousness is characteristic of a seizure or aortic stenosis. Arrhythmias and neurocardiogenic syncope are often associated with a brief period of syncope because the supine position reestablishes some blood flow to the brain.
H. **Recovery.** Nausea, pallor, and diaphoresis and a prolonged recovery from the episode suggest a vagal event caused by neurocardiogenic syncope. Syncope

caused by an arrhythmia is not associated with nausea or pallor. Neurologic changes or confusion during the recovery period is suggestive of a stroke or seizure.

I. **Witnesses** to the syncopal event may provide an account of any limb movements and the presence or absence of pallor or diaphoresis. The presence or absence of a pulse is also valuable information.

J. **Exertional syncope** may be caused by ventricular tachycardia and obstruction resulting from aortic stenosis or hypertrophic cardiomyopathy, and hypotension due to vagally-mediated vasodepression in patients with hypertrophic cardiomyopathy.

   1. Syncope associated with exercise also occurs in patients, usually young, who do not have underlying heart disease. Neurocardiogenic syncope, while not uncommon, is the diagnosis of exclusion if syncope occurred with exertion.

K. **Age.** Neurocardiogenic syncope is more likely to occur among young, otherwise healthy patients. The long QT syndrome or hypertrophic cardiomyopathy can also occur in young individuals.

L. **Preexisting medical conditions.** Hyperventilation or panic attacks can cause syncope. Diabetes mellitus may result from orthostatic hypotension secondary to autonomic neuropathy; antihypertensive medications can result in syncope; and heart disease can cause syncope.

M. **Medications or recreational drugs.** Antiarrhythmic (proarrhythmic effects) and antihypertensive agents (sympathetic blockers) can cause syncope. The abuse of illicit drugs or alcohol also has been associated with syncope

N. **Eating.** A vagal "surge" immediately upon swallowing can cause bradycardia and hypotension. Postprandial hypotension may be caused by meal-induced splanchnic pooling.

O. **Distinction of syncope from seizures.** Seizures cause of 5 to 15 percent of apparent syncopal episodes. Seizures can mimic syncope when the seizure is atypical and not associated with tonic-clonic movements.

   1. The postictal state is characterized by a slow and complete recovery. A seizure may cause soft tissue injury at multiple sites due to tonic-clonic movements.

III. **Physical examination**

A. **Abnormal vital signs.** Blood pressure obtained in the supine, sitting, and erect position may reveal orthostatic hypotension. Within two to five minutes of quiet standing, one or more of the following is present:

   1. At least a 20 mmHg fall in systolic pressure
   2. At least a 10 mmHg fall in diastolic pressure
   3. Symptoms of cerebral hypoperfusion

B. **Disturbances in heart rhythm or breathing.** The heart rate may be rapid or slow due to rhythm disturbances, or irregular due to atrial fibrillation. The pulse and blood pressure should be obtained when supine, setting, and erect. Hyperventilation can be seen with pulmonary embolism or panic disorder.

C. **Cardiac auscultation** may reveal the murmur of aortic stenosis, pulmonic stenosis, or atrial myxoma. Pulmonary hypertension may be suggested by a loud, palpable P2.

D. **Physiologic maneuvers.** Changes in an outflow murmur with the Valsalva maneuver indicate hypertrophic cardiomyopathy.

E. **Abnormal neurologic findings.** Unilateral weakness or neurologic deficits may be the result of a cerebral vascular accident.

F. **Gastrointestinal bleeding.** A positive stool guaiac generally indicates gastrointestinal blood loss, which can result in anemia, hypovolemia, and syncope.

G. Carotid sinus massage

1. Carotid sinus hypersensitivity is responsible for the carotid sinus syndrome, and it can be demonstrated by carotid sinus massage. Each carotid artery should be palpated and auscultated for bruits that indicate carotid artery disease.

2. In those without carotid disease, pressure is applied to one carotid sinus for two to three seconds with a vigorous and circular movement at the point at which the carotid artery meets the angle of the jaw, preferably with simultaneous electrocardiographic monitoring. The test is positive if there is a pause of three seconds or more. Carotid sinus pressure should be applied gently and with caution with carotid disease and the elderly.

Medications Associated with Syncope

Antihypertensives/anti-anginals
    Adrenergic antagonists
    Calcium channel blockers
    Diuretics
    Nitrates
    Vasodilators
Antidepressants
    Tricyclic antidepressants
    Phenothiazines

Antiarrhythmics
    Digoxin
    Quinidine
Insulin
Drugs of abuse
    Alcohol
    Cocaine
    Marijuana

Differential Diagnosis of Syncope

Non-cardiovascular	Cardiovascular

Metabolic
   Hyperventilation
   Hypoglycemia
   Hypoxia
Neurologic
   Cerebrovascular insufficiency
   Normal pressure hydrocephalus
   Seizure
   Subclavian steal syndrome
   Increased intracranial pressure
Psychiatric
   Hysteria
   Major depression
	Reflex syncope (heart structurally normal)
	   Neurocardiogenic (Vasovagal)
	   Situational
	   Cough
	   Defecation
	   Micturition
	   Postprandial
	   Sneeze
	   Swallow
	   Carotid sinus syncope
	Orthostatic hypotension
	Drug-induced
	Cardiac
	   Obstructive
	   Aortic dissection
	   Aortic stenosis
	   Cardiac tamponade
	   Hypertrophic cardiomyopathy
	   Left ventricular dysfunction
	   Myocardial infarction
	   Myxoma
	   Pulmonary embolism
	   Pulmonary hypertension
	   Pulmonary stenosis
	   Arrhythmias
	      Bradyarrhythmias
	         Sick sinus syndrome
	         Pacemaker failure
	      Supraventricular and ventricular
	         tachyarrhythmias

Clues to the Etiology of Syncope

Associated Feature	Etiology
Cough Micturition Defecation Swallowing	Situational syncope
Post-syncopal disorientation Urinary or fecal incontinence	Seizure
Syncope with arm exercise	Subclavian steal syndrome
Syncope with shaving	Carotid sinus syncope
Prodromal symptoms (nausea, diaphoresis)	Neurocardiogenic syncope (vasovagal)
Abrupt onset	Cardiac syncope
Syncope with exertion	Aortic stenosis, hypertrophic cardiomyopathy, arrhythmias

Associated Feature	Etiology
Syncope with change of position	Orthostatic hypotension
Blood pressure/pulse differential	Aortic dissection, subclavian steal syndrome
Abnormal postural vital signs	Orthostatic hypotension
Cardiac murmurs/rhythms	Aortic stenosis, hypertrophic cardiomyopathy, arrhythmias, pulmonary hypertension
Carotid bruit	Cerebrovascular insufficiency

IV. Testing

A. Electrocardiogram

1. **ECG findings that may suggest a cause for syncope:**
   a. Sinus bradycardia
   b. Atrioventricular nodal disease (second or third degree heart block)
   c. His-Purkinje system disease (Mobitz type II AV block)
   d. Bundle branch and/or fascicular block
   e. Prolonged QT interval
2. **Prolonged QT interval** implies torsade de pointes as a possible underlying cause for syncope. Patients with the long QT syndrome, however, may have a normal QT interval; however, the QT interval can fail to shorten or may increase during exercise.
3. Other possible causes of syncope that can be diagnosed from electrocardiogram include the Wolff-Parkinson-White syndrome, a myocardial infarction, chronic obstructive pulmonary disease, hypertrophic cardiomyopathy, arrhythmogenic right ventricular dysplasia, and Brugada syndrome. A prolonged rhythm strip of 30 to 60 seconds in length may be useful if the patient is symptomatic at the time of recording.

B. Ambulatory monitoring, either continuous monitoring for 24 to 48 hours or longer-term patient activated event recording, is commonly obtained in the assessment of syncope. Such techniques are of limited diagnostic value because they are useful only if symptoms occur during monitoring, which occurs rarely. Monitoring may be more helpful in excluding arrhythmia as the etiology of syncope if the patient has symptoms while wearing a monitor and no arrhythmia is recorded. Ambulatory monitoring establishes a diagnosis in only 2 to 3 percent of patients with syncope.

1. **Event recorders** appear to be somewhat more helpful than pure ambulatory monitoring in diagnosing the etiology of syncope or presyncope. Intermittent loop recorders have the ability to store several minutes of recording.
2. **Implantable loop recorder (ILR)** is a subcutaneous monitoring device for the detection of cardiac arrhythmias. Such a device is implanted in the left parasternal or pectoral region. It stores recorded ECG strips either when the device is activated automatically, or when the patient manually activates it with a magnet.
3. The ILR may be most useful in patients with infrequent symptoms and a suspected arrhythmia in whom noninvasive testing is negative or inconclusive.

C. Neurologic testing, including electroencephalogram, brain CT scan, brain magnetic resonance imaging, and carotid Doppler ultrasound, is rarely useful. An electroencephalogram may help to rule out epilepsy in patients with

syncope who have seizure-like activity, even though about 50 percent of those with seizures have a positive EEG.

D. **Exercise testing** has a role in patients with a history of exertion-related syncope or exercise-induced arrhythmias. Failure to shorten the QT interval with exercise may be a sign of congenital prolonged QT syndrome when this abnormality is not visible on regular electrocardiogram. Exercise testing may also be useful in patients with hypertrophic cardiomyopathy.

E. **Upright tilt table test** is a commonly performed test for the evaluation of syncope, particularly in young, otherwise healthy patients in whom the diagnosis of neurocardiogenic syncope is often entertained. It can be useful in older persons with suspected neurally mediated syncope.

F. **Brain natriuretic peptide** (BNP) is a hormone that is released from myocardial cells in response to volume expansion and possibly increased cardiac wall stress. Elevated plasma BNP concentrations are typically seen in patients with heart failure and other cardiovascular disorders. Measurement of plasma BNP may be useful in distinguishing cardiac from noncardiac causes of syncope.

G. **Signal-averaged electrocardiogram** (SAECG) may detect patients at risk for ventricular tachyarrhythmias (particularly sustained monomorphic ventricular tachycardia); it has no role in the evaluation of sinus or AV nodal dysfunction. The finding of late potentials on a SAECG has a sensitivity of 80 percent and a specificity of 90 percent for the prediction of inducible sustained ventricular tachycardia.

H. **Electrophysiology study (EPS)** is indicated in patients with unexplained syncope, particularly those with structural heart disease.
   1. Patients who may benefit from an EP study include those with:
      a. Left ventricular dysfunction
      b. Significant epicardial coronary artery disease
      c. A prior myocardial infarction
      d. Other structural heart disease
      e. Conduction system disease (eg, bundle branch block))
   2. In addition, patients without structural heart disease, but whose clinical picture suggests a tachyarrhythmic or bradyarrhythmic cause of syncope, should undergo EPS.

I. **Implantable cardio-defibrillator indications.** Patients with severe left ventricular dysfunction and unexplained syncope represent a unique subgroup who are at risk for sudden cardiac death. Such patients may be appropriate candidates for ICD therapy.

J. **Adenosine** or the related precursor compound adenosine triphosphate (ATP) provoke a short and potent cardioinhibitory response of vagal origin. The administration of these drugs can produce sinus bradycardia or pauses, atrioventricular (AV) block, and vasodepression.
   1. An abnormal response to adenosine (eg, asystole >6 seconds or AV block >10 seconds) can identify patients with a bradycardic cause of previously unexplained syncope.

V. **Indications for hospitalization of the patient with syncope**
   A. The presence of serious injury, or frequent and recurrent symptoms
   B. Old age
   C. The diagnosis or suspicion of a serious cardiovascular or neurologic etiology

VI. **Management of the patient with syncope**
   A. **Metabolic or iatrogenic syncope.** Metabolic abnormalities, anemia, and hypovolemia can be effectively managed by specific therapy which corrects these basic abnormalities. In addition, iatrogenic syncope resulting from drug therapy is a preventable and treatable condition.
   B. **Orthostatic hypotension** (ie, at least a 20 mmHg fall in systolic pressure, a 10 mmHg fall in diastolic pressure, or symptoms) in the absence of volume

depletion is most often due to an autonomic neuropathy or the administration of antidepressant drugs. Therapy for orthostatic hypotension is avoidance of volume depletion and sympathetic blockers and antidepressants. A major benefit may also be achieved from tensing the legs by crossing them while actively standing on both legs.

C. Other physical measures:
   1. Arising slowly in stages from supine to seated to standing
   2. Performing dorsiflexion of the feet or handgrip exercise before standing
   3. Wearing Jobst stockings, up to and including the thighs, to minimize venous pooling

D. Volume expansion with fludrocortisone (0.1 to 1.0 mg/day) and a high salt diet. Patients must be monitored for edema or hypertension. This drug is poorly tolerated in patients over the age of 65.

E. Alternatives to fludrocortisone
   1. **Alpha-1-adrenergic agonists**, such as midodrine (ProAmatine, 2.5 to 10 mg TID) or phenylephrine (Neo-Synephrine, 60 mg every 6 to 12 hours) are alternatives to fludrocortisone.
   2. **Nonsteroidal antiinflammatory drugs**
   3. **Caffeine**
   4. **Fluoxetine**

F. Cardiovascular disease with outflow obstruction generally require surgical correction or attenuation of the obstruction. Aortic valve replacement for aortic stenosis will alleviate symptoms, prevent syncope, and prolong survival.
   1. Dynamic outflow obstruction resulting from hypertrophic cardiomyopathy is treated with beta blockers or calcium channel blockers. Occasionally, right ventricular pacing, myomectomy, and/or mitral valve replacement may be effective in this setting.

G. Ventricular arrhythmias
   1. Patients with documented or inducible ventricular arrhythmias, primarily VT, with structural heart disease, long QT interval syndrome, Brugada syndrome, catecholaminergic polymorphic VT or other condition placing the patient at risk for cardiac arrest and recurrent syncopal episodes should receive an implantable cardioverter-defibrillator (ICD). Radiofrequency catheter ablation is effective especially in patients with idiopathic right or left ventricular monomorphic VT.
   2. Patients with the congenital long QT syndrome often respond to beta blockers; other options include pacing and an ICD.
   3. **Cardiomyopathy and unexplained syncope.** Patients with advanced heart failure due to nonischemic cardiomyopathy who also have syncope, regardless of cause, have a high one year risk of sudden death (45 percent).
   4. **Supraventricular arrhythmias.** Although supraventricular arrhythmias can be treated with antiarrhythmic drugs, radiofrequency ablation has become a preferred therapy for the majority of such arrhythmias, especially those that involve the AV node or an accessory pathway. Surgery or antitachycardia pacemakers are infrequently used.
   5. **Sinus bradycardia or AV block.** Permanent pacemaker implantation is indicated when sinus node dysfunction or AV block is the cause of syncope.

H. Indications for pacemaker insertion
   1. Bifascicular or trifascicular disease is present on the baseline electrocardiogram
   2. A prolonged HV interval or infranodal block occurs during atrial pacing, or there is evidence of significant AV nodal disease uncovered during EP testing.

3. Empiric pacemaker implantation is not indicated for patients with the triad of syncope of unknown etiology, no documented bradycardia, and a negative EP study.

I. **Neurocardiogenic syncope**
   1. Treatment is aimed at preventing conditions that contribute to syncope. In situational vasovagal syncope, the avoidance or modulation of the triggers responsible for syncope is curative. Patients should be advised to assume a supine position with legs raised at the onset of symptoms. Support features may include support stockings, volume expansion by liberalizing salt intake is encouraged, and occasionally fludrocortisone.
   2. **Beta blockers.** Midodrine, angiotensin converting enzyme inhibitors and other medical management has been tried. Pyridostigmine may be effective.
   3. Pacing can be considered for cardioinhibitory neurocardiogenic syncope in whom other medical therapy is ineffective.
   4. An orthostatic training program can be tried in young patients who respond poorly to medical therapy.
   5. Carotid sinus hypersensitivity is often considered to be a variant of neurocardiogenic syncope and is known as carotid sinus syndrome; many of the same therapies have been used. Pacemakers are of benefit for patients with only cardioinhibitory responses but not in those with a vasodepressor response.

References, see page 372.

Hypercholesterolemia

There is a direct relation between the plasma levels of total and low density lipoprotein (LDL) plasma cholesterol and the risk of CHD and coronary mortality. LDL cholesterol lowering in moderate to high-risk patients leads to a reduction in cardiovascular events.

I. **Pathophysiology**
   A. CHD remains the leading cause of death for both men and women of all races. In men over the age of 65, nearly one-half of all deaths are attributed to CHD, compared to less than 25 percent for all cancers and less than 2 percent for all infections. An even higher proportion of deaths are due to CHD in older women (56 percent), with less than 20 percent due to cancer.
   B. The optimal value for LDL cholesterol in both men and women is <100 mg/dL; a one standard deviation (38.5 mg/dL) LDL increase above the mean of 118 mg/dL was associated with relative risk for CHD of 1.42 for men and 1.37 for women.
   C. A one standard deviation increase in HDL (15.5 mg/dL) above the mean of 40 mg/dL in men and 51 mg/dL in women was associated with relative risk of 0.64 and 0.69, respectively.
   D. Triglycerides were an independent predictor of CHD only in women in whom a one standard deviation increase (62 mg/dL) above the mean of 115 mg/dL was associated with a relative risk of 1.31.
   E. When used in combination with blood pressure, smoking, and diabetes, LDL, HDL, Lp(a) and triglycerides (in women) provided a relative risk for CHD.

II. **Lipoprotein measurement**. A standard serum lipid profile consists of total cholesterol, triglycerides, and HDL-cholesterol. Lipoprotein analysis should be performed after 12 to 14 hours of fasting to minimize the influence of postprandial hyperlipidemia.

III. Risk stratification:

A. Obtain a fasting lipid profile

B. Identify the presence of CHD equivalents

C. Identify the presence of other major CHD risk factors

D. If two or more risk factors other than LDL (as defined in step 3) are present in a patient without CHD or a CHD equivalent (as defined in step 2), the 10-year risk of CHD is assessed using the ATP III modification of the Framingham risk tables.

E. **National Cholesterol Education Program guidelines.** Screening should be performed at least once every five years for all persons age 20 and over. A fasting lipid profile is recommended for screening, although if the testing opportunity is nonfasting, the total and HDL-cholesterol should be measured. In the latter circumstance, a total cholesterol >200 mg/dL or HDL cholesterol <40 mg/dL suggests the need for a follow-up fasting lipid profile.

F. **Individuals without known CHD** who have a desirable serum LDL cholesterol concentration (<160 mg/dL for 0 to one risk factor and <130 mg/dL for two or more risk factors) can be rescreened in five years. Patients with borderline-high cholesterol and less than two risk factors should be rescreened within one to two years.

G. The desirable LDL cholesterol level for those with CHD or CHD equivalent is <100 mg/dL; CHD equivalents include:
   1. Symptomatic carotid artery disease
   2. Peripheral arterial disease
   3. Abdominal aortic aneurysm
   4. Diabetes mellitus

H. **Elderly.** Screening and primary preventive drug therapy is recommended in some elderly subjects who are at very high risk, such as those with a serum LDL-cholesterol of 160 mg/dL or greater despite attempts at dietary modification plus two or more cardiac risk factors — cigarette smoking, hypertension, diabetes mellitus, or an HDL-cholesterol level below 35 mg/dL.

IV. Treatment of hypercholesterolemia

A. Identification of patients at risk

Step 1 — The first step in determining patient risk is to obtain a fasting lipid profile.

Classification of LDL, Total, and HDL Cholesterol (mg/dL)	
LDL Cholesterol	
<100	Optimal
100-129	Near optimal/above optimal
130-159	Borderline high
160-189	High
≥190	Very high
Total Cholesterol	
<200	Desirable
200-239	Borderline high

≥240	High
HDL Cholesterol	
<40	Low
≥60	High

Step 2 — CHD equivalents, that is, risk factors that place the patient at similar risk for CHD events as a history of CHD itself, are identified:
   a. Diabetes mellitus
   b. Symptomatic carotid artery disease
   c. Peripheral arterial disease
   d. Abdominal aortic aneurysm
   e. Multiple risk factors that confer a 10-year risk of CHD >20 percent.
B. In addition to the conditions identified as CHD equivalents, chronic renal insufficiency (defined by a plasma creatinine concentration that exceeds 1.5 mg/dL or an estimated glomerular filtration rate that is less than 60 mL/min per 1.73 m^2) to be a CHD equivalent.

Step 3 — Major CHD factors other than LDL are identified:
   Cigarette smoking
   Hypertension (BP ≥140/90 or antihypertensive medication)
   Low HDL-cholesterol (HDL-C) (<40 mg/dL)
   Family history of premature CHD (in male first degree relatives <55 years, in female first degree relative <65 years)
   Age (men ≥45 years, women ≥55 years)
   HDL-C ≥60 mg/dL counts as a "negative" risk factor; its presence removes one risk factor from the total count.

Step 4 — If two or more risk factors other than LDL (as defined in step 3) are present in a patient without CHD or a CHD equivalent, the 10-year risk of CHD is assessed using the ATP III modification of the Framingham risk tables.

Step 5 — The last step in risk assessment is to determine the risk category that establishes the LDL goal, when to initiate therapeutic lifestyle changes, and when to consider drug therapy.

LDL Cholesterol Goals for Therapeutic Lifestyle Changes and Drug Therapy in Different Risk Categories

Risk Category	LDL-C Goal	LDL Level at Which to Initiate Therapeutic Lifestyle Changes	LDL Level at Which to Consider Drug Therapy
CHD	<100 mg/dL	≥100 mg/dL	≥130 mg/dL (100-129 mg/dL: drug optional)
2+ Risk Factors	≤130 mg/dL	≥130 mg/dL	10-year risk 10-20%:≥130 mg/dL 10-year risk <10%:≥160 mg/dL
0-1 Risk Factor	≤160 mg/dL	≥160 mg/dL	≥190 mg/dL (160-189 mg/dL: LDL-lowering drug optional)

V. Summary and recommendations

A. All patients with an LDL-C above goal should undergo lifestyle modifications in an effort to reduce the serum cholesterol. These modifications include diet and exercise.

B. In patients with CHD or a CHD equivalent (diabetes mellitus, symptomatic carotid artery disease, peripheral arterial disease, abdominal aortic aneurysm, chronic renal insufficiency, or multiple risk factors that confer a 10-year risk of CHD greater than 20 percent) who are significantly above the goal LDL-C, drug therapy should not be delayed while waiting to see if lifestyle modifications are effective.

C. Patients who require drug therapy should almost always be treated with a statin.

D. Secondary prevention goals and therapy. Goals for LDL-C in patients with CHD or CHD equivalents being treated for secondary prevention:

1. Statin therapy with atorvastatin (Lipitor) 80 mg daily reduces mortality in patients with an acute coronary syndrome and is recommended as initial therapy. Given that benefit occurs earlier than the first cholesterol measurement on therapy would normally be obtained, patients should be started on atorvastatin 80 mg daily early in their hospital course.

2. Patients at very high risk for CHD events might also be expected to benefit from more intensive lipid lowering therapy. We suggest that such patients be treated with the lowest dose of a statin that reduces their LDL-C below 80 mg/dL. If such patients cannot achieve an LDL-C below 100 mg/dL with a statin alone, a second lipid-lowering agent should be added.

E. Primary prevention goals and therapy

1. Patients without CHD or a CHD equivalent should be assessed for major non-LDL risk factors (cigarette smoking, hypertension [BP $\geq$140/90 or antihypertensive medication], HDL-C <40 mg/dL, family history of premature CHD [male first degree relative <55 years; female first degree relative <65 years], age (men $\geq$45, women $\geq$55).

2. Count the number of risk factors, subtracting one risk factor if the HDL-C is $\geq$60 mg/dL. In patients with two or more risk factors, assess the 10-year risk of CHD using the ATP III modification of the Framingham risk tables.

3. Patients with no or one risk factor have a goal LDL-C of less than 160 mg/dL. Patients with two or more risk factors have a goal LDL-C of less than 130 mg/dL. Patients with a 10-year CHD risk of greater than 20 percent should be considered to have a CHD equivalent.

4. Drug therapy with a statin should be considered if after an adequate trial of lifestyle modification the LDL-C remains above 190 mg/dL in patients with no or one risk factor or above 160 mg/dL in patients with two or more risk factors.

Dose, Side Effects, and Drug Interactions of Lipid-Lowering Drugs

Drug class	Dose	Dosing	Major side effects and drug interactions
HMG CoA reductase inhibitors			
Atorvastatin (Lipitor) Lovastatin (generic, Mevacor) Extended-release lovastatin (Altocor) Pravastatin (Pravachol) Simvastatin (Zocor) Fluvastatin (Lescol, Lescol XL) Rosuvastatin (Crestor)	10-40 mg/day 20-80 mg/day 10-60 mg/day 10-40 mg/day 5-40 mg/day 10-40 mg/day 10-40 mg/day	Take at bedtime. Take BID if dose >20 mg/day.	Headache; nausea; sleep disturbance; elevations in liver enzymes and alkaline phosphatase. Myositis and rhabdomyolysis. Lovastatin and simvastatin potentiate warfarin and increase digoxin levels
Cholesterol absorption inhibitors			
Ezetimibe (Zetia)	10 mg/day	10 mg qd	Increased transaminases in combination with statins
Bile acid sequestrants			
Cholestyramine (Questran, Questran Lite) Colestipol (Colestid) Colesevelam (WelChol)	4-24 g/day 5-30 g/day 3.75 gm once or divided BID	Take within 30 min of meal. A double dose with dinner produces same effect as BID dosing	Nausea, bloating, cramping, constipation; elevations in hepatic transaminases and alkaline phosphatase. Impaired absorption of fat soluble vitamins, digoxin, warfarin, thiazides, beta-blockers, thyroxine, phenobarbital.
Nicotinic acid	1-12 g/day	Given with meals. Start with 100 mg BID and titrate to 500 mg TID. After 6 weeks, check lipids, glucose, liver function, and uric acid.	Prostaglandin-mediated cutaneous flushing, headache, pruritus; hyperpigmentation; acanthosis nigricans; dry skin; nausea; diarrhea; myositis.
Fibrates			
Gemfibrozil (Lopid)	600 mg BID	50 to 60 min before meals.	Potentiates warfarin. Absorption of gemfibrozil diminished by bile acid sequestrants.
Fenofibrate (Lofibra, micronized)	200 mg qd	Take with breakfast. Use lower dosage with renal insufficiency.	Skin rash, nausea, bloating, cramping, myalgia; lowers cyclosporin levels; nephrotoxic in cyclosporin-treated patients.
Fenofibrate (TriCor)	160 mg qd		

Drug class	Dose	Dosing	Major side effects and drug interactions
Probucol	500 mg BID		Loose stools; eosinophilia; QT prolongation; angioneurotic edema.
Extended-release niacin plus (immediate-release) lovastatin (Advicor)	1000 mg/40 mg/day	1000 mg + 40 mg h.s.3	markedly lowers LDL and triglycerides and raises HDL

VI. Approach to the patient with hypertriglyceridemia

A. Normal serum triglyceride concentration. The serum triglyceride concentration can be stratified in terms of coronary risk:

Normal <150 mg/dL
Borderline high — 150 to 199 mg/dL
High — 200 to 499 mg/dL
Very high $\geq$500 mg/dL).

B. General treatment guidelines

1. Nonpharmacologic therapy is recommended for serum triglyceride values above 200 mg/dL. Although the risk is enhanced at these levels, CHD risk begins to increase at a fasting triglyceride concentration of 160 to 190 mg/dL and, among patients with CHD, may begin to increase at values above 100 mg/dL.

Treatment of Hypertriglyceridemia*

Review medications	Laboratory studies	Diet
Change to lipid neutral or favorable agents (eg, alpha-blockers, biguanides, thiazolidinedione) Lower doses of drugs that increase triglycerides, such as beta-blockers, glucocorticoids, diuretics (thiazide and loop), ticlopidine, estrogens.	Exclude secondary disorders of lipid metabolism Fasting blood glucose Serum creatinine Thyroid function studies	Weight loss Avoid concentrated sugars Increase omega-3 fatty acid intake through fish consumption Exercise Aerobic exercise minimum of 3 hours weekly

*Hypertriglyceridemia is defined as a serum triglyceride concentration above 200 mg/dL

2. The National Cholesterol Education Program (Adult Treatment Panel [ATP] III) recommended that in all patients with borderline high or high triglycerides, the primary goal of therapy is to achieve the targets for LDL cholesterol. In addition, the following recommendations were made for various levels of elevated triglycerides:

a. When triglycerides are borderline high (150 to 199 mg/dL), emphasis should be upon weight reduction and increased physical activity.

b. When triglycerides are high (200 to 499 mg/dL), non-HDL cholesterol becomes a secondary target of therapy after LDL cholesterol. Drug therapy can be considered in high-risk patients, including those who have had an acute myocardial infarction, to reach the non-HDL cholesterol goals. These goals may be achieved by intensifying therapy with

> an LDL cholesterol lowering drug, or by adding nicotinic acid or a fibrate.
> c. When triglycerides are very high (>500 mg/dL), the initial goal is to prevent pancreatitis by lowering triglycerides with a fibrate or nicotinic acid. Once triglycerides are below 500 mg/dL, LDL cholesterol goals should be addressed.

References, see page 372.

Hypertriglyceridemia

Lipid disorders can occur as either a primary event or secondary to some underlying disease. The primary dyslipidemias are associated with overproduction and/or impaired removal of lipoproteins. Dyslipidemia is defined as total cholesterol, low-density lipoprotein (LDL)-cholesterol, triglyceride, apolipoprotein (apo)-B, or Lp(a) levels above the 90th percentile or high-density lipoprotein (HDL)-cholesterol or apo A-1 levels below the 10th percentile for the general population.

I. **Normal serum triglyceride concentration.** The serum triglyceride concentration can be stratified in terms of coronary risk:
   Normal <150 mg/dL
   Borderline high - 150 to 199 mg/dL
   High - 200 to 499 mg/dL
   Very high - >500 mg/dL

II. **Triglycerides and atherosclerosis**
   A. **CHD events.** Population-based studies and analyses of patients with CHD suggest that serum triglycerides are a risk factor for CHD.
      Hypertriglyceridemia is associated with increased mortality in patients with known CHD and both increased mortality and reduced event-free survival after coronary artery bypass graft surgery (CABG).
   B. **Coronary atherosclerosis.** The total triglyceride concentration is a risk factor for progression of low-grade but not high-grade coronary artery lesions.
   C. **Acquired disorders.** A number of acquired disorders raise serum triglycerides. These include:
      1. Obesity, often in association with an elevation in serum cholesterol.
      2. Diabetes mellitus, where there is a relationship to poor glycemic control and, in type 2 diabetes, obesity.
      3. Nephrotic syndrome, often is association with hypercholesterolemia, and renal failure.
      4. Hypothyroidism, often in association with hypercholesterolemia.
      5. Estrogen replacement, which is often associated with a fall in LDL cholesterol. The elevation in serum triglycerides may not be seen with transdermal estrogen delivery and is minimal with most oral contraceptives because of the lower estrogen dose.
      6. Tamoxifen can cause marked hypertriglyceridemia in a minority of women.
   D. **Mixed hypertriglyceridemia** (type V hyperlipoproteinemia) is characterized by triglyceride levels above the 99th percentile in association with a creamy plasma supernatant and increases in chylomicrons and VLDL. Clinical manifestations include hepatosplenomegaly and occasional eruptive xanthomas. However, patients with marked hypertriglyceridemia (>1000 mg/dL) may develop the chylomicronemia syndrome. Manifestations of this disorder include recent memory loss, abdominal pain and/or pancreatitis, dyspnea, eruptive xanthoma, flushing with alcohol, and lipemia retinalis. Mixed hypertriglyceridemia can be diagnosed by confirming the presence of

chylomicrons and excess VLDL on agarose gel electrophoresis or ultracentrifugal analysis.

E. Familial hypertriglyceridemia (type IV hyperlipoproteinemia phenotype) is an autosomal dominant disorder associated with moderate elevations in the serum triglyceride concentration (200 to 500 mg/dL). It is often accompanied by insulin resistance, obesity, hyperglycemia, hypertension, and hyperuricemia.

F. Familial combined hyperlipidemia (FCHL) is an autosomal disorder caused by overproduction of hepatically derived apolipoprotein B-100 associated with VLDL. It is associated with a clear increase in coronary risk and accounts for one-third to one-half of familial causes of CHD.

G. Familial dysbetalipoproteinemia (type III hyperlipoproteinemia) is a multifactorial disorder that is inherited as an autosomal recessive trait. It is characterized by the presence of two apo E2 alleles. Premature CHD and peripheral vascular disease are common. Physical findings include tuberoeruptive xanthomas and xanthomas of the palmar creases (xanthomata palmare striatum).

H. Hypertriglyceridemia and serum cholesterol. Hypertriglyceridemia reflects the accumulation of triglyceride-rich lipoproteins (chylomicrons, VLDL and remnant particles, beta-VLDL, and IDL) in plasma. Since triglyceride-rich lipoproteins also transport cholesterol, hypercholesterolemia of varying severity often accompanies hypertriglyceridemia.

III. General treatment guidelines

A. The epidemiologic data on the relationship between triglycerides and CHD provide strong evidence that hypertriglyceridemia promotes atherosclerosis.

B. Recommendations of expert groups. Nonpharmacologic therapy is recommended for serum triglyceride values above 200 mg/dL. Although the risk is enhanced at these levels, some studies suggest that CHD risk begins to increase at a fasting triglyceride concentration of 160 to 190 mg/dL and, among patients with CHD, may begin to increase at values above 100 mg/dL.

  1. The National Cholesterol Education Program (Adult Treatment Panel [ATP] III) recommends that in all patients with borderline high or high triglycerides, the primary goal of therapy is to achieve the targets for LDL cholesterol. In addition, the following recommendations were made for various levels of elevated triglycerides:

   a. When triglycerides are borderline high (150 to 199 mg/dL), emphasis should be upon weight reduction and increased physical activity.

   b. When triglycerides are high (200 to 499 mg/dL), non-HDL cholesterol becomes a secondary target of therapy after LDL cholesterol. In addition to nonpharmacologic therapy, drug therapy can be considered in high-risk patients, including those who have had an acute myocardial infarction, to reach the non-HDL cholesterol goals. These goals may be achieved by intensifying therapy with an LDL-cholesterol-lowering drug, or by adding nicotinic acid or a fibrate.

   c. When triglycerides are very high (>500 mg/dL), the initial goal is to prevent pancreatitis by lowering triglycerides with the combination of nonpharmacologic therapy and a triglyceride-lowering drug, such as a fibrate or nicotinic acid. Once triglycerides are below 500 mg/dL, LDL cholesterol goals should be addressed.

C. Nonpharmacologic therapy, such as weight loss in obese patients, aerobic exercise, avoidance of concentrated sugars and medications that raise serum triglyceride levels, and strict glycemic control in diabetics should be the first-line of therapy. Other risk factors for CHD, such as hypertension and smoking, should also be addressed. Alcohol abuse must be avoided as it can cause

large increases in triglyceride levels in patients with mixed or familial
hypertriglyceridemia and can precipitate pancreatitis in such patients.

D. Pharmacologic therapy

Treatment of hypertriglyceridemia*		
Review medications	**Laboratory studies**	**Diet**
Change to lipid neutral or favorable agents when possible (eg, alpha-blockers, biguanides, thiazolidinedione)	Exclude secondary disorders of lipid metabolism	Weight loss
	Fasting blood glucose	Avoid concentrated sugars
	Serum creatine	Increase omega-3 fatty acid intake through fish consumption
Lower doses of drugs that increase triglycerides, such as beta-blockers (particularly nonselective agents), glucocorticoids, diuretics (thiazide and loop), ticlopidine, estrogens.	Thyroid function studies	Exercise
		Aerobic exercise minimum of 3 hours weekly
*Hypertriglyceridemia is defined as a serum triglyceride concentration above 200 mg/dL		

1. **High-serum triglycerides with elevated LDL-C**
   a. The more potent statins (eg, atorvastatin [Lipitor] or rosuvastatin [Crestor]) will control the LDL-C and, if the LDL-C is proportionately more elevated than serum triglycerides, the hypertriglyceridemia as well. If additional triglyceride lowering is required, either a fibrate or nicotinic acid can be added. Nicotinic acid may worsen glucose tolerance in diabetic patients. Glycemic control should be monitored carefully in diabetic patients treated with nicotinic acid. Gemfibrozil increases the risk of muscle toxicity induced by statin therapy. The latter risk can be minimized by using pravastatin or fluvastatin, which are not metabolized by CYP3A4. Although rosuvastatin is also not metabolized by CYP3A4, it is recommended that the dosage be limited to 10 mg/day in patients being treated with gemfibrozil. Fenofibrate(TriCor) does not increase statin levels, and it is considered a safer agent for combined therapy with a statin.
   b. Bile acid sequestrants should be avoided until triglyceride levels have been normalized since they can increase VLDL synthesis and exacerbate the hypertriglyceridemia.
2. **High-serum triglycerides and LDL-C <130 mg/dL or low HDL**
   a. Possible indications for treatment of isolated hypertriglyceridemia include overt CHD, a strong family history of CHD, and multiple coexisting cardiac risk factors. The most effective triglyceride-lowering drugs

are fibric acid derivatives and nicotinic acid. These drugs have the added benefit of also being most effective in raising HDL-C, which is commonly reduced in these patients and may be associated with adverse cardiac outcomes.

   b. A fibrate is generally preferred in such patients, and combination therapy can be given in patients with marked hypertriglyceridemia or acute pancreatitis.

   c. Refractory cases may benefit from fish oil supplements (>3 g/day) which, by reducing VLDL production, can lower the serum triglyceride concentration by as much as 50 percent or more.

3. **Very-high-serum triglycerides.** Gemfibrozil therapy can lower the serum triglyceride concentration by 70 percent in patients with very-high-serum triglycerides, and reduce plasma viscosity, which may contribute to the clinical benefit. However, combination therapy with nicotinic acid is often given.

References, see page 372.

Pulmonary Disorders

Asthma

Asthma is the most common chronic disease among children. Asthma triggers include viral infections; environmental pollutants, such as tobacco smoke; aspirin, nonsteroidal anti-inflammatory drugs, and sustained exercise, particularly in cold environments.

I. **Diagnosis**
   A. Symptoms of asthma may include episodic complaints of breathing difficulties, seasonal or nighttime cough, prolonged shortness of breath after a respiratory infection, or difficulty sustaining exercise.
   B. Wheezing does not always represent asthma. Wheezing may persist for weeks after an acute bronchitis episode. Patients with chronic obstructive pulmonary disease may have a reversible component superimposed on their fixed obstruction. Etiologic clues include a personal history of allergic disease, such as rhinitis or atopic dermatitis, and a family history of allergic disease.
   C. The frequency of daytime and nighttime symptoms, duration of exacerbations and asthma triggers should be assessed.
   D. **Physical examination.** Hyperventilation, use of accessory muscles of respiration, audible wheezing, and a prolonged expiratory phase are common. Increased nasal secretions or congestion, polyps, and eczema may be present.
   E. **Measurement of lung function.** An increase in the forced expiratory volume in one second (FEV_1) of 12% after treatment with an inhaled beta$_2$ agonist is sufficient to make the diagnosis of asthma. A 12% change in peak expiratory flow rate (PEFR) measured on a peak-flow meter is also diagnostic.

II. **Treatment of asthma**
   A. **Beta$_2$ agonists**
      1. Inhaled short-acting beta$_2$-adrenergic agonists are the most effective drugs available for treatment of acute bronchospasm and for prevention of exercise-induced asthma. Levalbuterol (Xopenex), the R-isomer of racemic albuterol, offers no significant advantage over racemic albuterol.
      2. **Salmeterol (Serevent)**, a long-acting beta$_2$ agonist, has a relatively slow onset of action and a prolonged effect.
         a. Salmeterol should not be used in the treatment of acute bronchospasm. Patients taking salmeterol should use a short-acting beta$_2$ agonist as needed to control acute symptoms. Twice-daily inhalation of salmeterol has been effective for maintenance treatment in combination with inhaled corticosteroids.
         b. Fluticasone/Salmeterol (Advair Diskus) is a long-acting beta agonist and corticosteroid combination; dry-powder inhaler [100, 250 or 500 g/puff],1 puff q12h.
      3. **Formoterol (Foradil)** is a long-acting beta2 agonist. It should only be used in patients who already take an inhaled corticosteroid. Patients taking formoterol should use a short-acting beta$_2$ agonist as needed to control acute symptoms. For maintenance treatment of asthma in adults and children at least 5 years old, the dosage is 1 puff bid.
      4. **Adverse effects of beta$_2$ agonists.** Tachycardia, palpitations, tremor and paradoxical bronchospasm can occur. High doses can cause hypokalemia.

Drugs for Asthma

Drug	Formulation	Dosage
Inhaled beta$_2$-adrenergic agonists, short-acting		
Albuterol *Proventil* *Proventil-HFA* *Ventolin* *Ventolin Rotacaps*	metered-dose inhaler (90 µg/puff) dry-powder inhaler (200 µg/inhalation)	2 puffs q4-6h PRN 1-2 capsules q4-6h PRN
Albuterol *Proventil* multi-dose vials *Ventolin Nebules* *Ventolin*	nebulized	2.5 mg q4-6h PRN
Levalbuterol - *Xopenex*	nebulized	0.63-1.25 mg q6-8h PRN
Inhaled beta2-adrenergic agonist, long-acting		
Formoterol - *Foradil*	oral inhaler (12 µg/capsule)	1 cap q12h via inhaler
Salmeterol *Serevent* *Serevent Diskus*	metered-dose inhaler (21 µg/puff) dry-powder inhaler (50 µg/inhalation)	2 puffs q12h 1 inhalation q12h
Fluticasone/Salmeterol *Advair Diskus*	dry-powder inhaler (100, 250 or 500 µg/puff)	1 puff q12h
Inhaled Corticosteroids		
Beclomethasone dipropionate *Beclovent* *Vanceril* Vanceril Double-Strength	metered-dose inhaler (42 µg/puff) (84 µg/puff)	4-8 puffs bid 2-4 puffs bid
Budesonide *Pulmicort Turbuhaler*	dry-powder inhaler (200 µg/inhalation)	1-2 inhalations bid
Flunisolide - *AeroBid*	metered-dose inhaler (250 µg/puff)	2-4 puffs bid
Fluticasone Flovent *Flovent Rotadisk*	metered-dose inhaler (44, 110 or 220 µg/puff) dry-powder inhaler (50, 100 or 250 µg/inhalation)	2-4 puffs bid (44 µg/puff) 1 inhalation bid (100 µg/inhalation)
Triamcinolone acetonide *Azmacort*	metered-dose inhaler (100 µg/puff)	2 puffs tid-qid or 4 puffs bid

Drug	Formulation	Dosage
Leukotriene Modifiers		
Montelukast - *Singulair*	tablets	10 mg qhs
Zafirlukast - *Accolate*	tablets	20 mg bid
Zileuton - *Zyflo*	tablets	600 mg qid
Mast Cell Stabilizers		
Cromolyn *Intal*	metered-dose inhaler (800 µg/puff)	2-4 puffs tid-qid
Nedocromil *Tilade*	metered-dose inhaler (1.75 mg/puff)	2-4 puffs bid-qid
Phosphodiesterase Inhibitor		
Theophylline *Slo-Bid Gyrocaps, Theo-Dur, Unidur*	extended-release capsules or tablets	100-300 mg bid

   B. **Inhaled corticosteroids**
      1. Regular use of an inhaled corticosteroid can suppress inflammation and
         bronchial hyperresponsiveness. Inhaled corticosteroids are recommended
         for most patients.
      2. **Adverse effects.** Inhaled corticosteroids are usually free of toxicity.
         Slowing of linear growth may occur within 6-12 weeks in some children.
         Decreased bone density, glaucoma and cataract formation have been
         reported. Churg-Strauss vasculitis is rare. Dysphonia and oral candidiasis
         can occur. A spacer device and rinsing the mouth after inhalation de-
         creases the incidence of candidiasis.
   C. **Leukotriene modifiers**
      1. Leukotrienes increase production of mucus and edema of the airway and
         cause bronchoconstriction. Montelukast and zafirlukast are leukotriene
         receptor antagonists. Zileuton inhibits synthesis of leukotrienes.
      2. **Montelukast (Singulair)** is modestly effective for maintenance treatment.
         It is taken once daily in the evening. It is less effective than inhaled
         corticosteroids, but addition of montelukast may permit a reduction in
         corticosteroid dosage.
      3. **Zafirlukast (Accolate)** is modestly effective for mild-to-moderate asthma
         It is less effective than inhaled corticosteroids. Taking zafirlukast with food
         markedly decreases its bioavailability. Theophylline can decrease its
         effect. Zafirlukast increases serum concentrations of oral anticoagulants.
         Infrequent adverse effects include headache, gastrointestinal disturbances
         and increased serum aminotransferase activity. Lupus and Churg-Strauss
         vasculitis have been reported.
      4. **Zileuton (Zyflo)** is modestly effective, but it is taken four times a day and
         patients must be monitored for hepatic toxicity.
   D. **Cromolyn (Intal) and nedocromil (Tilade)**
      1. Cromolyn sodium, an inhibitor of mast cell degranulation, can decrease
         airway hyperresponsiveness in some patients. The drug has no

bronchodilating activity and is useful only for prophylaxis. Cromolyn has virtually no systemic toxicity.

2. Nedocromil (Tilade) has similar effects as cromolyn. Both cromolyn and nedocromil are much less effective than inhaled corticosteroids.

E. **Theophylline**
   1. Oral theophylline has a slower onset of action than inhaled beta$_2$ agonists and has limited usefulness for treatment of acute symptoms. It can, however, reduce the frequency and severity of symptoms, especially in nocturnal asthma, and can decrease inhaled corticosteroid requirements.
   2. When theophylline is used alone, serum concentrations between 8-12 mcg/mL provide a modest improvement is FEV_1. Serum levels of 15-20 mcg/mL are only minimally more effective and are associated with a higher incidence of cardiovascular adverse events.

F. **Oral corticosteroids** are the most effective drugs available for acute exacerbations of asthma unresponsive to bronchodilators.
   1. Oral corticosteroids decrease symptoms and may prevent an early relapse. Chronic use of oral corticosteroids can cause glucose intolerance, weight gain, increased blood pressure, osteoporosis, cataracts, immunosuppression and decreased growth in children. Alternate-day use of corticosteroids can decrease the incidence of adverse effects, but not of osteoporosis.
   2. **Prednisone, prednisolone or methylprednisolone** (Solu-Medrol), 40-60 mg qd; for children, 1-2 mg/kg/day to a maximum of 60 mg/day. Therapy is continued for 3-10 days. The oral steroid dosage does not need to be tapered after short-course "burst" therapy if the patient is receiving inhaled steroid therapy.

Pharmacotherapy for Asthma Based on Disease Classification		
Classification	**Long-term control medications**	**Quick-relief medications**
Mild intermittent		Short-acting beta$_2$ agonist as needed
Mild persistent	Low-dose inhaled corticosteroid or cromolyn sodium (Intal) or nedocromil (Tilade)	Short-acting beta$_2$ agonist as needed
Moderate persistent	Medium-dose inhaled corticosteroid plus a long-acting bronchodilator (long-acting beta$_2$ agonist)	Short-acting beta$_2$ agonist as needed
Severe persistent	High-dose inhaled corticosteroid plus a long-acting bronchodilator and systemic corticosteroid	Short-acting beta$_2$ agonist as needed

III. Management of acute exacerbations

A. High-dose, short-acting beta$_2$ agonists delivered by a metered-dose inhaler with a volume spacer or via a nebulizer remains the mainstay of urgent treatment.

B. Most patients require therapy with systemic corticosteroids to resolve symptoms and prevent relapse. Hospitalization should be considered if the PEFR remains less than 70% of predicted. Patients with a PEFR less than 50% of predicted who exhibit an increasing pCO_2 level and declining mental status are candidates for intubation.

    C. Non-invasive ventilation with bilevel positive airway pressure (BIPAP) may be used to relieve the work-of-breathing while awaiting the effects of acute treatment, provided that consciousness and the ability to protect the airway have not been compromised.

References, see page 372.

Chronic Obstructive Pulmonary Disease

Chronic obstructive pulmonary disease (COPD) is the fourth-ranked cause of death. Chronic obstructive pulmonary disease is defined as "disease state characterized by airflow limitation that is not fully reversible. Airflow limitation is usually progressive and associated with an abnormal inflammatory response of the lungs to noxious particles or gases."

I. Pathophysiology

    A. Airflow obstruction is the result of both small airway disease (obstructive bronchiolitis) and parenchymal destruction (emphysema). The relative contributions of each vary from person to person, and can be accompanied by partially reversible airways hyperreactivity.

    B. Chronic bronchitis is defined by the presence of chronic productive cough for three months in each of two successive years.

    C. Emphysema is the abnormal permanent enlargement of airspaces distal to the terminal bronchioles, accompanied by destruction of their walls without obvious fibrosis. Emphysema is frequently present in patients with moderate and severe COPD.

    D. Asthma is defined as an inflammatory disease of the airways characterized by an increased responsiveness of the trachea and bronchi to various stimuli, and manifested by a widespread narrowing of the airways.

    E. Cigarette smoking is the major cause of COPD. However, only about 15 to 20 percent of smokers develop COPD suggesting that host factors (most likely genetic) also contribute to pathogenesis of the disease.

    F. Alpha-1 antitrypsin deficiency. The only established genetic abnormality that predisposes to lung disease clinically and pathologically similar to COPD is alpha-1 antitrypsin [AAT] deficiency. Severe AAT deficiency has a frequency of about 1 in 3,000 live births. Persons with known COPD, or asthma with non-remittent airflow obstruction, should be screened for AAT deficiency.

II. Clinical features

    A. History. Patients with COPD have usually been smoking at least 20 cigarettes per day for 20 or more years before symptoms develop. Chronic productive cough, sometimes with wheezing, often begins when patients are in their forties.

    B. Dyspnea on effort does not usually begin until the mid sixties or early seventies. Sputum production is insidious, initially occurring only in the morning; the daily volume rarely exceeds 60 mL. Sputum is usually mucoid but becomes purulent with an exacerbation.

    C. Acute chest illnesses occur intermittently, and are characterized by increased cough, purulent sputum, wheezing, dyspnea, and occasionally fever.

    D. With disease progression, the intervals between acute exacerbations shorten. Late in the course of the illness, an exacerbation may give rise to hypoxemia with cyanosis. Associated findings also include:

        1. Weight loss - Approximately 20 percent of patients with moderate and severe disease experience weight loss and loss.

        2. Hypercapnia with more severe hypoxemia in the setting of end-stage disease.

3. **Morning headache**, which suggests hypercapnia.
4. **Cor pulmonale** with right heart failure and edema.
5. **Hemoptysis.** Since bronchogenic carcinoma occurs with increased frequency in smokers with COPD, an episode of hemoptysis raises the possibility that carcinoma has developed. However, most episodes of hemoptysis are due to bronchial mucosal erosion.

Diagnosis of chronic obstructive pulmonary disease

History
Smoking history
  Age at initiation
  Average amount smoked per day
  Date when stopped smoking or a current smoker
Environmental history
Cough
  Chronic productive cough for at least one quarter of the year for two successive years is the defining characteristic of chronic bronchitis. Sputum, blood or blood streaking in the sputum.
Wheezing
Acute chest illnesses
  Frequency of episodes of increased cough and sputum with wheezing.
Dyspnea
  Amount of effort required to induce uncomfortable breathing.

Physical examination
Chest
  The presence of severe emphysema is indicated by: overdistention of the lungs in the stable position; decreased intensity of breath and heart sounds and prolonged expiratory phase.
  Wheezes during auscultation on slow or forced breathing and prolongation of forced expiratory time.
  Severe disease is indicated by pursed-lip breathing, use of accessory respiratory muscles, retraction of lower interspaces.
Other
Unusual positions to relieve dyspnea at rest.
Digital clubbing suggests the possibility of lung cancer or bronchiectasis.
Mild dependent edema may be seen in the absence of right heart failure.

Differential diagnosis of COPD

Diagnosis	Features
COPD	Onset in mid-life
	Symptoms slowly progressive
	Long smoking history
	Dyspnea during exercise
	Largely irreversible airflow limitation

Diagnosis	Features
Asthma	Onset in childhood Symptoms vary from day to day Symptoms at night/early morning Allergy, rhinitis, and/or eczema also present Family history of asthma Largely reversible airflow limitation
Heart failure	Fine basilar crackles Chest X-ray shows dilated heart, pulmonary edema Pulmonary function tests indicate volume restriction, not airflow limitation
Bronchiectasis	Large volumes of purulent sputum Commonly associated with bacterial infection Coarse crackles/clubbing on auscultation Chest X-ray/CT shows bronchial dilation, bronchial wall thickening
Tuberculosis	Onset all ages Chest X-ray shows lung infiltrate Microbiological confirmation High local prevalence of tuberculosis
Obliterative bronchiolitis	Onset in younger age, nonsmokers May have history of rheumatoid arthritis or fume exposure CT on expiration shows hypodense areas
Diffuse panbronchiolitis	Most patients are male and non-smokers. Almost all have chronic sinusitis Chest X-ray and HRCT show diffuse small centrilobular nodular opacities and hyperinflation

Classification of Severity of Chronic Obstructive Pulmonary Disease

Stage	Characteristics
0: At risk	Normal spirometry Chronic symptoms (cough, sputum production)
I: Mild COPD	FEV_1/FVC <70 percent FEV_1 $\geq$80 percent predicted With or without chronic symptoms (cough, sputum production)
II: Moderate COPD	FEV_1/FVC <70 percent 30 percent $\leq$FEV1 <80 percent predicted IIA: 50 percent $\leq$FEV1 <80 percent predicted IIB: 30 percent $\leq$FEV1 <50 percent predicted

Stage	Characteristics
Severe COPD	FEV_1/FVC <70 percent FEV_1 30 percent predicted or FEV_1 <50 percent predicted plus respiratory failure or clinical signs of right heart failure

E. Physical examination

1. Early in the disease there is only prolonged expiration and wheezes on forced exhalation. As obstruction progresses, hyperinflation becomes evident, and the anteroposterior diameter of the chest increases. The diaphragm is depressed and limited in its motion. Breath sounds are decreased and heart sounds often become distant. Coarse crackles may be heard at the lung bases. Wheezes are frequently heard.

2. If the history and chest radiograph are compatible, a clinical diagnosis of COPD may be made. However, a forced expiratory spirogram before and after bronchodilator is always necessary for confirmation and quantification of the airflow obstruction.

3. Patients with end-stage COPD may adopt positions which relieve dyspnea, such as leaning forward with arms outstretched and weight supported on the palms. Other signs in a patient with end-stage disease may include:

   a. The full use of the accessory respiratory muscles of the neck and shoulder girdle.
   b. Expiration through pursed lips.
   c. Paradoxical retraction of the lower interspaces during inspiration (Hoover's sign).
   d. Cyanosis.
   e. An enlarged, tender liver secondary to right heart failure. Neck vein distention, especially during expiration.
   f. Asterixis due to severe hypercapnia.

4. **Plain chest radiography** is insensitive for diagnosing emphysema; only about half of the instances are detected when the disease is of moderate severity.

   a. Overdistention of the lungs is indicated by a low, flat diaphragm and a long, narrow heart shadow. Flattening of the diaphragmatic contour and an increased retrosternal airspace are observed on the lateral projection. Rapid tapering of the vascular shadows accompanied by hypertransradiancy of the lungs is a sign of emphysema.
   b. Bullae, presenting as radiolucent areas larger than one centimeter in diameter and surrounded by arcuate hairline shadows, are proof of the presence of emphysema. However, bullae reflect only locally severe disease and are not necessarily indicative of widespread emphysema.
   c. Pulmonary hypertension and right ventricular hypertrophy are indicated by prominent hilar vascular shadows and encroachment of the heart shadow on the retrosternal space as the right ventricle enlarges anteriorly.

5. **Pulmonary function tests** are necessary for diagnosing and assessing the severity of airflow obstruction, and are helpful in following its progress. The FEV1 has less variability than other measurements of airways dynamics.

   a. The FVC is also readily measured, although it is dependent on the expiratory time in severe COPD. In the mildest degree of airflow obstruction, the FEV1/FVC ratio falls below 0.70 and the FEV1 percent predicted is normal. The FEV1 and the FEV1/FVC ratio fall progressively as the severity of COPD increases. Up to 30 percent of patients have an increase of 15 percent or more in their FEV1 following inhalation of a beta-agonist aerosol.

    b. Lung volume measurements reveal an increase in total lung capacity, functional residual capacity, and residual volume, and often a decrease in the vital capacity. The single breath carbon monoxide diffusing capacity is decreased in proportion to the severity of emphysema.

  6. Arterial blood gases reveal mild or moderate hypoxemia without hypercapnia in the early stages. As the disease progresses, hypoxemia becomes more severe and hypercapnia supervenes. Hypercapnia is observed with increasing frequency as the FEV1 falls below one liter.

  7. Erythrocytosis increases as arterial PO2 falls below 55 mmHg.

  8. Sputum examination. In stable chronic bronchitis, sputum is mucoid and the predominant cell is the macrophage. During an exacerbation, sputum usually becomes purulent with an influx of neutrophils. The Gram stain usually shows a mixture of organisms. The most frequent pathogens cultured from the sputum are Streptococcus pneumoniae and Haemophilus influenzae. Other oropharyngeal flora such as Moraxella catarrhalis have been shown to cause exacerbations.

III. Management of stable chronic obstructive pulmonary disease

  A. Bronchodilators can improve symptoms and reduce airflow limitation in patients with COPD.

    1. Metered dose inhalers (MDI) result in a bronchodilator response equivalent to that of a nebulizer. However, nebulizer therapy may still be necessary if dyspnea and severe bronchospasm during exacerbations impair proper MDI technique.

    2. Beta agonists. The primary pharmacologic therapy of COPD is the sympathomimetic bronchodilator. Among these, short-acting selective beta-2 agonists (eg, albuterol) are the agents of choice. Beta-2 agonists can cause tremor and reflex tachycardia due to peripheral arterial dilation. Hypokalemia can also occur in extreme cases. There is no advantage of using short-acting beta-2 agonists on a regular basis instead of as-needed.

  B. Anticholinergics. Inhaled anticholinergic bronchodilators (eg, ipratropium and tiotropium) are an integral component of COPD treatment. Anticholinergic drugs reduce the frequency of severe exacerbations and respiratory deaths.

    1. Tiotropium (Spiriva), a long-acting inhaled anticholinergic agent, confers longer bronchodilation than ipratropium (Atrovent) and also appears to lessen the frequency of acute exacerbations.

    2. The effects of anticholinergics and beta-2 agonists are additive. Combination therapy may be simplified by the use of a single metered dose inhaler that delivers a combination of ipratropium and albuterol.

  C. Theophylline provides clear benefits to some patients with COPD. Theophylline is associated with decreased dyspnea, improved arterial blood gases, improved spirometry, and improved respiratory muscle function. Theophylline also has pulmonary vasodilator and cardiac inotropic effects, resulting in improvements in right ventricular performance in cor pulmonale.

    1. Serum levels should be maintained in the 8 to 12 mcg/mL range. The use of a long-acting preparation at night may reduce the nocturnal decrements in respiratory function and the morning respiratory symptoms.

  D. Systemic corticosteroids have long been used to treat patients with COPD; however, chronic use can have significant adverse effects. Inhaled corticosteroids have substantially fewer adverse consequences.

    1. Chronic corticosteroid administration does not benefit most patients with COPD. However, as many as 20 percent of stable patients with COPD demonstrate objective improvement in airflow with oral corticosteroid treatment.

2. Chronic steroid therapy should be considered only in patients who have continued symptoms or severe airflow limitation despite maximal therapy with other agents. Only patients with documented improvement in airflow should be considered for long-term therapy. Steroids should be reduced to the lowest dose possible. Alternate day or inhaled steroid usage should be considered.

3. **Inhaled corticosteroids** may benefit patients with COPD with chronic bronchitis and frequent exacerbations.

Therapy at each stage of COPD			
Stage	**Characteristics**	**Recommended treatments**	
ALL		Avoidance of risk factor(s) Influenza vaccination	
0: At risk	Chronic symptoms (cough, sputum) Exposure to risk factor(s)		
I: Mild COPD	FEV_1/FVC <70 percent $FEV_1 \geq 80$ percent predicted with or without symptoms	Short-acting bronchodilator when needed	
II: Moderate COPD	IIA		
	FEV_1/FVC <70 percent 50 percent $\leq FEV_1$ <80 percent With or without symptoms	Regular treatment with one or more bronchodialtors Rehabilitation	Inhaled glucorticosteroids if significant symptoms and lung function response
	IIB		
	FEV_1/FVC <70 percent 50 percent $\leq FEV_1$ <50 percent With our without symptoms	Regular treatment with one or more bronchodilators Rehabilitation	Inhaled glucortico-steroids if significant symptoms and lung function response or if repeated exacerbations
III: Severe COPD	FEV_1/FVC <70 percent FEV_1 <30 percent predicted or presence of respiratory or right heart failure	Regular treatment with one or more bronchodilators Inhaled glucocorticosteroids if significant symptoms and lung function response or if repeated exacerbations Treatment of complications Rehabilitation Long-term oxygen therapy if respiratory failure Surgical treatments	

E. Supplemental therapy

1. **Oxygen.** Assessment of arterial blood gases or pulse oximetry is the only reliable method for detecting hypoxemia. Arterial blood gas analysis is also helpful in assessing the presence and severity of hypercapnia.

2. **Surgery.** Selected patients may benefit from lung volume reduction surgery or lung transplantation. **Indications for lung transplantation**
   a. FEV1 is <25 percent of predicted, or
   b. $PaCO_2$ is >55 mmHg, or
   c. Cor pulmonale is present.
   d. Candidates must be under 65 years of age, not have dysfunction of major organs other than the lung, and not have active or recent malignancy or infection with HIV, hepatitis B, or hepatitis C viruses.

IV. Management of acute exacerbations of chronic obstructive pulmonary disease

A. An acute exacerbation of chronic obstructive pulmonary disease (COPD) is characterized by an acute worsening of symptoms accompanied by an impairment of lung function.

B. **Precipitants**. Acute exacerbations of COPD are most commonly precipitated by infection (bacterial or viral), air pollution or temperature.

C. Other medical conditions can mimic or cause COPD exacerbation include myocardial ischemia, congestive heart failure, pulmonary embolism, or aspiration

D. **Criteria for hospitalization:**
   1. High risk comorbidities including pneumonia, cardiac arrhythmia, congestive heart failure, diabetes mellitus, renal failure, or liver failure
   2. Inadequate response to outpatient management
   3. Marked increase in dyspnea
   4. Inability to eat or sleep due to symptoms
   5. Worsening hypoxemia
   6. Worsening hypercapnia
   7. Changes in mental status
   8. Inability to care for oneself
   9. Uncertain diagnosis
   10. Acute respiratory acidemia

E. **Pharmacologic treatment**
   1. The major components of managing an acute exacerbation of COPD include inhaled beta adrenergic agonists, anticholinergic bronchodilators, corticosteroids, and antibiotics.
   2. **Inhaled beta-2 adrenergic agonists** such as albuterol are the mainstay of therapy for an acute exacerbation of COPD. These medications may be administered via a nebulizer or a metered dose inhaler (MDI) with a spacer device. Nebulized therapy is preferred in this clinical setting.
      a. **Albuterol (Ventolin)** dosages are 180 mcg (two puffs) by metered dose inhaler, or 2.5 mg (diluted to a total of 3 mL) by nebulizer, given every one to two hours.
      b. Subcutaneous injection of beta adrenergic agonists is reserved for situations in which inhaled administration is not possible. Parenteral use may cause arrhythmias or myocardial ischemia.
   3. **Anticholinergic bronchodilators**, such as ipratropium bromide and glycopyrrolate, may be used in combination with beta adrenergic agonists to produce greater bronchodilation.
      a. **Ipratropium (Atrovent)** may be administered during acute exacerbations either by nebulizer (500 mcg every two to four hours) or via MDI (two puffs [36 mcg] every two to four hours with a spacer).

4. **Corticosteroids.** Methylprednisolone (60 to 125 mg intravenously, two to four times daily) is given to inpatients. Prednisone (40 to 60 mg orally, once daily) is given to outpatients.

5. **Antibiotics** are recommended for acute exacerbations of COPD with increased secretions. Outpatients should be prescribed a ten day course of amoxicillin, doxycycline, or trimethoprim-sulfamethoxazole. Beta-lactam antibiotics with a beta-lactamase inhibitor should be administered to hospitalized patients. Hospitalized patients at risk for infection with pseudomonas aeruginosa should receive a fluoroquinolone.

Choice of empirical antibiotic therapy for COPD exacerbation

First-line treatment	Dosage*
Amoxicillin (Amoxil, Trimox, Wymox)	500 mg tid
Trimethoprim-sulfamethoxazole (Bactrim, Cotrim, Septra)	1 tablet (80/400 mg) bid
Doxycycline	100 mg bid
Erythromycin	250-500 mg qid
Second-line treatment**	
Amoxicillin-clavulanate (Augmentin)	500-875 mg bid
Second- or third-generation cephalosporin (eg, cefuroxime [Ceftin])	250-500 mg bid
Macrolides	
Clarithromycin (Biaxin)	250-500 mg bid
Azithromycin (Zithromax)	500 mg on day 1, then 250 mg qd X 4 days
Quinolones	
Ciprofloxacin (Cipro)	500-750 mg bid
Levofloxacin (Levaquin)***	500 mg qd

*May need adjustment in patients with renal or hepatic insufficiency.
**For patients in whom first-line therapy has failed and those with moderate to severe disease or resistant or gram-negative pathogens.
***Although the newer quinolones have better activity against Streptococcus pneumoniae, ciprofloxacin may be preferable in patients with gram-negative organisms.

6. **Methylxanthines.** Aminophylline and theophylline are not recommended for the management of acute exacerbations of COPD. Randomized controlled trials of intravenous aminophylline in this setting have failed to show efficacy.

F. Oxygen therapy
1. Acute hypoxemia during an acute exacerbation of COPD may cause tissue hypoxia. Supplemental oxygen should be given to achieve a target PaO2 of 60 to 65 mmHg, with a hemoglobin saturation around 90 percent.
2. **Venturi masks** are the preferred means of oxygen delivery because they permit a precise delivered fraction of inspired oxygen (FiO2). Venturi masks can deliver an FiO2 of 24, 28, 31, 35, or 40 percent.
3. During oral feedings, nasal cannulae are also more comfortable and convenient for the patient. They can provide flow rates up to 6 L/min with FiO2 of approximately 44 percent.
4. When higher inspired concentrations of oxygen are needed, simple facemasks can provide an FiO2 up to 55 percent using flow rates of 6 to 10 L/min. Non-rebreather masks with a reservoir, one-way valves, and a tight face seal can deliver an inspired oxygen concentration up to 90 percent.
5. **Adequate oxygenation** must be assured, even if it results in acute hypercapnia due to altered ventilation-perfusion relationships, the Haldane effect of unloading CO2 from oxyhemoglobin, or decreased ventilatory drive. Hypercapnia is generally well tolerated in patients whose PaCO2 is chronically elevated; however, noninvasive positive pressure ventilation or intubation may be required when hypercapnia is associated with depressed mental status, profound acidemia, or cardiac dysrhythmias.

G. Noninvasive positive pressure ventilation (NIPPV) is effective and less morbid than intubation for selected patients with acute exacerbations of COPD. Early use of NIPPV is recommended when each of the following is present:
   a. Respiratory distress with moderate-to-severe dyspnea.
   b. pH less than 7.35 or $PaCO_2$ above 45 mm Hg.
   c. Respiratory rate of 25/minute or greater.
2. NIPPV is contraindicated in the presence of cardiovascular instability (eg, hypotension, serious dysrhythmias, myocardial ischemia), craniofacial trauma or burns, inability to protect the airway, or when indications for emergent intubation are present. Approximately 26 to 31 percent of patients initially treated with NIPPV ultimately require intubation and mechanical ventilation.

H. Surgical management
1. **Lung volume reduction surgery (LVRS)** is recommended in patients with upper lobe predominant disease and low exercise capacity.
2. **Indications for lung transplantation**
   a. FEV_1 is <25 percent of predicted, **OR**
   b. $PaCO_2$ is >55 mm Hg (7.3 kPa), **OR**
   c. Cor pulmonale is present.
   d. Candidates must be under 65 years of age, not have dysfunction of major organs other than the lung, and not have active or recent malignancy or infection with HIV, hepatitis B, or hepatitis C viruses.

References, see page 372.

Acute Bronchitis

Acute bronchitis is one of the most common diagnoses in ambulatory care medicine, accounting for 2.5 million physician visits per year. Viruses are the most common cause of acute bronchitis in otherwise healthy adults. Only a small portion of acute bronchitis infections are caused by nonviral agents, with the most common organisms being *Mycoplasma pneumoniae* and *Chlamydia pneumoniae*.

I. **Diagnosis**

   A. The cough in acute bronchitis may produce either clear or purulent sputum. This cough generally lasts seven to 10 days. Approximately 50 percent of patients with acute bronchitis have a cough that lasts up to three weeks, and 25 percent of patients have a cough that persists for over a month.

   B. **Physical examination.** Wheezing, rhonchi, or a prolonged expiratory phase may be present.

   C. **Diagnostic studies**

      1. The appearance of sputum is not predictive of bacterial infection. Purulent sputum is most often caused by viral infections. Microscopic examination or culture of sputum is not helpful. Since most cases of acute bronchitis are caused by viruses, cultures are usually negative or exhibit normal respiratory flora. M. pneumoniae or C. pneumoniae infection are not detectable on routine sputum culture.

      2. When pneumonia is suspected, chest radiographs and pulse oximetry may be helpful.

II. **Pathophysiology**

Selected Triggers of Acute Bronchitis

Viruses: adenovirus, coronavirus, coxsackievirus, enterovirus, influenza virus, parainfluenza virus, respiratory syncytial virus, rhinovirus

Bacteria: *Bordetella pertussis, Bordetella parapertussis, Branhamella catarrhalis, Haemophilus influenzae, Streptococcus pneumoniae,* atypical bacteria (eg, *Mycoplasma pneumoniae, Chlamydia pneumoniae,* Legionella species)

Yeast and fungi: *Blastomyces dermatitidis, Candida albicans, Candida tropicalis, Coccidioides immitis, Cryptococcus neoformans, Histoplasma capsulatum*

Noninfectious triggers: asthma, air pollutants, ammonia, cannabis, tobacco, trace metals, others

---

   A. Acute bronchitis is usually caused by a viral infection. In patients younger than one year, respiratory syncytial virus, parainfluenza virus, and coronavirus are the most common isolates. In patients one to 10 years of age, parainfluenza virus, enterovirus, respiratory syncytial virus, and rhinovirus predominate. In patients older than 10 years, influenza virus, respiratory syncytial virus, and adenovirus are most frequent.

   B. Parainfluenza virus, enterovirus, and rhinovirus infections most commonly occur in the fall. Influenza virus, respiratory syncytial virus, and coronavirus infections are most frequent in the winter and spring.

III. **Signs and symptoms**

   A. Cough is the most commonly observed symptom of acute bronchitis. Most patients have a cough for less than two weeks; however, 26 percent are still coughing after two weeks, and a few cough for six to eight weeks.

   B. Other signs and symptoms include sputum production, dyspnea, wheezing, chest pain, fever, hoarseness, malaise, rhonchi, and rales. Sputum may be clear, white, yellow, green, or tinged with blood. Color alone should not be considered indicative of bacterial infection.

IV. **Physical examination and diagnostic studies**

   A. **Fever, tachypnea, wheezing, rhonchi,** and prolonged expiration are comon. Consolidation is absent. High fever should prompt consideration of pneumonia or influenza.

   B. **Chest radiography** should be reserved for patients with possible pneumonia, heart failure, advanced age, chronic obstructive pulmonary disease, malignancy, tuberculosis, or immunocompromised or debilitated status.

V. Differential diagnosis

A. Acute bronchitis or pneumonia can present with fever, constitutional symptoms and a productive cough. Patients with pneumonia often have rales. When pneumonia is suspected on the basis of the presence of a high fever, constitutional symptoms or severe dyspnea, a chest radiograph should be obtained.

Differential Diagnosis of Acute Bronchitis	
Disease process	**Signs and symptoms**
Asthma	Evidence of reversible airway obstruction even when not infected
Allergic aspergillosis	Transient pulmonary infiltrates Eosinophilia in sputum and peripheral blood smear
Occupational exposures	Symptoms worse during the work week but tend to improve during weekends, holidays and vacations
Chronic bronchitis	Chronic cough with sputum production on a daily basis for a minimum of three months Typically occurs in smokers
Sinusitis	Tenderness over the sinuses, postnasal drainage
Common cold	Upper airway inflammation and no evidence of bronchial wheezing
Pneumonia	Evidence of infiltrate on the chest radiograph
Congestive heart failure	Basilar rales, orthopnea Cardiomegaly Evidence of increased interstitial or alveolar fluid on the chest radiograph S_3 gallop, tachycardia
Reflux esophagitis	Intermittent symptoms worse when lying down Heartburn
Bronchogenic tumor	Constitutional signs often present Cough chronic, sometimes with hemoptysis
Aspiration syndromes	Usually related to a precipitating event, such as smoke inhalation Vomiting Decreased level of consciousness

B. **Asthma** should be considered in patients with repetitive episodes of acute bronchitis. Patients who repeatedly present with cough and wheezing can be given spirometric testing with bronchodilation to help differentiate asthma from recurrent bronchitis.

C. **Congestive heart failure** may cause cough, shortness of breath and wheezing in older patients. Reflux esophagitis with chronic aspiration can cause bronchial inflammation with cough and wheezing. Bronchogenic tumors may produce a cough and obstructive symptoms.

VI. Treatment

A. **Protussives and antitussives**

1. Because acute bronchitis is most often caused by a viral infection, usually only symptomatic treatment is required. Treatment can focus on preventing or controlling the cough (antitussive therapy).

2. Antitussive therapy is indicated if cough is creating significant discomfort. Studies have reported success rates ranging from 68 to 98 percent. Nonspecific antitussives, such as hydrocodone (Hycodan), dextromethorphan

(Delsym), codeine (Robitussin A-C), carbetapentane (Rynatuss), and benzonatate (Tessalon), simply suppress cough.

Selected Nonspecific Antitussive Agents		
Preparation	**Dosage**	**Side effects**
Hydromorphone-guaifen-esin (Hycotuss)	5 mg per 100 mg per 5 mL (one teaspoon)	Sedation, nausea, vomiting, respiratory depression
Dextromethorphan (Delsym)	30 mg every 12 hours	Rarely, gastrointestinal upset or sedation
Hydrocodone (Hycodan syrup or tablets)	5 mg every 4 to 6 hours	Gastrointestinal upset, nausea, drowsiness, constipation
Codeine (Robitussin A-C)	10 to 20 mg every 4 to 6 hours	Gastrointestinal upset, nausea, drowsiness, constipation
Carbetapentane (Rynatuss)	60 to 120 mg every 12 hours	Drowsiness, gastrointestinal upset
Benzonatate (Tessalon)	100 to 200 mg three times daily	Hypersensitivity, gastrointestinal upset, sedation

B. Bronchodilators. Patients with acute bronchitis who used an albuterol metered-dose inhaler are less likely to be coughing at one week, compared with those who received placebo.

C. Antibiotics. Physicians often treat acute bronchitis with antibiotics, even though scant evidence exists that antibiotics offer any significant advantage over placebo. Antibiotic therapy is beneficial in patients with exacerbations of chronic bronchitis.

Oral Antibiotic Regimens for Bronchitis	
Drug	**Recommended regimen**
Azithromycin (Zithromax)	500 mg; then 250 mg qd
Erythromycin	250-500 mg q6h
Clarithromycin (Biaxin)	500 mg bid
Levofloxacin (Levaquin)	500 mg qd
Trovafloxacin (Trovan)	200 mg qd
Trimethoprim/sulfamethoxazole (Bactrim, Septra)	1 DS tablet bid
Doxycycline	100 mg bid

    D. Bronchodilators. Significant relief of symptoms occurs with inhaled albuterol (two puffs four times daily). When productive cough and wheezing are present, bronchodilator therapy may be useful.

References, see page 372.

Infectious Disorders

Community-acquired Pneumonia

Pneumonia is the sixth most common cause of death in the United States. Community-acquired pneumonia (CAP) is defined as an acute infection of the pulmonary parenchyma in a patient who has acquired the infection in the community.

I. **Clinical evaluation**
   A. Common clinical features of CAP include cough, fever, pleurisy, dyspnea and sputum production. Mucopurulent sputum production is most frequently found in association with bacterial pneumonia, while scant or watery sputum is suggestive of an atypical pathogen.
   B. Other common features are nausea, vomiting, diarrhea, and mental status changes. Chest pain occurs in 30 percent of cases, chills in 40 to 50 percent, and rigors in 15 percent.
   C. **Physical examination.** Fever is present in 80 percent, although frequently absent in older patients. A respiratory rate above 24 breaths/minute is noted in 45 to 70 percent of patients and may be the most sensitive sign in the elderly; tachycardia is also common. Chest examination reveals rales in most patients, while one-third have evidence of consolidation.
   D. The major blood test abnormality is leukocytosis (15,000 and 30,000 per mm^3) with a leftward shift. Leukopenia can occur, and generally has a poor prognosis.

II. **Radiologic evaluation.** An infiltrate on plain chest radiograph is considered the "gold standard" for diagnosing pneumonia and should be obtained in most patients. The radiographic appearances of CAP include lobar consolidation, interstitial infiltrates, and cavitation. Bacterial pneumonia and nonbacterial pneumonia can not be differentiated on the basis of the radiographic appearance.

III. **Diagnostic testing for microbial etiology**
   A. **Outpatients.** Culture and Gram's stain are usually not done in outpatients.
   B. **Hospitalized patients.** Blood cultures and sputum Gram's stain and culture should be obtained in hospitalized patients with suspected CAP.
   C. Blood cultures are positive for a pathogen in 7 to 16 percent of hospitalized patients. Streptococcus pneumoniae accounts for two-thirds of the positive blood cultures.
   D. The preferred tests for Legionella are culture on selective media and the urinary antigen assay. A new polymerase chain reaction (PCR) test that detects L. pneumophila (all serogroups) in respiratory secretions may become the preferred method to detect Legionella infection.
   E. **Urine antigen assays** are complementary methods to detect S. pneumoniae and Legionella. The advantages are:
      1. Results of urine antigen testing are immediately available.
      2. The test retains validity even after the initiation of antibiotic therapy.
      3. The test has high sensitivity compared to blood cultures and sputum studies.
   F. The pneumococcal urinary antigen assay is an acceptable test to augment blood culture and sputum Gram's stain and culture, with the potential advantage of rapid results similar to those for sputum Gram's stain.

Causes of Community-acquired Pneumonia	
Etiology	Prevalence (percent)
Streptococcus pneumoniae	20-60
Hemophilus influenzae	3-10
Staphylococcus aureus	3-5
Gram-negative bacilli	3-10
Aspiration	6-10
Miscellaneous	3-5
Legionella sp.	2-8
Mycoplasma pneumoniae	1-6
Chlamydia pneumoniae	4-6
Viruses	2-15

IV. **Organisms of special interest**
  A. **Streptococcus pneumoniae** accounts for about 65 percent of bacteremic pneumonia cases and is the most common identified pathogen in nearly all studies.
  B. **Staphylococcus aureus** is an infrequent pulmonary pathogen.
  C. **Influenza** is important to recognize because of the need for appropriate infection control in hospitalized patients, for public health reporting purposes, and for rapid treatment with antiviral agents. The rapid antigen assays provide results in 15 to 20 minutes.
  D. **Legionella spp** is implicated in 2 to 10 percent of CAP cases. Legionella is important to identify because of the potential to cause epidemics (usually in hospitals and hotels) and because Legionella spp infection has a relatively high mortality.
  E. **Chlamydia pneumoniae** is implicated in 10 to 30 percent of cases of CAP in adults. Diagnostic testing consists of PCR.
  F. **Mycoplasma pneumoniae** has historically been considered a pathogen primarily of children and adolescents, but there are reports of increasingly high rates of infection in adults, especially elderly adults.
  G. **Bioterrorism agents** that may be used for bioterrorism and can present as a CAP syndrome include Bacillus anthracis (inhalational anthrax), Yersinia pestis (pneumonic plague), Francisella tularensis (tularemia), Coxiella burnetii (Q fever), Legionella spp, Influenza virus, and hantavirus.

V. **Summary and recommendations**
  A. The combination of sputum specimen for Gram's stain and culture plus urinary pneumococcal antigen testing is likely to be most useful for the rapid diagnosis of CAP in hospitalized patients. In addition, hospitalized patients should have pretreatment blood cultures.
  B. The blood culture positivity rate is relatively low, but when positive establishes the microbial diagnosis.

VI. **Treatment of community-acquired pneumonia in adults**
  A. **Indications for hospitalization.** Inability to maintain oral intake, history of substance abuse, cognitive impairment, and poor functional status.
  B. Initial antimicrobial therapy should provide coverage for S. pneumoniae plus atypical pathogens (particularly M. pneumoniae or C. pneumoniae, which are common causes of outpatient CAP). The macrolides, which are effective against the atypical pathogens, are therefore recommended when there are no significant risk factors for macrolide-resistant S. pneumoniae.

C. Recommendations for outpatient therapy

1. Patients treated with an effective drug usually improve within 72 hours. Median time to resolution is three days for fever, six days for dyspnea, and 14 days for both cough and fatigue. Patients who do not improve within 72 hours are considered nonresponders.

2. **No comorbidities or recent antibiotic use.** For uncomplicated pneumonia in patients who do not require hospitalization, have no significant comorbidities, or use of antibiotics within the last three months, one of the following oral regimens is recommended:

   a. Azithromycin (Zithromax, 500 mg on day one followed by four days of 250 mg a day); 500 mg a day for three days or 2 g single dose (microsphere formulation).

   b. Clarithromycin XL (Biaxin XL, two 500 mg tablets daily) for five days or until afebrile for 48 to 72 hours.

   c. Doxycycline (100 mg twice a day) for seven to 10 days

3. **Comorbidities or recent antibiotic use.** For pneumonia in patients who do not require hospitalization, but who have significant comorbidities (ie, chronic obstructive pulmonary disease, liver or renal disease, cancer, diabetes, heart disease, alcoholism, asplenia, or immunosuppression), or use of antibiotics within prior three months, one of the following oral regimens is recommended:

   a. **A respiratory fluoroquinolone** (gemifloxacin [Factive] 320 mg daily or levofloxacin [Levaquin] 750 mg daily or moxifloxacin [Avelox] 400 mg daily).

   b. **Combination therapy** with a beta-lactam effective against S. pneumoniae (high-dose amoxicillin, 1 gm three times daily or amoxicillin clavulanate [Augmentin] 2 g twice daily or cefpodoxime [Vantin] 200 mg twice daily or cefuroxime [Ceftin] 500 mg twice daily) plus either a macrolide (azithromycin [Zithromax] 500 mg on day one followed by four days of 250 mg a day or clarithromycin [Biaxin] 250 mg twice daily or clarithromycin XL 1000 mg once daily) or doxycycline (100 mg twice daily).

   c. These regimens are also appropriate in patients without comorbidities or recent antimicrobial use in locations where the prevalence of "high-level" macrolide-resistant S. pneumoniae is high. When choosing between fluoroquinolones, moxifloxacin and gemifloxacin in vitro are progressively more active against penicillin-resistant pneumococci strains than levofloxacin. Gemifloxacin causes a mild rash in 2.8 percent of patients, but an unexpectedly higher rate (14 percent) in women under 40 years of age.

   d. Patients should be treated for a minimum of five days, and therapy should not be stopped until patients are afebrile for 48 to 72 hours. Longer duration of therapy is required if there is an extrapulmonary infection or for infections caused by S. aureus or Pseudomonas.

Recommended Empiric Drug Therapy for Patients with Community-Acquired Pneumonia

Clinical Situation	Primary Treatment	Alternative(s)
Younger (<60 yr) outpatients without underlying disease	Macrolide antibiotics (azithromycin, clarithromycin, dirithromycin, or erythromycin)	Levofloxacin or doxycycline
Older (>60 yr) outpatients with underlying disease	Levofloxacin or cefuroxime or Trimethoprim-sulfamethoxazole Add vancomycin in severe, life-threatening pneumonias	Beta-lactamase inhibitor (with macrolide if legionella infection suspected)
Gross aspiration suspected	Clindamycin IV	Cefotetan, ampicillin/sulbactam

Common Antimicrobial Agents for Community-Acquired Pneumonia in Adults

Type	Agent	Dosage
Oral therapy		
Macrolides	Erythromycin Clarithromycin (Biaxin) Azithromycin (Zithromax)	500 mg PO qid 500 mg PO bid 500 mg PO on day 1, then 250 mg qd x 4 days
Beta-lactam/beta-lactamase inhibitor	Amoxicillin-clavulanate (Augmentin) Augmentin XR	500 mg tid or 875 mg PO bid 2 tabs q12h
Quinolones	Ciprofloxacin (Cipro) Levofloxacin (Levaquin) Ofloxacin (Floxin)	500 mg PO bid 500 mg PO qd 400 mg PO bid
Tetracycline	Doxycycline	100 m g PO bid
Sulfonamide	Trimethoprim-sulfamethoxazole	160 mg/800 mg (DS) PO bid

Type	Agent	Dosage
Intravenous Therapy		
Cephalosporins Second-generation	Cefuroxime (Kefurox, Zinacef)	0.75-1.5 g IV q8h
Third-generation (anti-Pseudomonas aeruginosa)	Ceftizoxime (Cefizox)	1-2 g IV q8h
	Ceftazidime (Fortaz)	1-2 g IV q8h
	Cefoperazone (Cefobid)	1-2 g IV q8h
Beta-lactam/beta-lactamase inhibitors	Ampicillin-sulbactam (Unasyn)	1.5 g IV q6h
	Piperacillin/tazobactam (Zosyn)	3.375 g IV q6h
	Ticarcillin-clavulanate (Timentin)	3.1 g IV q6h
Quinolones	Ciprofloxacin (Cipro)	400 mg IV q12h
	Levofloxacin (Levaquin)	500 mg IV q24h
	Ofloxacin (Floxin)	400 mg IV q12h
Aminoglycosides	Gentamicin	Load 2.0 mg/kg IV, then 1.5 mg/kg q8h
	Amikacin	
Vancomycin	Vancomycin	1 gm IV q12h

A. Recommendations for hospitalized patients

1. Hospitalized patients with CAP are initially treated with empiric antibiotic therapy. When the etiology of CAP has been identified, treatment regimens may be simplified and directed to that pathogen.

2. **Not in the ICU.** For patients admitted to a general ward, one of the following regimens is recommended:

3. Combination therapy with ceftriaxone (Rocephin, 2 g IV daily; 1 g IV daily in patients >65 years of age) or cefotaxime (Claforan, 1 g IV every 8 hours) plus azithromycin (Zithromax, 500 mg IV daily) **OR**

4. Monotherapy with a respiratory fluoroquinolone given either IV or orally except as noted (levofloxacin, [Levaquin] 750 mg daily or moxifloxacin [Avelox] 400 mg daily or gemifloxacin [Factive] 320 mg daily (only available in oral formulation).

5. **Admitted to an intensive care unit.** Patients requiring admission to an ICU are more likely to have risk factors for resistant pathogens, including the possibility of community-associated MRSA. Treatment consists of an intravenous combination therapy with a potent anti-pneumococcal beta-lactam (ceftriaxone 2 g daily or cefotaxime 1 g every eight hours) plus either an advanced macrolide (azithromycin 500 mg daily) or a respiratory fluoroquinolone (levofloxacin 750 mg daily or moxifloxacin 400 mg daily).

6. **Patients who may be infected with Pseudomonas aeruginosa** or other resistant pathogens (particularly those with bronchiectasis or COPD with frequent antimicrobial or corticosteroid use) should be treated with agents that are effective against pneumococcus, P. aeruginosa, and Legionella spp. Regimens include the following:

   a. **Combination therapy with a beta-lactam antibiotic** such as piperacillin-tazobactam (Zosyn, 4.5 g every six hours) OR imipenem (Primaxin, 500 mg IV every six hours) OR meropenem (Merrem, 1 g every eight hours)

OR cefepime (Maxipime, 2 g every eight hours) OR ceftazidime (Fortaz, 2 g every 8 hours) PLUS either ciprofloxacin (Cipro, 400 mg every 8 hours) OR levofloxacin (Levaquin, 750 mg daily). For beta-lactam allergic patients, aztreonam (Azactam) plus levofloxacin (750 mg daily).

b. **For severely ill patients**, early Gram's stain of respiratory secretions should be completed. If S. aureus is suspected by Gram's stain, the addition of **vancomycin** (15 mg/kg every 12 hours, adjusted for renal function) or **linezolid (Zyvox**, 600 mg every 12 hours). In addition, we suggest empiric therapy of MRSA in patients with severe CAP who have risk factors for CA-MRSA, such as, prior antimicrobial therapy or recent influenza-like illness.

7. **Response to therapy.** With appropriate antibiotic therapy, some improvement in the patient's clinical course is usually seen within 48 to 72 hours. However, fever in patients with lobar pneumonia may take 72 hours or longer to improve. With pneumococcal pneumonia, the cough usually resolves within eight days and auscultatory crackles clear within three weeks.

8. **Duration of therapy.** Among hospitalized patients who have received initial therapy with intravenous antibiotics, switching to oral therapy may occur when the patient is improving, hemodynamically stable, and able to take oral medications.

9. **Treatment of hospitalized patients** should be continued for a minimum of five days. The patient should be afebrile for 48 to 72 hours, breathing without supplemental oxygen (unless required for preexisting disease), and have no more than one clinical instability factor (defined as heart rate [HR] >100 beats/min, respiratory rate [RR] >24 breaths/min, and systolic blood pressure [SBP] of ≤90 mm Hg) before stopping therapy.

References, see page 372.

Pulmonary Tuberculosis

Mycobacterium tuberculosis infection most commonly affects the lungs. Pulmonary manifestations of tuberculosis (TB) include primary, reactivation, endobronchial, and lower lung field infection.

I. **Primary tuberculosis**
   A. **Fever** is the most common symptom, occurring in 70 percent of patients. Fever is low grade but could be as high as 39ºC and usually last for14 to 21 days. Fever usually resolves in 10 weeks.
   B. Symptoms in addition to fever are present only in 25 percent of patients, and include chest pain and pleuritic chest pain.
   C. The physical examination is usually normal; pulmonary signs include pain to palpation and signs of an effusion.
   D. **Radiographic abnormalities.** The most common abnormality on chest radiography is hilar adenopathy, occurring in 65 percent. Hilar changes can be seen as early as one week after skin test conversion and within two months in all cases. These radiographic findings resolve slowly, often over a period of more than one year.
   E. One-third of converters developed pleural effusions. Pulmonary infiltrates occur in 27 percent. Perihilar and right sided infiltrates are the most common, with ipsilateral hilar enlargement. Lower and upper lobe infiltrates are observed in 33 and 13 percent of adults, respectively. Most infiltrates resolved over months to years.

II. Reactivation tuberculosis

A. Reactivation TB represents 90 percent of adult cases, and results from reactivation of a previously dormant focus seeded at the time of the primary infection. The apical posterior segments of the lung are frequently involved.

B. Symptoms typically began insidiously and are present for weeks or months before diagnosis. One-half to two-thirds of patients develop cough, weight loss and fatigue. Fever and night sweats or night sweats alone are present in one-half. Chest pain and dyspnea each are reported in one-third of patients, and hemoptysis in one-quarter.

C. The cough of TB may be mild initially and may be non-productive or productive of only scant sputum. Initially, it may be present only in the morning. As the disease progresses, cough becomes more continuous and productive of yellow or yellow-green sputum. Frank hemoptysis is present later.

D. Dyspnea can occur when patients have extensive parenchymal involvement, pleural effusions, or a pneumothorax. Pleuritic chest pain is not common.

E. **Physical findings of pulmonary TB** are usually absent in mild or moderate disease.

   1. Dullness with decreased fremitus may indicate pleural thickening or effusion. Rales may be heard only after a short cough (post-tussive rales).

   2. When large areas of the lung are involved, signs of consolidation, such as whispered pectoriloquy or tubular breath sounds, may be heard. Extrapulmonary signs include clubbing and findings at other sites of involvement.

F. **Laboratory findings** are usually normal in pulmonary TB. Late in the disease, hematologic changes may include normocytic anemia, leukocytosis, or, more rarely, monocytosis. Hyponatremia may be associated with the syndrome of inappropriate antidiuretic hormone secretion (SIADH) or rarely with adrenal insufficiency.

G. **Radiographic abnormalities**

   1. **Reactivation TB** typically involves the apical-posterior segments of the upper lobes (80 to 90 percent), followed in frequency by the superior segment of the lower lobes and the anterior segment of the upper lobes; 19 to 40 percent also have cavities, with visible air-fluid levels.

   2. **Computed tomographic (CT) scanning** is more sensitive than plain chest radiography for diagnosis. CT scan may show a cavity or centrilobular lesions, nodules and branching linear densities.

III. Targeted tuberculin testing and treatment of latent tuberculosis infection

A. **Targeted tuberculin testing** for latent tuberculosis infection (LTBI) identifies persons at high risk for developing TB who would benefit by treatment of LTBI, if detected. Persons with increased risk for developing TB include those who have had recent infection with Mycobacterium tuberculosis and those who have clinical conditions that are associated with an increased risk for progression of LTBI to active TB. Targeted tuberculin testing programs should be conducted only among groups at high risk.

B. For persons who are at highest risk for developing active TB (ie, HIV infection, immunosuppressive therapy, recent close contact with persons with infectious TB, or who have abnormal chest radiographs consistent with prior TB), ≥ 5 mm of induration is considered positive.

IV. Clinical and laboratory monitoring

A. Baseline laboratory testing is not routinely indicated for all patients at the start of treatment for LTBI. Patients whose initial evaluation suggests a liver disorder should have baseline hepatic measurements of serum aspartate aminotransferase (AST) or alanine aminotransferase(ALT) and bilirubin.

Groups at High Risk for Tuberculosis

Persons with recent Mycobacterium tuberculosis infection (within the past 2 years) or a history of inadequately treated tuberculosis

Close contacts of persons known or suspected to have tuberculosis

Persons infected with the human immunodeficiency virus

Persons who inject illicit drugs or use other locally identified high-risk substances (eg crack cocaine)

Residents and employees of high-risk congregate settings (eg correctional institutions, nursing homes, mental institutions or shelters for the homeless)

Health-care workers who serve high-risk clients

Foreign-born persons including children who have recently arrived (within 5 years) from countries that have a high incidence or prevalence of tuberculosis (Africa Asia and Latin America)

Some medically underserved low-income populations

High-risk racial or ethnic minority populations as defined locally

Elderly persons

Children less than 4 years of age or infants children and adolescents who have been exposed to adults in high-risk categories

Persons with medical conditions known to increase the risk of tuberculosis:

    Chest radiograph findings suggestive of previous tuberculosis in a person who received inadequate treatment or no treatment

    Diabetes mellitus

    Silicosis

    Organ transplantation

    Prolonged corticosteroid therapy (eg prednisone in a 15 mg or more per day for 1 month

    Other immunosuppressive therapy

    Cancer of the head and neck

    Hematologic and reticuloendothelial diseases (eg leukemia and lymphoma)

    End-stage renal disease

    Intestinal bypass or gastrectomy

    Chronic malabsorption syndromes

    Weight that is 10 percent or more below ideal body weight

Interpretation of the Purified Protein Derivative Tuberculin Skin Test

I. An induration of 5 mm or more is classified as positive in persons with any of the following:
    A. Human immunodeficiency virus infection
    B. Recent close contact with persons who have active tuberculosis
    C. Chest radiographs showing fibrosis (consistent with healed tuberculosis)

II. An induration of 10 mm or more is classified as positive in all persons who do not meet any of the criteria in section I but have other risk factors for tuberculosis

III. An induration of 15 mm or more is positive in persons who do not meet any of the criteria from sections I or II.

IV. Recent tuberculin skin test conversion is defined as an increase in induration of 10 mm or more within a two-year period, regardless of age.

V. In health-care workers, the recommendations in sections I, II and III generally should be followed. In facilities where tuberculosis patients frequently receive care, the optimal cut-off point for health-care workers with no other risk factors may be an induration of 10 mm or greater.

B. Baseline testing is also indicated for patients with HIV infection, pregnant women, and women in the immediate postpartum period (ie, within three months of delivery), persons with a history of chronic liver disease (eg, hepatitis B or C, alcoholic hepatitis, or cirrhosis), alcoholics, and persons at risk for chronic liver disease. Baseline testing is not routinely indicated in older persons. Hepatitis and end-stage liver disease are relative contraindications to the use of isoniazid or pyrazinamide for treatment of LTBI.

C. **Routine laboratory monitoring** during treatment of LTBI is indicated for persons whose baseline liver function tests are abnormal and other persons at risk for hepatic disease. Isoniazid should be withheld if transaminase levels exceed three times the upper limit of normal if associated with symptoms and five times the upper limit of normal if the patient is asymptomatic.

D. **Chest radiograph** is indicated for all persons being considered for treatment of LTBI to exclude active pulmonary TB.

E. If chest radiographs are normal and no symptoms consistent with active TB are present, tuberculin-positive persons may be candidates for treatment of LTBI. If radiographic or clinical findings are consistent with pulmonary or extrapulmonary TB, further studies (eg, medical evaluation, bacteriologic examinations, and a comparison of the current and old chest radiographs) should be done to determine if treatment for active TB is indicated.

F. Sputum examination is not indicated for most persons being considered for treatment of LTBI. However, persons with chest radiographic findings suggestive of prior, healed TB infections should have three consecutive sputum samples, obtained on different days, submitted for AFB smear and culture. HIV-infected persons with respiratory symptoms who are being considered for treatment of LTBI should also have sputum specimens submitted for mycobacterial examination, even if the chest radiograph is normal. If the results of sputum smears and cultures are negative, the person is a candidate for treatment of LTBI.

V. Treatment of tuberculosis

Drug regimens for culture-positive tuberculosis caused by drug-susceptible organisms					
Regimen	Drugs	Interval and doses, minimal duration	Regimen	Drugs	Interval and doses, minimal duration
1	INH RIF PZA EMB	Seven days per week for 56 doses (8 wk) or 5 d/wk for 40 doses (8 wk)	1a	INH/RIF	Seven days per week for 126 doses (18 wk) or 5 d/wk for 90 doses (18 wk)
			1b	INH/RIF	Twice weekly for 36 doses (18 wk)
			1c	INH/RPT	Once weekly for 18 doses (18 wk)
2	INH RIF PZA EMB	Seven days per week for 14 doses (2 wk), then twice weekly for 12 doses (6 wk) or 5 d/wk for 10 doses (2 wk), then twice weekly for 12 doses (6 wk)	2a	INH/RIF	Twice weekly for 36 doses (18 wk)
			2b	INH/RPT	Once weekly for 18 doses (18 wk)

Regimen	Drugs	Interval and doses, minimal duration	Regimen	Drugs	Interval and doses, minimal duration
3	INH RIF PZA EMB	Three times weekly for 24 doses (8 wk)	3a	INH/RIF	Three times weekly for 54 doses (18 wk)
4	INH RIF EMB	Seven days per week for 56 doses (8 wk) or 5 d/wk for 40 doses (8 wk)	4a	INH/RIF	Seven days per week for 217 doses (31 wk) or 5 d/wk for 155 doses (31 wk)
			4b	INH/RIF	Twice weekly for 62 doses (31 wk)

Treatment of latent tuberculosis infection				
Drugs	Duration (mo)	Interval	HIV-	HIV+
Isoniazid	9	Daily	preferred	preferred
		Twice weekly	acceptable alternative	acceptable alternative
Isoniazid	6	Daily	acceptable alternative	offer when others cannot be given
		Twice weekly	acceptable alternative	offer when others cannot be given
Rifampin-pyrazinamide	2	Daily	acceptable alternative	preferred
	2-3	Twice weekly	offer when others cannot be given	offer when others cannot be given
Rifampin	4	Daily	acceptable alternative	acceptable alternative

Treatment of Active Tuberculosis: First-Line Medications				
Drug	Daily dosing	Twice-weekly dosing	Thrice-weekly dosing	Adverse reactions
Isoniazid (INH)	Children: 10 mg per kg PO or IM Adults: 300 mg PO or IM Max: 300 mg Children: 20-40 mg/kg PO/IM	Adults: 15 mg per kg PO or IM Maximum: 300 mg Children: 20 to 40 mg per kg PO or IM	Adults: 15 mg per kg PO or IM Maximum: 300 mg	Elevation of hepatic enzyme levels, hepatitis, neuropathy, central nervous system effects
Rifampin (Rifadin)	Children: 10 to 20 mg per kg PO or IV Adults: 10 mg per kg PO or IV Maximum: 600 mg Children: 10 to 20 mg per kg PO or IV	Adults: 10 mg per kg PO or IV Maximum: 600 mg Children: 10 to 20 mg per kg PO or IV	Adults: 10 mg per kg PO or IV Maximum: 600 mg	Orange discoloration of secretions and urine, gastrointestinal tract upset, hepatitis, bleeding problems, flu-like symptoms, drug interactions, rash
Pyrazinamide	Children: 20 to 30 mg per kg PO Adults: 25 mg per kg PO	Maximum: 2 g Children: 50 to 70 mg per kg PO Adults: 50 to 70 mg per kg PO	Maximum: 4 g Children: 50 to 70 mg per kg PO Adults: 50 to 70 mg per kg PO Maximum: 3 g	Gastrointestinal tract upset, hepatitis, hyperuricemia, arthralgias
Ethambutol (Myambutol)	Children and adults: 15 to 25 mg per kg PO	Children and adults: 50 mg per kg PO	Children and adults: 25 to 30 mg per kg PO	Optic neuritis

VI. Monitoring

    A. Baseline and follow-up studies. Patients receiving combination antituberculous therapy with first-line drugs should undergo baseline measurement of hepatic enzymes (AST, bilirubin, alkaline phosphatase), platelet count, serum creatinine, and hepatitis B serology prior to the initiation of therapy. Testing of visual acuity and red-green color discrimination should be obtained when treatment includes EMB.

    B. Repeated monthly measurements should be obtained in the following settings:

        1. The baseline results are abnormal
        2. A drug reaction is suspected
        3. HIV infection
        4. Liver disease (eg, hepatitis B or C, alcohol abuse)
        5. Women who are pregnant or in the first three months postpartum
        6. Patients receiving combination therapy with pyrazinamide

    C. Response to treatment. The overall treatment success rate for tuberculosis worldwide is 82 percent.

    D. AFB smears. Patients being treated for pulmonary tuberculosis should submit a sputum specimen for microscopic examination and culture at a minimum of monthly intervals until two consecutive specimens are negative on culture.

References, see page 372.

Tonsillopharyngitis

In about a quarter of patients with a sore throat, the disorder is caused by group A beta-hemolytic streptococcus. Treatment of streptococcal tonsillopharyngitis reduces the occurrence of subsequent rheumatic fever, an inflammatory disease that affects the joints and heart, skin, central nervous system, and subcutaneous tissues.

I. **Prevalence of pharyngitis**
   A. Group A beta-hemolytic streptococcus (GABHS) typically occurs in patients 5-11 years of age, and it is uncommon in children under 3 years old. Most cases of GABHS occur in late winter and early spring.
   B. **Etiologic causes of sore throat**
      1. **Viral.** Rhinoviruses, influenza, Epstein-Barr virus
      2. **Bacterial.** GABHS (Streptococcus pyogenes), Streptococcus pneumoniae, Haemophilus influenzae, Moraxella catarrhalis, Staphylococcus aureus, anaerobes, Mycoplasma pneumoniae, Candida albicans.
   C. In patients who present with pharyngitis, the major goal is to detect GABHS infection because rheumatic fever may result. Severe GABHS infections may also cause a toxic-shock-like illness (toxic strep syndrome), bacteremia, streptococcal deep tissue infections (necrotizing fascitis), and streptococcal cellulitis.

II. **Clinical evaluation of sore throat**
   A. GABHS infection is characterized by sudden onset of sore throat, fever and tender swollen anterior cervical lymph nodes, typically in a child 5-11 years of age. Headache, nausea and vomiting may occur.
   B. Cough, rhinorrhea and hoarseness are generally absent.

III. **Physical examination**
   A. Streptococcal infection is suggested by erythema and swelling of the pharynx, enlarged and erythematous tonsils, tonsillar exudate, or palatal petechiae. The clinical diagnosis of GABHS infection is correct in only 50-75% of cases when based on clinical criteria alone.
   B. Unilateral inflammation and swelling of the pharynx suggests peritonsillar abscess. Distortion of the posterior pharyngeal wall suggests a retropharyngeal abscess. Corynebacterium diphtheriae is indicated by a dull membrane which bleeds on manipulation. Viral infections may cause oral vesicular eruptions.
   C. The tympanic membranes should be examined for erythema or a middle ear effusion.
   D. The lungs should be auscultated because viral infection occasionally causes pneumonia.

IV. **Diagnostic testing**
   A. Rapid streptococcal testing has a specificity of 90% and a sensitivity of 80%. A dry swab should be used to sample both the posterior wall and the tonsillar fossae, especially erythematous or exudative areas.
   B. **Throat culture** is the most accurate test available for the diagnosis of GABHS pharyngitis.
   C. **Clinical predictors.** Physicians are not able to reliably predict which patients will have a positive throat culture for GAS; sensitivity and specificity estimates range from 55 to 74 and 58 to 76 percent, respectively. The Centor criteria include:
      1. Tonsillar exudates.
      2. Tender anterior cervical adenopathy.
      3. Fever by history.

    4. Absence of cough.

    5. If three or four of these criteria are met, the positive predictive value are 40 to 60 percent. However, the absence of three or four of the criteria has a fairly high negative predictive value of 80 percent.

D. Diagnostic tests

    1. Throat cultures are the "gold standard" for diagnosing GAS pharyngitis. However, cultures take 24 to 48 hours to grow and thus cannot be used to decide which patients merit antibiotic therapy. Throat culture has a 90 percent and specificity of 95 to 99 percent.

    2. Rapid Antigen Test (RAT) uses enzyme or acid extraction of antigen from throat swabs. The diagnostic accuracy shows a sensitivity of 80 to 90 percent and specificity of 90 to 100 percent.

E. Reasons to treat a streptococcal pharyngitis with antibiotics:

    1. To prevent rheumatic fever — treatment works, but this complication has nearly disappeared in North America.

    2. To prevent peritonsillar abscess — again a vanishing complication.

    3. To reduce symptoms, there is a modest (approximately one day) reduction in symptoms with early treatment.

    4. To prevent transmission — this is important in pediatrics due to extensive exposures.

V. Recommendations: Using the Centor criteria and the rapid antigen test (RAT):

    A. Empirically treat patients who have all four clinical criteria (fever, tonsillar exudate, tender anterior cervical adenopathy, and absence of cough).

    B. Do not treat with antibiotics or perform diagnostic tests on patients with zero or one criterion.

    C. Perform RAT on those with two or three criteria and use antibiotic treatment only for patients with positive RAT results.

    D. Another approach is to treat empirically those adults with three or four of the clinical criteria.

VI. Antibiotic therapy

    A. Starting antibiotic therapy within the first 24-48 hours of illness decreases the duration of sore throat, fever and adenopathy by 12-24 hours. Treatment also minimizes risk of transmission and of rheumatic fever.

    B. Penicillin VK is the antibiotic of choice for GABHS; 250 mg PO qid or 500 mg PO bid x 10 days [250, 500 mg]. A 10-day regimen is recommended. Penicillin G benzathine (Bicillin LA) may be used as one-time therapy when compliance is a concern; 1.2 million units IM x 1 dose.

    C. Azithromycin (Zithromax) offers the advantage of once-a-day dosing for just 5 days; 500 mg x 1, then 250 mg qd x 4 days [6 pack].

    D. Clarithromycin (Biaxin), 500 mg PO bid; bacteriologic efficacy is similar to that of penicillin VK, and it may be taken twice a day.

    E. Erythromycin is also effective; 250 mg PO qid; or enteric coated delayed release tablet (PCE) 333 mg PO tid or 500 mg PO bid [250, 333, 500 mg]. **Erythromycin ethyl succinate (EES)** 400 PO qid or 800 mg PO bid [400 mg]. Gastrointestinal upset is common.

VII. Treatment of recurrent GABHS pharyngitis

    A. When patient compliance is an issue, an injection of penicillin G benzathine may be appropriate. When patient compliance is not an issue, therapy should be changed to a broader spectrum agent.

        1. Cephalexin (Keflex) 250-500 mg tid x 5 days [250, 500 mg]

        2. Cefadroxil (Duricef) 500 mg bid x 5 days [500 mg]

        3. Loracarbef (Lorabid) 200-400 mg bid x 5 days [200, 400 mg]

        4. Cefixime (Suprax) 400 mg qd x 5 days [200, 400 mg]

        5. Ceftibuten (Cedax) 400 mg qd x 5 days [400 mg]

        6. Cefuroxime axetil (Ceftin) 250-500 mg bid x 5 days [125, 250, 500 mg]

    B. Amoxicillin-clavulanate (Augmentin) has demonstrated superior results in comparison with penicillin; 250-500 mg tid or 875 mg bid [250, 500, 875 mg].
    C. Sulfonamides, trimethoprim, and the tetracyclines are not effective for the treatment of GABHS pharyngitis.
References, see page 372.

Acute Sinusitis and Rhinosinusitis

Acute sinusitis is caused by infection of one or more of the paranasal sinuses. Viral infection is the most frequent causes of acute sinusitis. Only two percent of viral rhinosinusitis is complicated by acute bacterial sinusitis. Uncomplicated viral rhinosinusitis usually resolves in seven to ten days. Complications of untreated acute bacterial sinusitis include intracranial and orbital complications, and chronic sinus disease.

I. Microbial etiology
    A. Viral. Rhinovirus, parainfluenza, and influenza viruses have all been recovered from sinus aspirates of patients with colds and influenza-like illnesses.
    B. Bacterial. Bacterial sinusitis can be divided into community-acquired and nosocomial infections.
    C. Community-acquired bacterial sinusitis is usually a complication of viral rhinosinusitis, occurring in 0.5 to 2 percent of cases. Other risk factors include nasal allergy, swimming, intranasal cocaine use, problems with mucociliary clearance (eg, cystic fibrosis, cilial dysfunction), and immunodeficiency states (eg, HIV). Patients with nasal obstruction due to polyps, foreign bodies or tumors are also at risk.
    D. The most common bacterial organisms are Streptococcus pneumoniae and Haemophilus influenzae. S. pneumoniae and H. influenzae are each responsible for 35 percent of cases in adults.

II. Clinical manifestations
    A. Symptoms of acute sinusitis include nasal congestion, purulent nasal discharge, maxillary tooth discomfort, hyposmia, and facial pain or pressure that is worse when bending forward. Headache, fever (nonacute), halitosis, fatigue, cough, ear pain, and ear fullness are symptoms of rhinosinusitis.

Microbial causes of acute sinusitis
Viral
Rhinovirus Parainfluenza virus Influenza virus Coronavirus Respiratory syncytial virus Adenovirus
Bacterial
Community-acquired Streptococcus pneumoniae Haemophilus influenzae Moraxella catarrhalis Other streptococcal species Staphylococcus aureus Anaerobic bacteria

Nosocomial
Staphylococcus aureus
Streptococcal species
Pseudomonas species
Escherichia coli
Klebsiella species
Other Gram negative bacteria
Anaerobic bacteria
Candida species
Fungal
Aspergillus species
Pseudallescheria boydii
Sporothrix schenckii
Homobasidiomycetes
Phaeohyphomycosis
Zygomycetes

    B. Diagnosis. Since rhinoviral infection typically improves in seven to ten days, a patient with a cold or influenza-like illness that has persisted without improvement or has worsened over seven to ten days may have developed bacterial sinusitis. The presence of nasal discharge, particularly if purulent, and/or maxillary pain or tenderness in the face or teeth, particularly if unilateral, is suggestive of acute bacterial sinusitis. Fever with facial pain, swelling, and erythema may develop.

    C. Patients with acute bacterial sinusitis may give a history of tooth pain, foul odor to the breath, and other signs of dental infection.

    D. Sinus aspirate culture is the gold standard for making a microbial diagnosis in sinus infection. However, this procedure is not appropriate for use in routine medical practice. Sinus aspirate culture should be considered if there is a suspicion of intracranial extension of the infection or other serious complications.

    E. Radiologic tests. Imaging studies are not indicated in the usual case of acute community-acquired sinusitis, unless intracranial or orbital complications are suspected. CT scanning is the imaging procedure of choice as it provides better sensitivity than plain x-ray. However, neither test can distinguish viral from bacterial infection. One limitation of CT scanning is that it is frequently abnormal in patients with the common cold.

        1. Magnetic resonance imaging (MRI) can be used to demonstrate intracranial spread of infection but is not as good as CT scanning for the diagnosis of acute sinusitis.

        2. Plain films of the sinuses are not recommended. If imaging is performed, CT is the usual test of choice.

III. Treatment of acute bacterial sinusitis

    A. Treatment for acute bacterial sinusitis should be considered in patients with persistent symptoms after seven to ten days and at least one of the following:

        1. Maxillary pain or tenderness/pressure in the face or teeth

        2. Purulent nasal discharge

        3. Postnasal discharge

        4. Cough

    B. Viral rhinosinusitis

        1. Used in combination, chlorpheniramine (12 mg sustained release) and ibuprofen (400 mg) are effective in reducing nasal mucus and the severity of sneezing, rhinorrhea, sore throat, cough, malaise, and headache.

C. Community-acquired bacterial sinusitis

1. **Choice of antibiotics**. The development of beta-lactamase production by H. influenzae and M. catarrhalis and of multiple antibiotic resistance by S. pneumoniae has limited the selection of antimicrobials that provide adequate coverage of these common bacteria in community-acquired sinusitis. Cephalexin and the macrolides generally either do not provide the necessary antibacterial spectrum or are associated with too much resistance among pneumococci.

2. **Amoxicillin** is recommended at the higher end of the dose range (eg, 1 g three times per day). Contact in children with daycare centers or recent antibiotic use warrents broader spectrum antibiotics.

3. Antibiotics that cover resistant S. pneumoniae, H. influenzae, and M. catarrhalis: amoxicillin-clavulanate (Augmentin, 875-125 mg every 12 hours) for 7 to 10 days, cefpodoxime (Vantin, 200 mg every 12 hours), cefdinir (Omnicef, 600 mg once daily), levofloxacin (Levaquin, 500 mg once daily) or moxifloxacin (Avelox, 400 mg once daily).

Antibiotics for acute community-acquired bacterial sinusitis	
Drug	**Dose**
Amoxicillin-clavulanate (Augmentin)	875/125 mg q12h
Cefpodoxime proxetil (Vantin)	200 mg q12h
Cefdinir (Omnicef)	600 mg qd
Levofloxacin (Levaquin)	500 mg qd
Moxifloxacin (Avelox)	400 mg qd

4. A seven to ten day course of antimicrobial treatment is recommended. This duration of therapy can be expected to provide a 90 percent or better bacterial eradication rate in cases of acute community-acquired sinusitis.

5. **Treatment failure.** One alternative is to give a second, more prolonged course of treatment with another antibiotic (particularly if a narrow spectrum antibiotic was used as first-line therapy). Another approach is to obtain a sinus CT scan and refer the patient to an otolaryngologist for sinus aspirate culture and sinus washing, followed by another course of antibiotics.

6. **Sinus surgery** should be strongly considered in patients with CT-confirmed sinus disease persisting over several months despite adequate medical management. Endoscopic sinus surgery is successful in 85 percent of cases.

7. **Nosocomial bacterial sinusitis**. Treatment should be based upon sinus aspirate culture and sensitivity data when available. If such information is not available, antimicrobial coverage should be directed at S. aureus and the Gram negative bacteria which commonly infect the respiratory tract.

8. **Complications of acute bacterial sinusitis**, which now rarely occur, include meningitis, orbital cellulitis, and osteitis of the sinus bones.

References, see page 372.

Conjunctivitis

Conjunctivitis is the most likely diagnosis in a patient with a red eye and discharge. Most infectious conjunctivitis is viral in adults and children.

I. Etiology and clinical manifestations

A. Acute conjunctivitis can be classified as infectious or noninfectious and further divided into four main types:

1. **Infectious:** Bacterial or viral
2. **Noninfectious:** Allergic nonallergic

Differential Diagnosis of Red Eye	
Conjunctivitis 　**Infectious** 　　Viral 　　Bacterial (eg, staphylococcus, 　　Chlamydia) 　**Noninfectious** 　　Allergic conjunctivitis 　　Dry eye 　　Toxic or chemical reaction 　　Contact lens use 　　Foreign body 　　Factitious conjunctivitis	**Keratitis** 　**Infectious.** Bacterial, viral, fungal 　**Noninfectious.** Recurrent epithelial erosion, foreign body **Uveitis** **Episcleritis/scleritis** **Acute glaucoma** **Eyelid abnormalities** **Orbital disorders** 　Preseptal and orbital cellulitis 　Idiopathic orbital inflammation (pseudotumor)

B. **Bacterial conjunctivitis** is commonly caused by Staphylococcus aureus, Streptococcus pneumoniae, Haemophilus influenzae, and Moraxella catarrhalis.

1. Bacterial conjunctivitis is highly contagious; it is spread by direct contact with the patient and his secretions or with contaminated objects.
2. Bacterial conjunctivitis usually causes unilateral redness and discharge. Similar to viral and allergic conjunctivitis, the affected eye often is "stuck shut" in the morning. The purulent discharge continues throughout the day. The discharge is thick and globular; it may be yellow, white, or green. The appearance differs from that of viral or allergic conjunctivitis, which presents with a mostly watery discharge during the day, with a scanty, stringy component that is mucus rather than pus.

C. **Hyperacute bacterial conjunctivitis**

1. N. gonorrhoeae can cause a hyperacute bacterial conjunctivitis that is severe and sight-threatening, requiring immediate ophthalmologic referral. Concurrent urethritis is typically present.
2. The eye infection is characterized by a profuse purulent discharge. Other symptoms include redness, irritation, and tenderness to palpation. There is typically marked chemosis, lid swelling, and tender preauricular adenopathy. Gram negative diplococci can be identified on Gram stain of the discharge. These patients require hospitalization for systemic and topical therapy.

D. **Viral conjunctivitis** is typically caused by adenovirus. The conjunctivitis may be followed by adenopathy, fever, pharyngitis, and upper respiratory tract infection. Viral conjunctivitis is highly contagious; it is spread by direct contact with the patient and his or her secretions or with contaminated objects and surfaces.

1. Viral conjunctivitis presents as injection, watery or mucoserous discharge, and a burning, sandy, or gritty feeling in one eye. Patients may have morning crusting followed by watery discharge with some scanty mucus throughout the day. The second eye usually becomes involved within 24 to 48 hours.
2. On examination there typically is only mucoid discharge on the lower lid in the corner of the eye. Usually there is profuse tearing rather than dis-

charge. The tarsal conjunctiva may have a follicular or "bumpy" appearance. An enlarged and tender preauricular node may be present.

3. Viral conjunctivitis is a self-limited process. The symptoms frequently get worse for the first three to five days, with very gradual resolution over the following one to two weeks.

E. Allergic conjunctivitis is caused by airborne allergens, which cause local mast cell degranulation and the release of histamine.

1. It typically presents as bilateral redness, watery discharge, and itching. Itching is the cardinal symptom of allergy, distinguishing it from a viral etiology, which is more typically described as grittiness, burning, or irritation. Eye rubbing can worsen symptoms. Patients with allergic conjunctivitis often have a history of atopy, seasonal allergy, or specific allergy (eg, to cats).

2. Similar to viral conjunctivitis, allergic conjunctivitis causes diffuse injection with a follicular appearance to the tarsal conjunctiva and profuse watery or mucoserous discharge. There may be morning crusting. It is the complaint of itching and the history of allergy or hay fever and a recent exposure allows the distinction between allergic and viral conjunctivitis; the clinical findings are the same.

II. Diagnosis

A. Conjunctivitis is a diagnosis of exclusion. Conjunctivitis causes red eye and discharge; however, the vision is normal and there is no evidence of keratitis, iritis, or glaucoma.

B. Patients with all types of conjunctivitis complain of morning crusting and daytime redness and discharge. On examination, there should be no focal pathology in the lids such as hordeolum (stye), cancerous mound or ulceration, or blepharitis (diffuse eyelid margin thickening and hyperemia with lash crusts). The redness or injection should be diffuse. Foreign body, pterygium, or episcleritis should be considered if the conjunctival injection is localized rather than diffuse.

C. Cultures are not necessary for the initial diagnosis and therapy of conjunctivitis.

D. **Red flags** for more serious problems that should prompt evaluation by an ophthalmologist:

1. Reduction of visual acuity

2. **Ciliary flush:** A pattern of injection in which the redness is most pronounced in a ring at the limbus (the limbus is the transition zone between the cornea and the sclera).

3. Photophobia.

4. Severe foreign body sensation that prevents the patient from keeping the eye open.

5. Corneal opacity.

6. Fixed pupil.

7. Severe headache with nausea.

III. Therapy. Bacterial conjunctivitis is likely to be self-limited, although treatment shortens the clinical course and reduces person-to-person spread.

A. **Bacterial conjunctivitis** is treated with erythromycin ophthalmic ointment (Ilotycin and generic), or sulfa ophthalmic drops (Sulf-10, Bleph-10, Sulamyd, or as a 10% generic solution). The dose is 1/2" (1.25 cm) of ointment deposited inside the lower lid or 1 to 2 drops instilled four times daily for five to seven days. The dose may be reduced from four times daily to twice daily, if there is improvement in symptoms after three days.

1. Ointment is preferred over drops for children, drops are preferable for adults because ointments blur vision for 20 minutes after the dose is administered.

2. Alternative therapies include bacitracin ointment, sulfacetamide ointment, polymyxin-bacitracin ointment (Polysporin), or fluoroquinolone drops (Ciloxan, Ocuflox, Quixin, Zymar, Vigamox). Aminoglycosides are poor choices since they are toxic to the corneal epithelium and can cause a reactive keratoconjunctivitis.

3. The fluoroquinolones are effective and well tolerated; they are the treatment of choice for corneal ulcers and are extremely effective against pseudomonas. Conjunctivitis in a contact lens wearer should be treated with a fluoroquinolone because of the high incidence of pseudomonas infection.

4. Contact lens wearers with a red eye should discontinue contact lens wear. Contact lens wear can resume when the eye is white and has no discharge for 24 hours after the completion of antibiotic therapy. The lens case should be discarded and the lenses subjected to overnight disinfection or replaced if disposable.

B. **Viral conjunctivitis.** Some patients derive symptomatic relief from topical antihistamine/decongestants. These are available over the counter (Naphcon-A, OcuHist, generics). Warm or cool compresses may provide additional symptomatic relief.

C. **Allergic conjunctivitis.** There are numerous therapies available for allergic conjunctivitis (see below).

References, see page 372.

Allergic Conjunctivitis

Allergic conjunctivitis is estimated to affect 20 percent of the population on an annual basis. Allergic conjunctivitis is associated with itching, tearing, redness, burning, photophobia, and mucus discharge.

I. **Pathophysiology**
   A. Allergic conjunctivitis has an average age of onset of 20 years of age, and is principally a disease of young adults. Symptoms tend to decrease with age.
   B. **Acute allergic conjunctivitis** is an acute, hypersensitivity reaction caused by environmental exposure to allergens. It is characterized by intense episodes of itching, hyperemia, tearing, chemosis, and eyelid edema. It resolves in less than 24 hours.
   C. **Seasonal allergic conjunctivitis** (SAC) is also known as allergic conjunctivitis. It is frequently associated with rhinitis. It occurs in the spring and late summer, and it is caused by exposure to pollen, grasses, and ragweed.
   D. **Perennial allergic conjunctivitis** (PAC) is a mild, chronic, allergic conjunctivitis related to environmental exposure to year-round allergens such as dust mites and mold.
   E. Acute allergic conjunctivitis, seasonal allergic conjunctivitis (SAC), and perennial allergic conjunctivitis (PAC) are referred to as "allergic conjunctivitis," and result from allergens.

II. **Clinical evaluation**
   A. Allergic conjunctivitis is frequently associated with atopy, allergic rhinitis, skin allergies, and asthma.
   B. **Signs and symptoms of allergic conjunctivitis** include itching, tearing, conjunctival edema, hyperemia, eyelid edema, watery discharge, burning, and photophobia. Symptoms are usually bilateral. The differential diagnosis includes infectious conjunctivitis, blepharitis, and dry eye.
   C. Acute allergic conjunctivitis occurs rapidly upon exposure to an allergen, such as cat dander. Symptoms can be severe and debilitating but resolve quickly,

usually within 24 hours of removal of the allergen. Seasonal allergic conjunctivitis typically has a less dramatic onset; it will have a more predictable and chronic course that corresponds to the ragweed (late summer and early fall), grass (summer), and pollen (spring) seasons.

D. Laboratory findings. The diagnosis of allergic conjunctivitis is usually made clinically; therefore, laboratory testing is not typically performed.

III. Treatment of allergic conjunctivitis

A. Avoidance of the allergen is recommended. Preventive steps to reduce symptoms of SAC include limiting outdoor exposure during high "counts" of pollen and ragweed, use of air conditioning, and keeping windows closed. For those with PAC, prevention includes replacement of old pillows and mattresses, covers for pillows and mattresses, frequent washing of beddings, reducing humidity, and frequent vacuuming and dusting. Old curtains or drapes should be removed. When the allergen is animal dander, the animal may need to be removed from the home.

B. In all types of allergic conjunctivitis, patients should not rub their eyes because that can cause mast cell degranulation. Patients should use topical antihistamines, frequent artificial tears, and cool compresses.

C. Mast cell stabilizers

1. Mast cell stabilizers include Crolom (cromolyn 4.0 percent), Opticrom (cromolyn), and Alomide (lodoxamide). These drugs are particularly useful for allergic conjunctivitis. Dosing is four times per day. Since the onset of action is 5 to 14 days after therapy has been initiated, these medicines are not useful for acute conjunctivitis. These drops cause burning and stinging.

2. These drugs are well tolerated, non-toxic, and can be used in contact lens wearers. However disadvantages include delayed onset of action, maintenance therapy, and multiple daily dosing.

D. Antihistamines

1. **Oral antihistamines** and combinations of antihistamines plus decongestants include Allegra (fexofenadine, 60 mg bid or tab ER: 180 mg qd), Allegra D (fexofenadine plus pseudoephedrine, 1 tab bid), Claritin (loratadine, 10 mg qd), Claritin-D (loratadine plus pseudoephedrine, 1 tab qd), and Zyrtec (cetirizine, 5-10 mg qd) or Zyrtec-D (cetirizine plus pseudoephedrine, 1 tab bid).

2. The full effect of oral administration of antihistamines occurs hours after initiating therapy. Since oral antihistamine use is associated with drying of mucosal membranes, the use of oral antihistamines may worsen allergic symptoms. This effect is not observed with topical antihistamines.

3. **Topical antihistamines** include Emadine (emedastine) and Livostin (levocabastine), which are used as one drop up to 4 times daily. The advantages of topical antihistamine usage include a more rapid onset of action and reduced drowsiness and dry eyes. Emadine and Livostin are topical, highly specific, H1-receptor antagonists, and their onset of action is within minutes.

4. **Topical, antihistamine/vasoconstrictor combinations** have been shown to be effective. Examples of such combination drugs include Naphcon-A (naphazoline/pheniramine), Vasocon-A (naphazoline/pheniramine), OcuHist (naphazoline/pheniramine), and Opcon-A (naphazoline/pheniramine). Dosing is up to four times daily. However, chronic use can lead to rebound hyperemia.

5. **Olopatadine (Patanol)** is a combination antihistamine and mast cell stabilizer. It is the most commonly prescribed drug for allergic conjunctivitis. The H1-receptor selectivity is superior to that of other antihistamines. Patanol is very safe and effective. Side effects include stinging and headache. Dosing is two to four times daily of the 0.1% drops.

E. Corticosteroids

1. Topical corticosteroid use should only be used for short "pulse therapy" when antihistamines and mast cell stabilizers provide inadequate therapy. Side effects from corticosteroids include cataract formation, elevated intraocular pressure (IOP), glaucoma, and secondary infections. Ocular steroids should only be administered by ophthalmologists.

2. Prednisolone and dexamethasone have the greatest risk of raising IOP. "Soft" steroids are a group of topical corticosteroids that have a greatly reduced risk of causing increased IOP, since they undergo rapid inactivation upon penetration of the cornea. These drugs include Pred Mild (prednisolone), FML (fluorometholone), HMS (medrysone), Lotemax (loteprednol), and Vexol (rimexolone). They are administered two to four times per day for two weeks.

F. Treatment recommendations

1. **Acute allergic conjunctivitis**

   a. Topical antihistamine/vasoconstrictors are usually sufficient in treating short exacerbations of symptoms. Combination drugs include Naphcon-A (naphazoline/pheniramine), Vasocon-A (naphazoline/pheniramine), OcuHist (naphazoline/pheniramine), and Opcon-A (naphazoline/pheniramine). Dosing is up to four times daily. Chronic use (greater than two weeks) can lead to rebound hyperemia.

   b. For frequent attacks of acute allergic conjunctivitis (occurring more than two days per month), mast cell stabilizers can be added. Olopatadine (Patanol), a combination drug consisting of an antihistamine and mast cell stabilizer, is a good agent for treating more frequent attacks. It can be used up to four times per day.

   c. If these are ineffective, oral antihistamines may be helpful. Oral antihistamines and combinations of antihistamines plus decongestants include Allegra (fexofenadine, 60 mg bid or tab ER: 180 mg qd), Allegra D (fexofenadine plus pseudoephedrine, 1 tab bid), Claritin (loratadine, 10 mg qd), Claritin-D (loratadine plus pseudoephedrine, 1 tab qd), and Zyrtec (cetirizine, 5-10 mg qd) or Zyrtec-D (cetirizine plus pseudoephedrine, 1 tab bid). Frequent use of artificial tears is recommended while using oral antihistamines.

2. **Seasonal allergic conjunctivitis and perennial allergic conjunctivitis**

   a. **Olopatadine (Patanol)** should be initiated two weeks before the onset of symptoms is anticipated. Patanol, a combination mast cell stabilizer and antihistamine, has become the first-line drug of choice in treating SAC and PAC. It is approved for children older than five years of age and adults. Dosing is two to four times daily.

   b. Oral antihistamines may be helpful; however, these agents cause decreased tear production. These patients are frequently using oral antihistamines for systemic symptoms; therefore, artificial tears should be used.

   c. A short two-week course of topical steroids can be helpful in resistant cases. Pred Mild (prednisolone), FML (fluorometholone), HMS (medrysone), Lotemax (loteprednol), or Vexol (rimexolone) are administered two to four times per day for two to three weeks.

References, see page 372.

Bacterial Meningitis

Meningitis is an infection of the meninges and the cerebrospinal fluid (CSF) of the subarachnoid space and the cerebral ventricles. Meningitis is one of the ten most common infectious causes of death. Neurologic sequelae are common among survivors.

I. Epidemiology

A. Causative organisms in adults

1. Up to age 60, S. pneumoniae is responsible for 60 percent of cases, followed by N. meningitidis (20 percent), H. influenzae (10 percent), L. monocytogenes (6 percent), and group B streptococcus (4 percent).

2. Age 60 and above, almost 70 percent of cases are caused by S. pneumoniae, 20 percent to L. monocytogenes, and 3 to 4 percent each to N. meningitidis, group B streptococcus, and H. influenzae. An increased prevalence of L. monocytogenes occurs in the elderly.

B. Predisposing factors. Major mechanisms for developing meningitis:

1. Colonization of the nasopharynx with subsequent bloodstream invasion and subsequent central nervous system (CNS) invasion

2. Invasion of the CNS following bacteremia due to a localized source, such as infective endocarditis or a urinary tract infection

3. Direct entry of organisms into the CNS from a contiguous infection (eg, sinuses, mastoid), trauma, neurosurgery, or medical devices (eg, shunts or intracerebral pressure monitors).

C. Host factors that can predispose to meningitis include asplenia, complement deficiency, corticosteroid excess, and HIV infection. Other predisposing factors for meningitis include:

1. Recent exposure to someone with meningitis

2. A recent infection (especially respiratory or otic infection)

3. Recent travel, particularly to areas with endemic meningococcal disease such as sub-Saharan Africa

4. Injection drug use

5. Recent head trauma

6. Otorrhea or rhinorrhea

II. Clinical features. Patients with bacterial meningitis appear ill and often present soon after symptom onset.

A. Presenting manifestations. The classic triad of acute bacterial meningitis consists of fever, nuchal rigidity, and a change in mental status, although many patients do not have all three features. Most patients have high fevers, often greater than 38°C, but a small percentage have hypothermia.

B. Headache is also common. The headache is severe and generalized. It is not easily confused with normal headaches.

C. Fever is present in 95 percent at presentation and developed in another 4 percent within the first 24 hours.

D. Nuchal rigidity is present in 88 percent.

E. Mental status is altered in 78 percent. Most were confused or lethargic, but 22 percent are responsive only to pain and 6 percent are unresponsive to all stimuli.

F. Significant photophobia is common.

G. Neurologic complications such as seizures, focal neurologic deficits (including cranial nerve palsies), and papilledema, may be present early or occur later in the course. Seizures occur in 15 to 30 percent and focal neurologic deficits in 20 to 30 percent. Hearing loss is a late complication. Dexamethasone therapy may reduce the rate of neurologic sequelae.

H. N. meningitidis can cause petechiae and palpable purpura.

I. Examination for nuchal rigidity. Passive or active flexion of the neck will usually result in an inability to touch the chin to the chest.

1. Brudzinski sign refers to spontaneous flexion of the hips during flexion of the neck.

2. The Kernig sign refers to the inability or reluctance to allow full extension of the knee when the hip is flexed 90°.
3. The sensitivity of meningeal signs is extremely low (5 percent for each sign and 30 percent for nuchal rigidity); the specificity was 95 percent for each sign and 68 percent for nuchal rigidity.

J. **Initial blood tests** should include a complete blood count with differential and platelet count, and two sets of blood cultures. Most often the white blood cell count is elevated with a shift toward immature forms. Severe infection can be associated with leukopenia.

K. **Blood cultures** are often positive. Approximately 50 to 75 percent of patients with bacterial meningitis have positive blood cultures. Cultures obtained after antimicrobial therapy are much less likely to be positive.

L. **Lumbar puncture.** Every patient with suspected meningitis should have CSF obtained unless contraindicated. Risk factors for an occult mass lesion on CT scan include the presence of impaired cellular immunity, history of previous central nervous system disease, a seizure within the previous week, reduced level of consciousness, and focal motor or cranial abnormalities. A CT scan is recommended before an LP only in patients with suspected bacterial meningitis who have one or more risk factors for a mass lesion.

1. **Opening pressure** is typically elevated in patients with bacterial meningitis. The mean opening pressure is 350 mm H_2O (normal up to 200 mm H_2O).
2. **CSF analysis.** When the clinical diagnosis strongly suggests meningitis, CSF cell count and differential, glucose and protein concentration Gram stain, culture, and analysis can distinguish between bacterial and viral infection. A Gram stain should be obtained whenever there is suspicion of bacterial meningitis.
3. Characteristic findings in bacterial meningitis include a CSF glucose concentration below 45 mg/dL, a protein concentration above 500 mg/dL, and a white blood cell count above 1000/microL, usually composed primarily of neutrophils.
4. Gram positive diplococci suggest pneumococcal infection.
5. Gram negative diplococci suggest meningococcal infection.
6. Small pleomorphic Gram negative coccobacilli suggest Haemophilus influenzae.
7. Gram positive rods and coccobacilli suggest listerial infection.

III. **Treatment of bacterial meningitis in adults**

A. Antibiotic therapy should be initiated immediately after the results of lumbar puncture (LP) or immediately after LP alone if the clinical suspicion is high. A screening CT scan is not necessary in the majority of patients.

B. Risk factors for cerebral herniation include impaired cellular immunity, central nervous system disease, a seizure within the previous week, reduced consciousness, focal motor or cranial abnormalities, and papilledema. Should LP be delayed by the need for cranial imaging, blood cultures should be obtained and antibiotics should be administered empirically before the imaging study, followed by the LP.

C. **Empiric drug regimen.** Selected third-generation cephalosporins, such as cefotaxime and ceftriaxone, are the beta-lactams of choice in the empiric treatment of meningitis.

1. Cefotaxime and ceftriaxone are equivalent or superior to penicillin and ampicillin because of their consistent CSF penetration and their activity against the major pathogens of meningitis with one notable exception, some penicillin-resistant S. pneumoniae. Ceftazidime, another third-generation cephalosporin, is much less active against penicillin-resistant pneumococci than cefotaxime and ceftriaxone.

Utility of CSF Analysis in Infectious Causes of CNS Infection

	Glucose		Protein		Total WBC		
	<10 mg/dL	10-45 mg/dL	>500 mg/dL	50-500 mg/dL	>1000	100-1000	5-100
More common	Bacterial meningitis	Bacterial meningitis	Bacterial meningitis	Viral meningitis	Bacterial meningitis	Bacterial or viral meningitis	Early bacterial meningitis
				Lyme disease			Viral meningitis
				Meningeal syphilis			Meningeal syphilis
							TB meningitis
Less common	TB meningitis	Meningeal syphilis	TB meningitis		Some cases of mumps	Encephalitis (including West Nile virus)	Encephalitis (including Herpes simplex virus)

Common self-limited forms of viral meningitis usually have a CSF protein concentration below 100 mg/dL (1 g/L) and a total WBC less than 100/μL. In addition to the total WBC, the percent neutrophils also may be helpful: more than 50 percent suggests bacterial meningitis while a value below 10 percent is compatible with viral infection

Empiric antibiotic therapy in adults with suspected bacterial meningitis and a nondiagnostic CSF gram stain

Suggested antibiotics	Most likely pathogens
Immunocompetent adults	
Age 18 to 60 years Ceftriaxone (2 g twice daily) **OR**, less preferably, cefotaxime (2 g every four to six or six to eight hours) **AND** vancomycin (2 g/day in two to four divided doses) if cephalosporin-resistant pneumococci in community	S. Pneumoniae, N. Meningitis H. influenzae, and, much less often, L. monocytogenes and group B streptococci

Suggested antibiotics	Most likely pathogens
Age ≥60 years As above plus ampicillin (200 mg/kg per day in six divided doses)	S. Pneumoniae, L. monocytogenes, and, less often, group B streptococci, N. Meningitis, H. influenzae

Impaired cellular immunity
  Ceftazidime (2 g every eight hours)
  PLUS Ampicillin (2 g every four hours)
  AND vancomycin (2 g/day in two to four divided doses) if cephalosporin-resistant pneumococci in community
	L. Monocytogenes, gram negative bacilli

2. Intravenous antibiotics should be directed at the presumed pathogen if the Gram stain is diagnostic. Antibiotic therapy should then be modified once the CSF culture results are available.
   a. If Gram positive cocci are seen in community-acquired meningitis, S. pneumoniae should be the suspected pathogen. However, in the setting of neurosurgery or head trauma within the past month, a neurosurgical device, or a CSF leak, Staphylococcus aureus and coagulase negative staphylococci are more common and vancomycin is required.
   b. If Gram negative cocci are seen, N. meningitidis is the probable pathogen.
   c. Gram positive bacilli suggest Listeria.
   d. Gram negative bacilli usually represent Enterobacteriaceae (eg, Klebsiella, Escherichia coli) in cases of community-acquired meningitis.
   e. If there is a history of neurosurgery or head trauma within the past month, a neurosurgical device, or a CSF leak in patients with Gram negative rods, ceftriaxone should be replaced with ceftazidime since such patients are at greater risk for Pseudomonas and Acinetobacter infection.
D. **Adjuvant dexamethasone.** Permanent neurologic sequelae, such as hearing loss and focal neurologic deficits, are not uncommon in survivors of bacterial meningitis, particularly with pneumococcal meningitis. Intravenous dexamethasone (0.15 mg/kg every six hours) should be given shortly before or at the time of initiation of antibiotic therapy in adults with suspected bacterial meningitis who have a Glasgow coma score of 8 to 11. Dexamethasone should be continued for four days if the Gram stain or the CSF culture reveals S. pneumoniae. Dexamethasone should be discontinued if the Gram stain and/or culture reveal another pathogen or no meningitis.
E. **Choice of agent when pathogen is unknown**
   1. In adults up to age 60, S. pneumoniae was responsible for 60 percent of cases, followed by N. meningitidis (20 percent), H. influenzae (10 percent), L. monocytogenes (6 percent), and group B streptococcus (4 percent).
   2. In adults ≥60 years of age, almost 70 percent of cases are caused by S. pneumoniae, 20 percent to L. monocytogenes, and 3 to 4 percent each to N. meningitidis, group B streptococcus, and H. influenzae.
   3. **No known immune deficiency**
      a. Meningococcus, pneumococcus, and, less often, H. influenzae and group B streptococcus are the most likely causes of community-acquired bacterial meningitis in adolescents and adults up to the age of 60.
      b. Initiate IV ceftriaxone (2 g BID) or cefotaxime (2 g every six to eight hours). If cephalosporin resistance occurs in more than 3 percent S. pneumoniae isolates, vancomycin should be added (2 g/day intravenously in two to four divided doses if renal function is normal).

c. Beta-lactams should be continued even if in vitro tests suggest resistant organisms, since they will provide synergy with vancomycin.

d. Adults ≥60 years of age, in whom 20 percent of cases are due to listeria, should receive ampicillin (200 mg/kg per day IV in six divided doses).

Antibiotic recommendations for adults with suspected meningitis with a positive cerebrospinal fluid gram stain or culture	
Bacterial type	**Recommended antibiotic regimen**
Morphology on CSF Gram stain	
Gram positive cocci	Vancomycin (500 mg Q6h)‡ **PLUS** either ceftriaxone (2 g Q12h) or, less preferably, cefotaxime (2 g Q4-6h or Q6-8h)
Gram negative cocci	Penicillin G (4 million U Q4h) or, if H. Influenzae (which typically appears as small, pleomorphic rods) is suspected, ceftriaxone (2 g Q12h) or cefotaxime (2 g Q6-8h)
Gram positive bacilli	Ampicillin (2 g Q4h) **PLUS** gentamicin (1-2 mg/kg Q8h)
Gram negative bacilli	Ceftriaxone (2 g Q12h) or cefotaxime (2 g Q6-8h) **PLUS** gentamicin (1-2 mg/kg Q8h)
Growth in CSF culture	
S. pneumoniae	Vancomycin (500 mg Q6h)‡ **PLUS** either ceftriaxone (2 g Q12h) or, less preferably, cefotaxime (2 g Q4-6h or Q6-8h) for 14 days; vancomycin can be discontinued if the isolate is not cephalosporin-resistant
N. meningitis	Penicillin G (4 million units Q4h) for seven days
H. influenzae	Ceftriaxone (2 g Q12h) or cefotaxime (2 g Q6h) for seven days
L. Monocytogenes	Ampicillin (2 g Q4h) or penicillin G (3-4 million U Q4h) **PLUS** gentamicin (1-2 mg/kg Q8h); ampicillin is given for two to four weeks in immunocompetent patients and for at lease six to eight weeks in immunocompromised patients; gentamicin is gen until the patient improves (usually 10 to 14 days) or, in poor responders, for up to three weeks if there are no signs of nephrotoxicity and ototoxicity

Bacterial type	Recommended antibiotic regimen
Group B streptococci	Penicillin G (4 million U Q4h) for two to three weeks
Enterobacteriaceae	Ceftriaxone (2 g Q12h) or cefotaxime (2 g Q6h-8h) **PLUS** gentamicin (1-2 mg/kg Q8h) for three weeks
Pseudomonas or acinetobacter	ceftazidime (2 g Q8h) **PLUS** gentamicin (1-2 mg/kg Q8h) for 21 days

4. **Impaired cellular immunity** due to lymphoma, cytotoxic chemotherapy, or high-dose glucocorticoids requires coverage against L. monocytogenes and Gram negative bacilli as well as S. pneumoniae. Patients should receive ceftazidime (2 g every eight hours) and ampicillin (200 mg/kg per day IV in six divided doses). Vancomycin should be added (2 g/day intravenously in two to four divided doses if renal function is normal) if there is possible cephalosporin-resistant pneumococci.
5. **Nosocomial infection.** Empiric therapy must cover both Gram negative (K pneumoniae, P aeruginosa) and Gram positive nosocomial pathogens. Ceftazidime (2 g every eight hours) plus vancomycin (2 g/day intravenously in two to four divided doses if renal function is normal) is recommended.

F. **Prevention**
1. **Vaccines** are available for S. pneumoniae, N. meningitidis, and H. influenzae.
   a. **Pneumococcal vaccine** is administered to chronically ill and older adults (over age 65).
   b. **Meningococcal vaccine** is not warranted as postexposure prophylaxis unless the strain is documented to have a capsular serotype represented in the vaccine (type A, C, Y or W-135). Meningococcal vaccination is indicated for patients with asplenia and complement deficiencies.
   c. **H. influenzae vaccine.** A marked reduction in H. influenzae meningitis has been associated with the near universal use of a H. influenzae vaccine.
2. **Chemoprophylaxis**
   a. **Neisseria meningitidis.** Chemoprophylaxis of close contacts consists of rifampin (600 mg PO every 12 h for a total of four doses in adults), ciprofloxacin (500 mg PO once), and ceftriaxone (250 mg IM once).

Antimicrobial chemoprophylaxis regimens for meningococcal infection			
Drug	**Age group**	**Dose**	**Duration**
Rifampin (oral)	Children <1 month Children >1 month Adults	5 mg/kg every 12 hours 20 mg/kg every 12 hours 600 mg every 12 hours	Two days Two days Two days
Ciprofloxacin (IM)	Adults	500 mg	Single dose

Drug	Age group	Dose	Duration
Ceftriaxone (IM)	Children ≤12 years	125 mg	Single dose
	Older children and adults	250 mg	Single dose

   b. H. influenzae. Unvaccinated, young children (less than four years of age)
   who have close contact with patients with H. influenzae type b meningitis
   require rifampin (20 mg/kg with a max of 600 mg/day PO for four days).
References, see page 372.

Shock

Shock is characterized by a reduction in tissue perfusion, resulting in decreased
tissue oxygen delivery. These abnormalities may cause end-organ damage, failure
of multiple organ systems, and death. The mortality from shock is 35 to 40 percent

I. **Stages of shock.** The shock syndrome is characterized by physiologic stages
   beginning with an initial event which causes a systemic circulatory disturbance;
   shock may subsequently progress through three stages, culminating in irreversible end-organ damage and death.
   A. **Preshock.** During this stage, the homeostatic mechanisms of the body com-
      pensate for diminished perfusion. Tachycardia, peripheral vasoconstriction, and
      a modest decrease in systemic blood pressure may be the only clinical signs of
      hypovolemic or low preload shock. By comparison, distributive or low afterload
      shock is frequently characterized by peripheral vasodilation and a
      hyperdynamic state.
   B. **Shock.** During this stage, the regulatory mechanisms are overwhelmed and
      signs and symptoms of organ dysfunction appear, including tachycardia,
      tachypnea, metabolic acidosis, oliguria, and cool and clammy skin. The
      emergence of these signs and symptoms corresponds to one or more of the
      following:
      1. A 20 to 25 percent reduction in effective blood volume in low preload shock.
      2. A fall in the cardiac index to less than 2.5 L/min/M^2.
      3. Activation of mediators of the sepsis syndrome.
   C. **End-organ dysfunction.** During this stage, progressive end-organ dysfunction
      leads to irreversible organ damage and death:
      1. Urine output declines, culminating in anuria.
      2. Restlessness evolves into agitation, obtundation, and coma.
      3. Acidosis further decreases cardiac output and alters cellular metabolic
         processes.
      4. Multiple organ system failure proceeds to cause the demise of the patient.
II. **Classification of shock.** Three broad types of shock states are recognized:
    hypovolemic, cardiogenic, and distributive. Each type is characterized by one
    primary physiologic derangement.
    A. **Hypovolemic shock** results from decreased preload. Cardiac output falls.
       Hypovolemic shock can be further divided into hemorrhagic and fluid loss.
       Causes of hemorrhage include trauma, gastrointestinal bleeding, ruptured
       aortic or ventricular aneurysm, hematoma, pancreatitis, and fractures. Fluid
       loss can be a result of diarrhea, vomiting, heat stroke, inadequate repletion of
       insensible losses, burns, intestinal obstruction, pancreatitis, and cirrhosis.

B. **Cardiogenic shock** results from pump failure, manifested as decreased systolic function and cardiac output. The causes can be divided into four broad categories: myopathic, arrhythmic, mechanical, and extracardiac (obstructive).

C. **Distributive (vasodilatory) shock** results from a severe decrease in SVR, often associated with an increased cardiac output. Causes include:
   1. Septic shock.
   2. Activation of the systemic inflammatory response (eg, by pancreatitis, burns, or multiple traumatic injuries).
   3. Toxic shock syndrome.
   4. Anaphylaxis and anaphylactoid reactions.
   5. Drug or toxin reactions, including insect bites, transfusion reactions, and heavy metal poisoning.
   6. Addisonian crisis (which should be considered if clinical signs of sepsis exist without evidence of infection).
   7. Myxedema coma.
   8. Neurogenic shock after a central nervous system or spinal cord injury.
   9. Some patients after acute myocardial infarction who develop cardiogenic shock accompanied by a systemic inflammatory state.
   10. Post-cardiopulmonary bypass.

III. **Common features of shock**

A. **Hypotension** (systolic BP <90 mm Hg) occurs in most shock patients. However, early in the development of shock (preshock), the hypotension may only be relative to the patient's baseline blood pressure. As a result, a drop in systolic blood pressure of greater than 40 mm Hg suggests impending shock. As shock advances toward irreversible stages, profound hypotension may occur, and vasopressors are often necessary to maintain adequate perfusion.

B. **Cool, clammy skin,** regulatory processes may compensate for decreased effective tissue perfusion. Potent vasoconstrictive mechanisms redirect blood from the periphery to the vital organs, thus maintaining coronary, cerebral, and splanchnic perfusion but causing cool, clammy skin of shock. Notable exceptions are the flushed, hyperemic skin of early distributive shock, and the peripheral vasodilation of terminal shock states associated with failure of the mechanisms maintaining increased peripheral vascular resistance.

C. **Oliguria** reflects shunting of renal blood flow to other vital organs and is an objective measure of intravascular volume depletion. Other signs of hypovolemia in patients with shock include tachycardia, orthostatic hypotension, poor skin turgor, absent axillary sweat, and dry mucous membranes.

D. **Change in mental status.** Mental status changes in shock begin with agitation, progressing to confusion or delirium, and ending in obtundation or frank coma.

E. **Metabolic acidosis.** Initially, shock patients may have a respiratory alkalosis. However, as shock progresses, a metabolic acidosis develops, reflecting decreased clearance of lactate. If shock progresses to produce circulatory failure and tissue hypoxia, lactate production is increased due to anaerobic metabolism.

IV. **Initial examination in shock**

A. **History.** The patient's general condition, recent complaints, and activities prior to presentation may suggest a cause of shock. Additional clues include:
   1. Food and medicine allergies.
   2. Recent changes in medications.
   3. Potential acute or chronic drug intoxication.
   4. Pre-existing diseases.
   5. Immunosuppressed states.
   6. Hypercoagulable conditions.

B. Physical examination
1. **HEENT.** Scleral icterus; dry conjunctivae; dry mucous membranes; pinpoint pupils; dilated and fixed pupils; nystagmus.
2. **Neck.** Jugular venous distention; delayed carotid upstroke (pulsus parvus et tardus); carotid bruits; meningeal signs.
3. **Chest.** Tachypnea; shallow breaths; crackles (rales); consolidation; egophony; absent breath sounds; rub.
4. **Cardiovascular system.** Irregular rhythm; tachycardia; bradycardia; S3 gallop; diffuse PMI; right or left ventricular heave; murmurs; distant heart sounds; rub; pulsus paradoxus.
5. **Abdomen.** Tenseness; distention; tenderness; rebound; guarding; absence of or high-pitched bowel sounds; pulsatile masses; hepatosplenomegaly; ascites.
6. **Rectal exam.** Decreased tone; bright red blood; melena; Hemoccult positive stool.
7. **Extremities.** Swollen calf; palpable cord; unequal intensity of pulses or disparity of blood pressure between upper extremities.
8. **Neurologic exam.** Agitation; confusion; delirium; obtundation; coma.
9. **Skin.** Cold, clammy or warm, hyperemic skin; rashes; petechiae; urticaria; cellulitis.

C. Laboratory evaluation.
Complete blood count with differential; basic chemistry tests; liver function test; amylase and lipase; fibrinogen and fibrin split products; lactate; cardiac enzymes; arterial blood gases; toxicology screen; chest x-ray; abdominal x-ray for intestinal obstruction; electrocardiogram; urinalysis.

D. Pulmonary artery catheterization
is frequently used to provide hemodynamic measurements in shock patients, including CO, pulmonary artery wedge (pulmonary capillary wedge) pressure, and SVR. Right heart catheterization with a Swan-Ganz catheter is potentially useful in monitoring fluid resuscitation, titrating vasoconstrictive agents, and measuring the effects of changes in mechanical ventilatory settings (including PEEP) on hemodynamics.

References, see page 372.

Sepsis

Sepsis is a syndrome that complicates severe infection. Sepsis is characterized by systemic inflammation and widespread tissue injury, characterized by vasodilation, increased microvascular permeability, and leukocyte accumulation. More than 650,000 cases of sepsis are diagnosed annually. Sepsis occurs in approximately two percent of hospitalized patients, with a mortality rate of 20 to 50 percent.

I. Definitions
A. **Infection** is characterized by an inflammatory response to microorganisms, or the invasion of normally sterile host tissue by those organisms.
B. **Bacteremia** is defined as the presence of viable bacteria in the blood.
C. **Systemic inflammatory response syndrome (SIRS)** refers to the consequences of a dysregulated host inflammatory response when infection is absent.
   1. Systemic inflammatory response syndrome is diagnosed in the presence of two or more of the following:
      a. Temperature >38°C or <35°C
      b. Heart rate >90 beats/min
      c. Respiratory rate >20 breaths/min or PaCO2 <32 mmHg
      d. WBC >12,000 cells/mm^3, <4000 cells/mm^3, or >10% immature (band) forms

2. SIRS can result from autoimmune disorders, pancreatitis, vasculitis, thromboembolism, burns, or surgery.

D. **Sepsis.** In sepsis, the clinical signs that define SIRS are present and are due to either a culture-proven infection or an infection identified by visual inspection.

E. **Severe sepsis** exists if there is sepsis plus at least one of the following signs of organ hypoperfusion or dysfunction:

1. Areas of mottled skin
2. Capillary refilling requires three seconds or longer
3. Urine output <0.5 mL/kg for at least one hour, or renal replacement therapy
4. Lactate >2 mmol/L
5. Abrupt change in mental status
6. Abnormal electroencephalographic (EEG) findings
7. Platelet count <100,000 platelets/mL
8. Disseminated intravascular coagulation
9. Acute lung injury or acute respiratory distress syndrome (ARDS)
10. Cardiac dysfunction, as defined by echocardiography or direct measurement of the cardiac index

F. **Septic shock**

1. **Diagnostic criteria for septic shock:** There is severe sepsis plus one or both of the following:
   a. Systemic mean blood pressure is <60 mmHg (or <80 mmHg if the patient has baseline hypertension) despite adequate fluid resuscitation.
   b. Maintaining the systemic mean blood pressure >60 mmHg (or >80 mmHg if the patient has baseline hypertension) requires dopamine <5 mcg/kg per min, norepinephrine <0.25 mcg/kg per min, or epinephrine <0.25 mcg/kg per min despite adequate fluid resuscitation.
2. Septic shock is one type of vasodilatory or distributive shock. It results from a marked reduction in systemic vascular resistance, often associated with an increase in cardiac output.
3. **Refractory septic shock** exists if maintaining the systemic mean blood pressure >60 mmHg (or >80 mmHg if the patient has baseline hypertension) requires dopamine >5 mcg/kg per min, norepinephrine >0.25 mcg/kg per min, or epinephrine >0.25 mcg/kg per min despite adequate fluid resuscitation.

G. **Multiple organ failure** refers to the presence of altered organ function in an acutely ill patient such that homeostasis cannot be maintained without intervention. The multiple organ dysfunction syndrome (MODS) is classified as either primary or secondary.

1. Primary MODS is the result of a well-defined insult in which organ dysfunction occurs early and can be directly attributable to the insult itself (eg, renal failure due to rhabdomyolysis).
2. Secondary MODS is organ failure not in direct response to the insult itself, but as a consequence of a host response (eg, acute respiratory distress syndrome in pancreatitis). MODS represents the more severe end of the severity of illness characterized by SIRS/sepsis.

Noninfectious Disorders That May Resemble Sepsis

Myocardial infarction
Pulmonary embolus
Acute pancreatitis
Fat emboli syndrome
Acute adrenal insufficiency

Acute gastrointestinal hemorrhage
Overzealous diuresis
Transfusion reactions
Adverse drug reactions
Transient bacteremia after procedures
Amniotic fluid embolism

Defining sepsis and related disorders	
Term	**Definition**
Systemic inflammatory response syndrome (SIRS)	The systemic inflammatory response to a severe clinical insult manifested by >2 of the following conditions: Temperature >38°C or <36°C, heart rate >90 beats/min, respiratory rate >20 breaths/min or $PaCO_2$ <32 mm Hg, white blood cell count >12,000 cells/mm^3, <4000 cells/mm^3, or >10% band cells
Sepsis	The presence of SIRS caused by an infectious process; sepsis is considered severe if hypotension or systemic manifestations of hypoperfusion (lactic acidosis, oliguria, change in mental status) is present.
Septic shock	Sepsis-induced hypotension despite adequate fluid resuscitation, along with the presence of perfusion abnormalities that may induce lactic acidosis, oliguria, or an alteration in mental status.
Multiple organ dysfunction syndrome (MODS)	The presence of altered organ function in an acutely ill patient such that homeostasis cannot be maintained without intervention

Manifestations of Sepsis	
Clinical features	**Laboratory findings**
Temperature instability	Respiratory alkaloses
Tachypnea	Hypoxemia
Hyperventilation	Increased serum lactate levels
Altered mental status	Leukocytosis and increased neutrophil concentration
Oliguria	Eosinopenia
Tachycardia	Thrombocytopenia
Peripheral vasodilation	Anemia
	Proteinuria
	Mildly elevated serum bilirubin levels

II. **Management of severe sepsis and septic shock in adults**
   A. **Organisms.** Although the number of cases of Gram negative sepsis remains substantial, Gram positive bacteria are more frequently identified.
   B. **Early management.** The first priority in severe sepsis or septic shock is stabilization of their airway and breathing. Next, perfusion to the peripheral tissues should be restored.
      1. **Stabilize respiration.** Supplemental oxygen should be administered, and oxygenation should be monitored continuously with pulse oximetry. Intubation and mechanical ventilation may be required to support the increased work of breathing or for airway protection since encephalopathy and a depressed level of consciousness frequently complicate sepsis.

a. Etomidate (an ultrashort-acting nonbarbiturate hypnotic)should be avoided in septic patients because it can cause adrenal insufficiency via inhibition of glucocorticoid synthesis.

b. Chest radiographs and arterial blood analysis should be obtained following initial stabilization.

2. **Assess perfusion.** The adequacy of perfusion should be assessed. Hypotension is the most common indicator that perfusion is inadequate. An arterial catheter may be inserted if blood pressure is labile or restoration of arterial perfusion pressures is expected to be a protracted process, because a sphygmomanometer may be unreliable in hypotensive patients.

a. Critical hypoperfusion can also occur in the absence of hypotension. All patients with sepsis should be evaluated for evidence of impaired perfusion.

b. Common signs of hypoperfusion include cool, vasoconstricted skin due to redirection of blood flow to core organs (although warm, flushed skin may be present in the early phases of sepsis), obtundation or restlessness, oliguria or anuria, and lactic acidosis.

c. **Catheters.** A central venous catheter (CVC) should be inserted in most patients with severe sepsis or septic shock. A CVC can be used to infuse intravenous fluids, infuse medications, infuse blood products, and draw blood. It can be used for hemodynamic monitoring by measuring the central venous pressure (CVP) and the central venous oxyhemoglobin saturation (ScvO2).

d. Pulmonary artery catheters (PACs) should not be used in the routine management of patients with severe sepsis or septic shock. PACs can measure the pulmonary artery occlusion pressure (PAOP) and mixed venous oxyhemoglobin saturation (SvO2). The PAOP is a poor predictor of fluid responsiveness in sepsis and the SvO2 is similar to the ScvO2, which can be obtained from a CVC. PACs increase complications and have not been shown to improve outcome.

3. **Restore perfusion.** Early restoration of perfusion is necessary to prevent multiple organ dysfunction and reduce mortality. Hypoperfusion results from loss of plasma volume into the interstitial space, decreased vascular tone, and myocardial depression.

a. Resuscitation of the circulation should target a ScvO2 or SvO2 of 70% within six hours of presentation. Other goals include a central venous pressure 8 to 12 mmHg, a mean arterial pressure (MAP) 65 mmHg, and a urine output 0.5 mL/kg per hour.

b. **Intravenous fluids.** Relative intravascular hypovolemia is typical and may be severe. Early goal-directed therapy may require an infusion volume of five liters within the initial six hours of therapy. Rapid, large volume infusions of intravenous fluids are indicated as initial therapy for severe sepsis or septic shock, unless there is clinical or radiographic evidence of congestive heart failure.

   (1) Fluid therapy should be administered in 500 mL, rapidly infused boluses. Volume status, tissue perfusion, blood pressure, and the presence or absence of pulmonary edema must be assessed before and after each bolus. Intravenous fluid challenges can be repeated until blood pressure is acceptable, tissue perfusion is acceptable, pulmonary edema ensues, or fluid fails to augment perfusion.

   (2) Careful monitoring is essential because patients with sepsis typically develop noncardiogenic pulmonary edema.

4. **Crystalloid** is recommended because of the higher cost of albumin.

5. **Vasopressors** are second line agents in the treatment of severe sepsis and septic shock. Vasopressors are useful in patients who remain

hypotensive despite adequate fluid resuscitation or who develop cardiogenic pulmonary edema.

   a. Norepinephrine is recommended, although dopamine is also a reasonable first-choice among vasopressors. Phenylephrine, a pure alpha-adrenergic agonist, may be useful when tachycardia or arrhythmias preclude the use of agents with beta-adrenergic activity.

   b. Vasopressin (antidiuretic hormone) may be useful in vasodilatory septic shock. It is a reasonable choice for refractory septic shock despite adequate fluid resuscitation and high-dose conventional vasopressors. It is not recommended as a first-choice agent because it may reduce stroke volume and cause harmful vasoconstriction.

Hemodynamic effects of vasoactive agents				
Agent	Dose	Effect		
		CO	MAP	SVR
Dopamine (Intropin)	5-20 mcg/kg/min	2+	1+	3+
Norepinephrine (Levophed)	0.05-0.5 mcg/kg/min	-/0/+	2+	4+
Dobutamine (Dobutrex)	10 mcg/kg/min	2+	-/0/+	-/0
Epinephrine	0.05-2 mcg/kg/min	3+	2+	4+
Phenylephrine (Neo-Synephrine)	2-10 mcg/kg/min	0	2+	4+

1. **Additional therapies.** When the ScvO2 remains <70 percent after optimization of intravenous fluid and vasopressor therapy, it is reasonable to consider additional therapies, such as inotropic therapy or red blood cell transfusion.

   a. Inotropic therapy. A trial of inotropic therapy (usually dobutamine) is warranted if ScvO2 remains <70 percent after all of the prior interventions. At low doses, dobutamine may cause the blood pressure to decrease because it can dilate the systemic arteries. However, as the dose is increased, blood pressure usually rises because cardiac output increases.

   b. Red blood cell transfusions. Early goal-directed therapy should aggressively utilize red blood cell transfusions to raise the ScvO2.

B. Ongoing management

1. **If hypoperfusion persists** and progressive organ failure continues despite aggressive therapy, reassess of the adequacy of the above therapies, antimicrobial regimen, control of the septic focus, and the possibility of complications or coexisting problems (eg, pneumothorax).

2. **If the patient may has responded** to the above interventions with restored perfusion and a ScvO2 >70%, continue to monitor blood pressure, arterial lactate, urine output, creatinine, platelet count, Glasgow coma score, serum bilirubin, liver enzymes, oxygenation, and gut function (gastric tonometry).

3. In early sepsis, most lactate is probably a byproduct of anaerobic metabolism due to organ hypoperfusion. Early goal-directed therapy decreases lactate levels faster than conventional therapy.

C. Control of the septic focus

1. **Identification of the septic focus.** History and physical examination may identify the source of sepsis. Gram stain of infected fluids may give early clues to the etiology of infection while cultures are incubating. Urine should be Gram stained and cultured, sputum should be examined in a patient with a productive cough, and postoperative patients with intra-abdominal fluid should be percutaneously sampled under radiologic guidance.

2. **Blood cultures** should be obtained from two different venipuncture sites. Blood cultures should be incubated both aerobically and anaerobically.

3. **Eradication of infection.** Source control should be undertaken since undrained foci of infection may not respond to antibiotics. Infected foreign bodies (eg, vascular access devices) should be removed, and abscesses should undergo drainage.

Source Control for Common Infections	
Site	**Interventions**
Sinusitis	Surgical decompression of the sinuses
Pneumonia	Chest physiotherapy, suctioning
Empyema thoracis	Drainage, decortication
Mediastinitis	Drainage, debridement, diversion
Peritonitis	Resection, repair, or diversion of ongoing sources of contamination, drainage of abscesses, debridement of necrotic tissue
Cholangitis	Bile duct decompression
Pancreatic infection	Drainage or debridement
Urinary tract	Drainage of abscesses, relief of obstruction, removal or changing of infected catheters
Catheter-related bacteremia	Removal of catheter
Endocarditis	Valve replacement
Septic arthritis	Joint drainage and debridement
Soft tissue infection	Debridement of necrotic tissue and drainage of discrete abscesses
Prosthetic device infection	Device removal

4. **Intravenous antibiotic therapy** should be initiated after obtaining cultures.
   a. Cephalosporin, 3rd or 4th generation (eg, ceftriaxone, cefotaxime, or cefepime), or
      (1) Beta-lactam/beta-lactamase inhibitor (eg, piperacillin-tazobactam, ticarcillin-clavulanate, or ampicillin-sulbactam), or
      (2) Carbapenem (eg, imipenem or meropenem).
      (3) Alternatively, if Pseudomonas is a possible pathogen, vancomycin should e combined with two of the following:

      (a) Antipseudomonal cephalosporin (eg, cefepime, ceftazidime, or cefoperazone), or

      (b) Antipseudomonal carbapenem (eg, imipenem, meropenem), or

      (c) Antipseudomonal beta-lactam/beta-lactamase inhibitor (eg, piperacillin-tazobactam,ticarcillin-clavulanate), or

      (d) Fluoroquinolone with good anti-pseudomonal activity (eg, ciprofloxacin), or

      (e) Aminoglycoside (eg, gentamicin, amikacin), or

      (f) Monobactam (eg, aztreonam)

      (g) Selection of two agents from the same class (two beta-lactams) should be avoided.

  b. Staphylococcus aureus is associated with significant morbidity if not treated. Methicillin-resistant S. aureus (MRSA) is a cause of sepsis in hospitalized patients and in community dwelling individuals. Many of these Staphylococci have the Panton-Valentine leucocidin virulence factor, which causes severe, necrotizing infections. Severely ill patients presenting with sepsis of unclear etiology should be treated with intravenous vancomycin (adjusted for renal function) until the possibility of MRSA sepsis has been excluded.

Recommended Antibiotics in Septic Shock	
Suspected source	**Recommended antibiotics**
Pneumonia	Third or 4th-generation cephalosporin (cefepime, ceftazidime, cefotaxime, ceftizoxime) *plus* macrolide (antipseudomonal beta lactam *plus* aminoglycoside if hospital-acquired) + anaerobic coverage with metronidazole or clindamycin).
Urinary tract	Ampicillin *plus* gentamicin (Garamycin) or third-generation cephalosporin (ceftazidime, cefotaxime, ceftizoxime) or a quinolone (ciprofloxacin, levofloxacin).
Skin or soft tissue	Nafcillin (add metronidazole [Flagyl] or clindamycin if anaerobic infection suspected)
Meningitis	Third-generation cephalosporin (ceftazidime, cefotaxime, ceftizoxime)
Intra-abdominal	Third-generation cephalosporin (ceftazidime, cefotaxime, ceftizoxime) *plus* metronidazole or clindamycin
Primary bacteremia	Ticarcillin/clavulanate (Timentin) *or* piperacillin/tazobactam(Zosyn)

Dosages of Antibiotics Used in Sepsis	
Agent	**Dosage**
Cefepime (Maxipime)	2 gm IV q12h; if neutropenic, use 2 gm q8h
Cefti zoxime (Cef izox)	2 gm IV q8h
Cef tazidime (For taz)	2 g IV q8h
Cefot axime (Cla foran)	2 gm q4-6h
Cefuroxime (Kefurox, Zinacef)	1.5 g IV q8h
Cefox itin (Mefoxin)	2 gm q6h

Dosages of Antibiotics Used in Sepsis	
Cefotetan (Cefotan)	2 gm IV q12h
Piperacillin/tazobactam (Zosyn)	3.375-4.5 gm IV q6h
Ticarcillin/clavulanate (Timen tin)	3.1 gm IV q4-6h (200-300 mg/kg/d)
Ampicillin	1-3.0 gm IV q6h
Ampicillin/sulbac tam (Unasyn)	3.0 gm IV q6h
Nafcillin (Nafcil)	2 gm IV q4-6h
Piperacillin, ticarcillin, mezlocill in	3 gm IV q4-6h
Meropenem (Merrem)	1 gm IV q8h
Imipenem/cilastatin (Primaxin)	1.0 gm IV q6h
Gentamicin or tobramyci n	2 mg/kg IV loading dose, then 1.7 mg/kg IV q8h
Amikacin (Amikin)	7.5 mg/kg IV loading dose, then 5 mg/kg IV q8h
Vancomycin	1 gm IV q12h
Metronid azole (Flagyl)	500 mg IV q6-8h
Clindamycin (Cleocin)	600-900 mg IV q8h
Linezolid (Zyvox)	600 mg IV/PO q12h
Quinupristin/dalfopristin (Synercid)	7.5 mg/kg IV q8h

A. **Recombinant human activated protein C (drotrecogin alfa; Xigris)**
supplementation may produce clinical benefit in the setting of purpura
fulminans. In patients with septic shock or severe sepsis with a high risk of
death, defined as an APACHE II score >25, multiple organ dysfunction, or
sepsis-induced acute respiratory distress syndrome, recombinant human
activated protein C should be administered unless contraindicated. The
infusion should be initiated within 24 hours of the first-sepsis induced organ
dysfunction; 24 mcg/kg per hour for 96 hours.

Parameters for monitoring organ system function in sepsis	
Organ system	**Parameter**
Respiratory system	PaO2/FiO2 ratio
Renal system	Urine output and serum creatinine
Hematologic system	Platelet count
Central nervous system	Glasgow coma score
Hepatobiliary system	Serum bilirubin and liver enzymes
Cardiovascular system	Blood pressure, arterial lactate
Gastrointestinal system	Gastric intramucosal pH (pHi), ileus, blood in nasogastric aspirate

References, see page 372.

Colonic Diverticulitis

The prevalence colonic diverticular disease increases from less than 5 percent at age 40, to 30 percent by age 60, to 65 percent by age 85. Among all patients with diverticulosis, 70 percent remain asymptomatic, 15 to 25 percent develop diverticulitis, and 5 to 15 percent develop diverticular bleeding.

I. **Pathophysiology**
   A. Diverticulitis represents micro- or macroscopic perforation of a diverticulum. The inflammation is frequently mild. Complications may include development of an abscess, fistula, obstruction, perforation and peritonitis.
   B. **Complicated diverticulitis** refers to the presence of an abscess, fistula, obstruction, or perforation while simple diverticulitis refers to inflammation in the absence of these complications.

II. **Clinical evaluation**
   A. **Left lower quadrant pain** is the most common complaint, occurring in 70 percent of patients. Pain is often present for several days prior to admission. Up to one-half have had one or more previous episodes of similar pain. Other possible symptoms include nausea and vomiting in 20 to 62 percent, constipation in 50 percent, diarrhea in 25 to 35 percent, and urinary symptoms (eg, dysuria, urgency and frequency) in 10 to 15 percent.
   B. Right-sided diverticulitis occurs in only 1.5 percent of patients
   C. **Physical examination** usually reveals abdominal tenderness in the left lower quadrant. A tender mass is palpable in 20 percent and abdominal distention is common. Right lower quadrant tenderness usually results from redundant sigmoid colon or right-sided diverticulitis which is rare in the west but common in Asia. Generalized tenderness suggests free perforation and peritonitis.
   D. **Low grade fever and mild leukocytosis** are common. However, the absence of these findings does not exclude the diagnosis; a normal white count occurs in 45 percent. Liver function tests are usually normal and amylase is either normal or mildly elevated, especially in the patient with perforation and peritonitis. The urinalysis may reveal sterile pyuria; the presence of colonic flora on culture suggests a colovesical fistula.

Differential Diagnosis of Diverticulitis	
Elderly	**Middle Aged and Young**
Ischemic colitis Carcinoma Volvulus Colonic Obstruction Penetrating ulcer Nephrolithiasis/urosepsis	Appendicitis Salpingitis Inflammatory bowel disease Penetrating ulcer Urosepsis

III. **Diagnosis of diverticulitis**
   A. **Radiologic evaluation** in the acute setting. Routine abdominal and chest radiographs are commonly performed in the patient with acute abdominal pain, and are most useful in excluding other causes, such as intestinal obstruction, rather than in making the diagnosis of diverticulitis. Free air may be present in patients with a perforated diverticulum.

B. **Computer tomographic (CT) scanning** is the optimal method of investigation in suspected acute diverticulitis. The sensitivity and specificity of helical CT (with colonic contrast) are 97 and 100 percent, respectively.
   1. CT features of acute diverticulitis:
      a. Increased soft tissue density within pericolic fat, secondary to inflammation — 98 percent
      b. Colonic diverticula — 84 percent
      c. Bowel wall thickening — 70 percent
      d. Soft tissue masses representing phlegmon, and pericolic fluid collections, representing abscesses — 35 percent
   2. CT can permit percutaneous drainage of abscesses, thereby downstaging complicated diverticulitis, avoiding emergent surgery, and permitting single-stage elective surgical resection.
C. **Contrast enema** is safe in the acute phase if performed by the single contrast technique and if there is no evidence of complications. In the presence of complications, such as pneumoperitoneum or generalized peritonitis, barium is absolutely contraindicated. Water soluble contrast should be used in any patient suspected of having acute diverticulitis.
D. **Evaluation in the elective setting.** After resolution of an episode of acute diverticulitis, the colon requires full evaluation to establish the extent of disease and to rule out coexistent lesions, such as polyps or carcinoma. This can be accomplished either with colonoscopy, or with the combination of barium enema plus flexible sigmoidoscopy.

IV. **Treatment of acute diverticulitis**
A. **Uncomplicated diverticulitis**
   1. Conservative treatment (with bowel rest and antibiotics) is successful in 70 to 100 percent of patients with acute uncomplicated diverticulitis.
   2. Selection for outpatient management. The elderly, immunosuppressed, those with significant comorbidities, and those unable to tolerate oral intake, those with high fever or significant leukocytosis should be hospitalized.
   3. Causative bacteria are principally Gram negative rods and anaerobes (particularly E. coli and B. fragilis). Reasonable antibiotic choices include a quinolone with metronidazole, amoxicillin-clavulanate, or sulfamethoxazole-trimethoprim with metronidazole.
   4. Outpatient treatment of diverticulitis
      a. Ciprofloxacin (Cipro), 500 mg PO twice daily plus metronidazole, 500 mg PO three times daily.
      b. An alternative is amoxicillin-clavulanate (Augmentin, 875/125 mg twice daily) is an acceptable alternative. Treatment should be continued for 7 to 10 days. Oral ciprofloxacin achieves levels similar to those with intravenous administration, has broad coverage of enteric Gram negative pathogens, and requires only twice daily dosing.
      c. Patients requiring hospitalization should receive empiric broad-spectrum intravenous antibiotics directed at colonic anaerobic and gram-negative flora. Metronidazole is the antibiotic of choice for anaerobic coverage, while gram-negative coverage can be achieved with a third-generation cephalosporin (ceftriaxone 1 to 2 g daily or cefotaxime 1 to 2 g every six hours) or a fluoroquinolone (ciprofloxacin 400 mg IV every 12 hours or levofloxacin 500 mg IV daily).
      d. Single agent coverage is also reasonable with the following alternative agents:
         (1) **Ampicillin-sulbactam (Unasyn)** (3 g every six hours), piperacillin-tazobactam (3.375 g or 4.5 g every six hours), or ticarcillin-clavulanate (3.1 g every four hours)

        (2) Carbapenem such as imipenem (Primaxin, 500 mg every six hours) or meropenem (1 g every eight hours).

5. **Dietary recommendations.** Outpatients should be instructed to consume clear liquids only. Clinical improvement should be evident after two to three days, after which the diet can be advanced slowly. Patients requiring hospitalization should receive clear liquids or NPO with intravenous hydration. Patients should consume a high fiber diet once the acute phase has resolved.

6. **Abscesses** amenable to percutaneous drainage should be treated. Laparotomy is necessary if abscesses cannot be drained or if drainage does not result in improvement. Surgery should proceed without delay if a patient's condition deteriorates (increased pain, more localized peritonitis or diffuse tenderness, increased white count).

7. **Two to six weeks after recovery**, patients should undergo an evaluation of the colon to exclude other diagnostic considerations (colon cancer) and to evaluate the extent of the diverticulosis. This is usually accomplished with a colonoscopy, although a flexible sigmoidoscopy plus barium enema is a reasonable alternative. Patients should be advised to consume a diet high in fiber.

8. **Prognosis.** Following successful conservative therapy for a first attack of diverticulitis, 30 to 40 percent of patients will remain asymptomatic, 30 to 40 percent will have episodic abdominal cramps without frank diverticulitis, and one-third will proceed to a second attack of diverticulitis.

9. After a second attack, elective surgery is not necessary for all patients who respond to medical therapy.Patients in whom elective surgery has been recommended following a single attack of diverticulitis include young patients (less than 40 or 50 years of age) and those who are immunosuppressed.

B. **Complicated diverticulitis**
1. **Peritonitis.** Diffuse peritonitis mandates resuscitation, broad-spectrum antibiotics, and emergency exploration.
   a. Ampicillin (2 g IV every six hours), gentamicin (1.5 to 2 mg/kg IV every 8 hours), and metronidazole (500 mg IV every 8 hours)
   b. Imipenem/cilastin (500 mg IV every six hours)
   c. Piperacillin-tazobactam (3.375 g IV every six hours)
2. **Obstruction.** Resection with primary anastomosis is usually possible; a colostomy is required if the bowel preparation is inadequate or on-table colonic lavage can be considered to permit primary anastomosis.
3. **Perforation.** Free intraperitoneal rupture of diverticulitis is unusual; however, such patients have high mortality rates of 20 to 30 percent. Treatment usually involves a two-stage procedure.
4. **Abscesses** occur in 16 percent of patients with acute diverticulitis without peritonitis and in 31 to 56 percent of those requiring surgery for diverticulitis. Percutaneous drainage now permits elective single stage surgery in 60 to 80 percent of patients; furthermore, in selected patients with contraindications to surgery, catheter drainage may be sufficient to relieve symptoms.

C. **Surgery.** Up to 30 percent of patients with uncomplicated diverticulitis require surgical intervention during the initial attack. Surgery is advised after a first attack of complicated diverticulitis or after two or more episodes of uncomplicated diverticulitis.

Indications for Surgery in Acute Diverticulitis

Absolute
  Complications of diverticulitis: peritonitis, abscess (failed percutaneous drainage), fistula, obstruction
  Clinical deterioration or failure to improve with medical therapy
  Recurrent episodes
  Intractable symptoms
  Inability to exclude carcinoma

Relative Indications
  Symptomatic stricture
  Immunosuppression
  Right-sided diverticulitis
  Young patient

1. **Preoperative preparation.** A second- or third generation cephalosporin is administered or more broad-spectrum antibiotics, depending upon the degree of contamination. Regimens include cefazolin (Ancef [1 g IV every eight hours]) plus metronidazole (Flagyl [500 mg IV every 8 hours]); ampicillin-sulbactam (Unasyn [1.5 g IV every six hours]); or ticarcillin-clavulanate (Timentin 3.1 g IV every six hours]). Bowel preparation is often possible in nonemergent situations.
2. **Emergency sigmoid colectomy** with proximal colostomy is indicated for attacks of diverticulitis associated with sepsis, peritonitis, obstruction, or perforation.
3. **Elective sigmoid resection** is indicated for second or subsequent attacks of diverticulitis, or for attacks with complications managed nonoperatively (eg, percutaneous CT-guided drainage of an abscess), or carcinoma.
4. **Operative procedures**
   a. **Single-stage procedure.** This procedure is usually performed as an elective procedure after resolution of the acute attack of diverticulitis. The segment containing inflamed diverticulum (usually sigmoid colon) is resected with primary anastomosis. A bowel prep is required.
   b. **Two-stage procedure.** This procedure is indicated for acute diverticulitis with obstruction or perforation and an unprepared bowel. The first stage consists of resection of the involved segment of colon with end colostomy and either a mucous fistula or a Hartmann rectal pouch. The second stage consists of a colostomy take-down and reanastomosis after 2-3 months.

References, see page 372.

Acute Cystitis

Cystitis is an infection of the bladder. Acute cystitis in the healthy nonpregnant adult woman is considered to be uncomplicated. A complicated infection is associated with a condition that increases the risk of failing therapy. About 7.8% of girls and 1.6% of boys have had a symptomatic UTI. Approximately 50 to 60% of adult women have had a UTI at some time during their life. Young sexually active women have 0.5 episodes of acute cystitis per year.

I. Microbiology Clinical features

A. Escherichia coli is the causative pathogen in 80 to 85% of episodes of acute uncomplicated cystitis. Staphylococcus saprophyticus is responsible for most other episodes, while Proteus mirabilis, Klebsiella species, enterococci or other uropathogens are isolated from a small proportion of patients.

B. Acute uncomplicated cystitis is characterized by dysuria, usually in combination with frequency, urgency, suprapubic pain, and/or hematuria. Fever (>38°C), flank pain, costovertebral angle tenderness, and nausea or vomiting suggest pyelonephritis

C. Vaginitis should be considered if there is vaginal discharge or odor, pruritus, dyspareunia, external dysuria, and the absence of frequency or urgency.

II. Diagnosis

A. **Physical examination** should include temperature, abdominal examination, and assessment for costovertebral angle tenderness. A pelvic examination is indicated if symptoms of urethritis or vaginitis are present.

B. **Urinalysis.** Pyuria is usually present with acute cystitis; its absence strongly suggests a noninfectious cause for the symptoms. An unspun voided midstream urine specimen should be examined with a hemocytometer; 10 or more leukocytes per mm^3 is considered abnormal. White blood cell casts in the urine are diagnostic of upper tract infection. Hematuria is common with UTI but not in urethritis or vaginitis. Microscopic evaluation of the urine for bacteriuria is generally not recommended for acute uncomplicated cystitis because pathogens in low quantities ($\leq 10^4$ CFU/mL) are difficult to find on the wet mount or Gram stain.

C. **Indications for voided midstream urine cultures**
1. Suspected complicated infection.
2. The symptoms are not characteristic of UTI.
3. The patient has persistent symptoms of UTI following treatment.
4. UTI symptoms recur less than one month after treatment of a previous UTI.

D. **Acute urethral syndrome.** A CFU count $\geq 10^2$/mL should be considered positive on a midstream urine specimen in women with acute symptoms and pyuria. Some women with acute dysuria have neither bacteriuria nor pyuria. The symptoms usually resolve after antimicrobial therapy.

E. **Urine dipsticks**
1. Dipsticks detect the presence of leukocyte esterase and nitrite; the former detect pyuria and the latter Enterobacteriaceae which convert urinary nitrate to nitrite. The leukocyte esterase test is a practical screening test with a sensitivity of 75 to 96% and specificity of 94 to 98%. A microscopic evaluation for pyuria or a culture is indicated with a negative leukocyte esterase test with urinary symptoms.
2. The nitrite test is fairly sensitive and specific for detecting $\geq 10^5$ Enterobacteriaceae CFU per mL of urine. However, it lacks adequate sensitivity for detection of "low count" UTIs, or, in some cases, infections caused by common uropathogenic species.

III. Treatment

A. **E. coli Resistance**
1. One-third or more of isolates demonstrate resistance to ampicillin and sulfonamides; these agents should not be used for empiric therapy. An increasing proportion of uropathogens demonstrate resistance to trimethoprim and/or TMP-SMX.
2. The prevalence of resistance to nitrofurantoin among E. coli is less than 5%, although non-E. coli uropathogens are often resistant.
3. Resistance to the fluoroquinolones remains well below 5%.

B. **S. saprophyticus resistance.** Three% are resistant to TMP-SMX, 1% to cephalothin, 0% to nitrofurantoin, and 0.4% to ciprofloxacin.

C. Recommendation
1. Because of increasing fluoroquinolone resistance, TMP-SMX should be the first-line treatment for acute cystitis if the woman:
   a. Has no history of allergy to the drug.
   b. Has not been on antibiotics, especially TMP-SMX, in the past three months.
   c. Has not been hospitalized recently.
   d. If the prevalence of E. coli resistance to TMP-SMX in the area is not known to be more than 20% among women with acute uncomplicated cystitis.
2. **A fluoroquinolone** is an appropriate choice for women who have an allergy to TMP-SMX or risk factors for TMP-SMX resistance and who have moderate to severe symptoms.

Oral Antibiotics for Acute Uncomplicated Cystitis		
Drug, dose	**Dose and interval**	**Duration**
Levofloxacin (Levaquin)	250 mg q24h	3 days
Ciprofloxacin (Cipro)	100 to 250 mg q12h **OR** 500 mg q24h	3 days 3 days
Gatifloxacin (Tequin)	400 mg single dose **OR** 200 mg q24h	3 days
Trimethoprim-sulfamethoxazole (Bactrim)	160/800 mg q12h	3 days
Trimethoprim	100 mg q12h	3 days
Cefpodoxime proxetil (Vantin)	100 mg q12h	3-7days
Nitrofurantoin macrocrystals (Macrobid)	50 mg q6h	7 days
Nitrofurantoin monohydrate macrocrystals (Macrobid)	100 mg q12h	7 days
Amoxicillin-clavulanate (Augmentin)	500 mg q12h	7 days

3. **Nitrofurantoin (Macrodantin** [for seven days]) should be used for women with mild-to-moderate symptoms who have allergy to TMP-SMX or risk factors for TMP-SMX resistance.
4. Urinary analgesia (phenazopyridine [Pyrimidine] 200 mg orally TID) is offered to those with severe dysuria (10%). Phenazopyridine is usually given for only one to two days.
5. Routine post-treatment cultures in non-pregnant women who have become asymptomatic after an episode of cystitis are not indicated. In patients whose symptoms do not resolve, urine culture and antimicrobial susceptibil-

ity testing should be performed. Empiric therapy should include a fluoroquinolone unless such an agent was used initially.

IV. Acute complicated cystitis

A. Urinary tract infection may lead to serious complications in the person who is pregnant, very young or old, diabetic, immunocompromised, or who has an abnormal genitourinary tract.

B. **Clinical presentation.** Acute complicated cystitis generally presents with dysuria, frequency, urgency, suprapubic pain, and/or hematuria. Fever (>38ºC), flank pain, costovertebral angle tenderness, and nausea or vomiting suggest the infection has extended beyond the bladder.

C. **Bacteriology.** The spectrum of uropathogens causing complicated cystitis is much broader than that causing uncomplicated cystitis. Infection with Proteus, Klebsiella, Pseudomonas, Serratia, and Providencia species, and enterococci, staphylococci and fungi is more common in complicated cystitis. These uropathogens, including E. coli, are much more likely to be resistant to common antimicrobials.

D. **Diagnosis.** Pyuria is present in almost all patients with complicated cystitis. Urine cultures with susceptibility testing should be obtained in complicated cystitis. A Gram stain may be helpful since the presence of Gram positive cocci, suggestive of enterococci, may influence the choice of empiric antibiotics.

E. **Treatment**

1. Complicated cystitis should be treated with an oral fluoroquinolone such as ciprofloxacin, levofloxacin, or gatifloxacin. The fluoroquinolones are well tolerated, provide a broad spectrum of activity covering most expected pathogens (including P. aeruginosa), and achieve high levels in the urine and urinary tract tissue. The recommended dose for ciprofloxacin (Cipro) is 500 mg PO twice daily, for levofloxacin (Levaquin) is 500 mg PO once daily, and for gatifloxacin (Tequin) is 400 mg PO once daily, each for 7 to 14 days.

2. Amoxicillin, nitrofurantoin and sulfa drugs are poor choices for empiric therapy in complicated cystitis because of the high prevalence of resistance.

3. Parenteral therapy is occasionally indicated for the treatment of complicated cystitis caused by multiply-resistant uropathogens, or for those patients who are allergic or intolerant to fluoroquinolones. Parenteral levofloxacin (500 mg) or gatifloxacin (400 mg), ceftriaxone (1 g), or an aminoglycoside (3 to 5 mg/kg of gentamicin or tobramycin) can be administered once daily. Patients initially given parenteral therapy can be switched to oral agents, usually a fluoroquinolone, after clinical improvement.

4. Gram positive cocci, suggestive of enterococci, may require the addition of ampicillin (1 g every six hours) or amoxicillin (500 mg PO every eight hours) to a treatment regimen.

5. If the patient does not show improvement within 24 to 48 hours, a repeat urine culture and ultrasound or computerized tomography should be considered to rule out urinary tract pathology.

6. The recommended duration of treatment for acute complicated cystitis is 7 to 14 days. A follow-up urine culture is not indicated in the asymptomatic patient.

V. Cystitis in young men. A small number of 15- to 50-year-old men suffer acute uncomplicated UTIs. Risk factors include homosexuality, intercourse with an infected female partner, and lack of circumcision.

A. Dysuria, frequency, urgency, suprapubic pain, or hematuria are typical of cystitis in men. The absence of pyuria suggests a non-infectious diagnosis. A midstream urine culture is recommended.

B. **Other causes of infection.** Urethritis must be considered in sexually active men; examination for penile ulcerations and urethral discharge, evaluation of a urethral swab specimen Gram stain, and diagnostic tests for N. gonorrheae and C. trachomatis are warranted. A urethral Gram stain demonstrating leukocytes and predominant Gram negative rods suggests E. coli urethritis.

C. Chronic prostatitis should also be considered, particularly in men who have had recurrent UTIs.

D. Treatment of cystitis. The etiologic agents causing uncomplicated urinary tract infections in men are similar to those in women. Thus, the TMP-SMX (Bactrim) is appropriate for empiric use in men, although 7-day regimens are recommended. Nitrofurantoin and beta-lactams should not be used in men with cystitis since they do not achieve reliable tissue concentrations and would be ineffective for occult prostatitis. Fluoroquinolones provide the best antimicrobial spectrum and prostatic penetration.

References, see page 372.

Acute Pyelonephritis

Urinary tract infections (UTIs) are common, especially in young children and sexually active women. UTI is defined either as a lower tract (acute cystitis) or upper tract (acute pyelonephritis) infection.

I. Clinical features

  A. Acute uncomplicated pyelonephritis is suggested by flank pain, nausea/vomiting, fever (>38ºC) and/or costovertebral angle tenderness. Frequency, dysuria, and suprapubic pain are found in the majority of patients whether infection is localized to the upper or lower tract.

  B. Fever $\geq$37.8ºC is strongly correlated with acute pyelonephritis. The examination should focus on temperature, abdomen, and costovertebral angle tenderness.

  C. Pelvic examination may be indicated since pelvic inflammatory disease is a condition often mistaken for acute uncomplicated pyelonephritis. Pelvic examination does not need to be performed, however, in a woman with unilateral CVA pain and tenderness, fever, pyuria, and no vaginal symptoms.

Risk Factors for Occult Renal Infection or a Complicated Urinary Tract Infection	
Male sex	Functional or anatomic abnormality of the urinary tract
Elderly	
Presentation in emergency department	Recent antimicrobial use
	Symptoms for more than seven days at presentation
Hospital-acquired infection	Diabetes mellitus
Pregnancy	Immunosuppression
Indwelling urinary catheter	
Recent urinary tract instrumentation	
Childhood urinary tract infection	

II. Laboratory features

  A. Pyuria is present in virtually all women with acute pyelonephritis; its absence strongly suggests an alternative diagnosis. Hematuria is common with urinary tract infection but not in urethritis or vaginitis. Most patients with acute pyelonephritis have leukocytosis and an elevated erythrocyte sedimentation rate and serum C-reactive protein.

B. Some patients with pyelonephritis may have colony counts of 10^3 to 10^4 CFU per mL. Blood cultures are positive in 10 to 20% of women with acute uncomplicated pyelonephritis.

C. A urinalysis should be performed to look for pyuria. White cell casts indicate a renal origin for the pyuria. Gram stain, usually performed on spun urine, may distinguish Gram negative from Gram positive infections. A pregnancy test should be performed if there is missed menses or lack of contraception.

D. Urine culture and antimicrobial susceptibility testing should be performed routinely in acute pyelonephritis.

E. Rapid methods for detection of bacteriuria, such as the nitrite test, should not be relied upon in the evaluation of patients with suspected pyelonephritis because tests lack adequate sensitivity for detection of "low count" urinary tract infection and common uropathogenic species. The nitrite test has a sensitivity of 35 to 80% and does not detect organisms unable to reduce nitrate to nitrite, such as enterococci and staphylococci.

F. Blood cultures are limited to those patients who warrant hospitalization.

III. Treatment. Microbiology of acute uncomplicated upper and lower urinary tract infection is rather limited with Escherichia coli accounting for 70 to 95% of infections and Staphylococcus saprophyticus 5 to 20%.

A. Indications for admission to the hospital include:

  1. Inability to maintain oral hydration or take medications.

  2. Patient noncompliance.

  3. Uncertainty about the diagnosis.

  4. Severe illness with high fevers, pain, and marked debility.

  5. Outpatient therapy should generally be reserved for nonpregnant women with mild-to-moderate uncomplicated pyelonephritis who are compliant.

B. Empiric antibiotic therapy

  1. Ampicillin and sulfonamides should not be used for empiric therapy because of the high rate of resistance. An increasing proportion of uropathogens demonstrate resistance to trimethoprim-sulfamethoxazole. In comparison, resistance to the fluoroquinolones and aminoglycosides is very low in uncomplicated UTIs.

  2. Oral agents. In patients with acute uncomplicated pyelonephritis, an oral fluoroquinolone, such as ciprofloxacin (500 mg PO BID), levofloxacin (Levaquin [250 to 500 mg PO QD]), or gatifloxacin (Tequin [400 mg PO QD]), is recommended for outpatients as initial empiric treatment of infection caused by Gram negative bacilli. The newer fluoroquinolones, sparfloxacin, trovafloxacin and moxifloxacin, should be avoided because they may not achieve adequate concentrations in urine.

   a. Trimethoprim, trimethoprim-sulfamethoxazole or other agents can be used if the infecting strain is known to be susceptible. If enterococcus is suspected by the presence of small Gram positive cocci on Gram stain, amoxicillin (500 mg PO TID) should be added to the treatment regimen until the causative organism is identified.

   b. Cefixime (Suprax) and cefpodoxime proxetil (Vantin) also appear to be effective for the treatment of acute uncomplicated pyelonephritis. Cefixime is less effective against S. saprophyticus. Nitrofurantoin should not be used for the treatment of pyelonephritis since it does not achieve reliable tissue levels.

Parenteral Regimens for Empiric Treatment of Acute Uncomplicated Pyelonephritis	
Antibiotic, dose	**Interval**
Ceftriaxone (Rocephin), 1 g	q24h
Ciprofloxacin (Cipro), 200-400 mg	q12h
Levofloxacin (Levaquin), 250-500 mg	q24h
Ofloxacin (Floxin), 200-400 mg	q12 h
Gatifloxacin (Tequin), 400 mg	q24h
Gentamicin, 3-5 mg/kg (±ampicillin)	q24h
Gentamicin, 1 mg per kg (±ampicillin)	q8h
Ampicillin, 1-2 g (plus gentamicin)*	q6h
Aztreonam (Azactam), 1 g	q8-12h
*Recommended regimen if enterococcus suspected.	

3. **Parenteral therapy.** For hospitalized patients, ceftriaxone (Rocephin [1 gram IV QD]) is recommended if enterococcus is not suspected. Aminoglycosides (3 to 5 mg/kg) given once daily provide a therapeutic advantage compared with beta lactams because of their marked and sustained concentration in renal tissue.
   a. Ciprofloxacin, ofloxacin, levofloxacin and gatifloxacin are also effective for the parenteral treatment of uncomplicated pyelonephritis but should be used orally if the patient is able to tolerate oral medications since the costs are lower and serum levels are equivalent.
   b. If enterococcus is suspected based upon the Gram stain, ampicillin (1 to 2 g IV Q6h) plus gentamicin (1.0 mg/kg IV Q8h) or piperacillin-tazobactam (3.375 g IV Q8h) are reasonable broad spectrum empiric choices. Once-daily dosing of aminoglycosides is not recommended for serious probable enterococcal infection since this regimen may not provide adequate synergy against the organism.
C. **Duration.** Patients with acute uncomplicated pyelonephritis can often be switched to oral therapy at 24 to 48 hours. Patients should be evaluated for complicated pyelonephritis if they fail to defervesce or if bacteremia persists. A 14-day regimen is recommended. In sicker patients, a longer duration of treatment may be required (14 to 21 days).
D. **Posttreatment follow-up cultures** in an asymptomatic patient are not indicated. In women whose pyelonephritis symptoms resolve but recur within two weeks, a repeat urine culture and antimicrobial susceptibility testing should be performed. If the initially infecting species is isolated again with the same susceptibility profile, a renal ultrasound or computed tomographic (CT) scan should be performed. Retreatment with a two-week regimen using another agent should be considered.

  E. **Urologic evaluation**
    1. Routine urologic investigation of young healthy women with acute uncompli-
       cated pyelonephritis is generally not recommended. Ultrasound or CT scan
       should be considered if the patient remains febrile or has not shown clinical
       improvement after 72 hours of treatment. CT scan or renal ultrasound
       should be performed after two recurrences of pyelonephritis.
IV. **Acute complicated pyelonephritis**
  A. **Clinical features.** In addition to flank pain, dysuria and fever, complicated
     urinary tract infections may also be associated with malaise, fatigue, nausea,
     or abdominal pain.
  B. A urine Gram stain and culture should always be performed in patients with
     suspected complicated UTI. A colony count threshold of $\geq 10^3$ CFU per mL
     should be used to diagnose symptomatic complicated infection except when
     urine cultures are obtained through a newly-inserted catheter in which case a
     level of $\geq 10^{(2)}$ CFU per mL is evidence of infection.
  C. **Microbiology.** E. coli is still the predominant uropathogen, but other
     uropathogens, including Citrobacter sp, Enterobacter sp, Pseudomonas
     aeruginosa, enterococci, Staphylococcus aureus, and fungi account for a
     higher proportion of cases compared with uncomplicated urinary tract infec-
     tions.
  D. **Treatment.** Patients with complicated pyelonephritis, including pregnant
     women, should be managed as inpatients. Underlying anatomic (eg, stones,
     obstruction), functional (eg, neurogenic bladder), or metabolic (eg, poorly
     controlled diabetes) defects must be corrected.
    1. In contrast to uncomplicated UTI, S. aureus is relatively more likely to be
       found. For those patients with mild to moderate illness who can be treated
       with oral medication, a fluoroquinolone is the best choice for empiric
       therapy. Fluoroquinolones are comparable or superior to other broad
       spectrum regimens, including parenteral therapy. Sparfloxacin,
       trovafloxacin and moxifloxacin are not effective.
    2. Antimicrobial regimen can be modified when the infecting strain susceptibili-
       ties are known. Patients on parenteral regimens can be switched to oral
       treatment, generally a fluoroquinolone, after clinical improvement. Patients
       undergoing effective treatment with an antimicrobial to which the infecting
       pathogen is susceptible should have definite improvement within 24 to 48
       hours and, if not, a repeat urine culture and imaging studies should be
       performed.
    3. At least 10 to 14 days of therapy is recommended. Urine culture should be
       repeated one to two weeks after the completion of therapy. Suppressive
       antibiotics may be considered with complicated pyelonephritis and a
       positive follow-up urine culture.

Parenteral Regimens for Empiric Treatment of Acute Complicated Pyelonephritis	
Antibiotic, dose	**Interval**
Cefepime (Maxipime) , 1 g	q12 hours
Ciprofloxacin (Cipro), 400 mg	q12 hours
Levofloxacin (Levaquin), 500 mg	q24 hours
Ofloxacin (Floxin), 400 mg	q12 hours
Gatifloxacin (Tequin), 400 mg	q24 hours
Gentamicin, 3-5 mg/kg (+ ampicillin)*	q24 hours
Gentamicin, 1 mg per kg (+ ampicillin)*	q8 hours
Ampicillin, 1-2 g (+ gentamicin)*	q6 hours
Ticarcillin-clavulante (Timentin), 3.2 g	q8 hours
Piperacilin-tazobactam (Zosyn), 3.375 g*	q6-8 hours
Imipenem-cilastatin, 250-500 mg	q6-8 hours

*Recommended regimen if enterococcus suspected

References, see page 372.

Early Syphilis

Syphilis is a chronic infection caused by the bacterium Treponema pallidum (Tp). Early syphilis is defined as the stages of syphilis that typically occur within the first year after infection. Early latent syphilis is defined as asymptomatic infection, with positive serology and a negative physical examination, when the date of infection can be established as having occurred within one year's time. Early syphilis is a reportable infection.

I. Clinical manifestations
   A. Early syphilis begins when an uninfected person acquires Tp, usually via direct contact with an infectious lesion during sex. The spirochete gains access at sites of minor trauma. Transmission occurs in one-third of patients exposed to early syphilis.
   B. Primary syphilis. After an average incubation period of two to three weeks, a painless papule appears at the site of inoculation. This soon ulcerates to produce the classic chancre of primary syphilis, a one to two centimeter ulcer with a raised, indurated margin. The ulcer has a non-exudative base and is associated with regional lymphadenopathy. Most lesions are seen on the genitalia. Chancres heal spontaneously within three to six weeks.
   C. Secondary syphilis. Weeks to a few months later, 25% of individuals with untreated infection will develop a systemic illness that represents secondary syphilis. Secondary syphilis can produce a wide variety of symptoms.
      1. Rash is the most characteristic finding of secondary syphilis. The rash is classically a symmetric papular eruption involving the entire trunk and extremities including the palms and soles. Individual lesions are discrete red or reddish-brown and measure 0.5 to 2 cm. They are often scaly but may be smooth and rarely pustular. The involvement of the palms and soles is an important clue to the diagnosis of secondary syphilis.
      2. Large, raised, gray to white lesions, involving warm, moist areas such as mucous membranes in the mouth or perineum, may develop in some patients during secondary syphilis. These are referred to as condyloma lata.

3. **Systemic symptoms** include fever, headache, malaise, anorexia, sore throat, myalgias, and weight loss.

4. **Diffuse lymphadenopathy.** Most patients with secondary syphilis have lymph node enlargement with palpable nodes present in the inguinal, axillary, posterior cervical, femoral, and/or epitrochlear regions. These nodes are generally minimally tender, firm, and rubbery in consistency.

5. **Alopecia.** "Moth-eaten" alopecia is occasionally seen among patients presenting with secondary syphilis. This condition is usually reversible with treatment.

6. **Neurologic abnormalities.** Central nervous system (CNS) syphilis may occur within the first few weeks after initial infection or up to 25 years later.

   a. The acute manifestations of secondary syphilis (including the neurologic abnormalities) typically resolve spontaneously, even in the absence of therapy.

   b. Indications for lumbar puncture are symptoms of meningitis or focal neurologic findings.

   c. **Early syphilis in HIV-infected patients.** There is a strong association between syphilis and the human immunodeficiency virus (HIV) infection.

   d. **Latent syphilis** refers to the period during which patients infected with Tp have no symptoms but have infection demonstrable by serologic testing. Early latent syphilis is defined as infection of one year's duration or less. All other cases are referred to as late latent syphilis or latent syphilis of unknown duration. A longer duration of therapy is recommended for patients with late latent syphilis.

II. **Diagnosis.** The chancre of primary syphilis is best diagnosed by darkfield microscopy, while secondary syphilis is reliably diagnosed by serologic testing.

A. **Serologic testing for syphilis**

1. **Darkfield microscopy.** The most rapid method for diagnosing primary and secondary syphilis is direct visualization of the spirochete from moist lesions by darkfield microscopy.

2. **Serologic tests.** Most patients suspected of having syphilis must be diagnosed by serologic testing. There are two types of serologic tests for syphilis: nontreponemal tests such as the Venereal Disease Research Laboratory (VDRL) test and the Rapid Plasma Reagin (RPR) test, and treponemal tests such as the fluorescent treponemal antibody absorption (FTA-ABS) test, the microhemagglutination test for antibodies to Treponema pallidum (MHA-TP), and the Treponema pallidum particle agglutination assay (TPPA).

   a. **Nontreponemal tests** are based upon the reactivity of serum from patients with syphilis to a cardiolipin-cholesterol-lecithin antigen. These tests measure IgG and IgM antibodies and are used as the screening test for syphilis. Positive tests are usually reported as a titer of antibody, and they can be used to follow the response to treatment in many patients.

   b. **Treponemal tests** are used as confirmatory tests when the nontreponemal tests are reactive. These tests all use T. pallidum antigens and are based upon the detection of antibodies directed against treponemal cellular components.

3. **Algorithm for screening and testing.** Serologic testing to diagnose syphilis is performed in two settings: screening of patients at increased risk and evaluation of patients with suspected disease.

   a. Screening is recommended for all pregnant women and people at higher risk of acquiring syphilis (MSM who engage in high risk behaviors, commercial sex workers, persons who exchange sex for drugs, and those in adult correctional facilities).

   b. Screening begins with a nontreponemal test such as the VDRL; a reactive specimen is then confirmed with a treponemal test such as the FTA-ABS.

    c. The most common cause of a false negative syphilis serologic test is performance prior to the development of antibodies. Twenty to 30 percent of patients presenting with a chancre will not yet have developed a reactive serologic test for syphilis.

4. **Monitoring the response to therapy.** The following reductions in reagin antibody titers are noted after recommended antibiotic therapy:

    a. Among patients with primary and secondary syphilis, a fourfold decline by six months and an eightfold decline by 12 months.

    b. Compared to those with primary and secondary syphilis, the rate of decline is slower among patients with early latent syphilis — fourfold decline by 12 months.

Causes of False-positive Tests for Syphilis		
Nontreponemal tests (VDRL, RPR) - acute	**Nontreponemal tests (VDRL, RPR) - chronic**	**Treponemal tests (FTA-ABS, MHA-TP)**
Pneumococcal pneumonia Scarlet fever Leprosy Lymphogranuloma venereum Relapsing fever infective endocarditis Malaria Rickettsial infections Psittacosis Leptospirosis Chancroid Tuberculosis Mycoplasma infections Trypanosomiasis Varicella infections HIV Measles Infectious mononucleosis Mumps Viral hepatitis Pregnancy	Chronic liver disease Malignancy (advanced) Injection drug use Myeloma Advanced age Connective tissue disease Multiple transfusions	Lyme borreliosis Leprosy Malaria Infectious mononucleosis Relapsing fever Leptospirosis Systemic lupus erythematosus

Indications for cerebrospinal fluid examination in patients with reactive syphilis serologic tests

Signs of neurosyphilis
    Weakness, pain, paresthesias, sensory changes in the legs
    Hyperactive deep tendon reflexes (later, absent DTRs)
    Loss of vibratory and position sense in the legs
    Broad-based, stamping gait
    Fecal or urinary incontinence
    Confusion, psychotic behavior, dementia

Signs of ophthalmic syphilis
    Chorioretinitis
    Acute optic neuritis
    Optic atrophy
    Pupillary abnormalities (small, fixed pupils that do not react to light)

Evidence of active tertiary syphilis
    Cardiovascular syphilis (aortic aneurysm, aortic regurgitation)
    Late benign syphilis (gummatous syphilis): most frequently involving bones, skin

Treatment failure
    In primary and secondary syphilis:
        Failure of non-treponemal test titer to decline fourfold after six months
        Failure of non-treponemal test titer to decline eightfold after twelve months
    In early latent syphilis
        Failure of non-treponemal test titer to decline fourfold after twelve months

HIV-infected patients with late latent syphilis or latent syphilis of unknown duration

III. Treatment of early syphilis

A. A single dose of benzathine penicillin G (2.4 million units IM) is standard therapy for all forms of early syphilis.

B. The single dose of benzathine penicillin as therapy is only appropriate when it is possible to document that there was a non-reactive syphilis serologic within the past year or if there is good documentation of the chancre of primary syphilis serology within the past year. Otherwise it should be referred to as latent syphilis of unknown duration for which three doses of benzathine penicillin at weekly intervals are recommended.

C. Some patients do not respond, based upon failure of serum VDRL titers to decrease at least fourfold over 6 to 12 months of follow-up. Some of these cases may be due to reinfection. Such treatment failures are managed by giving another course of benzathine penicillin, and all sexual contacts.

D. Patients with early syphilis who are allergic to penicillin may be treated with 14 days of either doxycycline (100 mg PO BID) or tetracycline (500 mg PO QID).

E. Azithromycin has also been considered as an option for penicillin-allergic patients. Azithromycin should be avoided in regions where azithromycin resistance is relatively common and in patients with frequent macrolide use (eg, MAC prophylaxis in HIV-infected patients).

F. There is no alternative to penicillin for the treatment of syphilis during pregnancy; penicillin allergic pregnant patients should be desensitized to penicillin.

Stages of Syphilitic Infection

Stage	Clinical manifestations	Diagnosis (sensitivity)	Treatment
Primary syphilis	Chancre	Dark-field microscopy of skin lesion (80%) Nontreponemal tests (78% to 86%) Treponemal-specific tests (76% to 84%)	Penicillin G benzathine, 2.4 million units IM (single dose) Alternatives in nonpregnant patients with penicillin allergy: doxycycline (Vibramycin), 100 mg orally twice daily for 2 weeks; tetracycline, 500 mg orally four times daily for 2 weeks; ceftriaxone (Rocephin), 1 g once daily IM or IV for 8 to 10 days; or azithromycin (Zithromax), 2 g orally (single dose)

Stage	Clinical manifestations	Diagnosis (sensitivity)	Treatment
Secondary syphilis	Skin and mucous membranes: diffuse rash, condyloma latum, other lesions Renal system: glomerulonephritis, nephrotic syndrome Liver: hepatitis Central nervous system: headache, meningismus, cranial neuropathy, iritis and uveitis Constitutional symptoms: fever, malaise, generalized lymphadenopathy, arthralgias, weight loss, others	Dark-field microscopy of skin lesion (80%) Nontreponemal tests (100%) Treponemal-specific tests (100%)	Same treatments as for primary syphilis
Latent syphilis	None	Nontreponemal tests (95% to 100%) Treponemal-specific tests (97% to 100%)	Early latent syphilis: same treatments as for primary and secondary syphilis Late latent syphilis: penicillin G benzathine, 2.4 million units IM once weekly for 3 weeks Alternatives in nonpregnant patients with penicillin allergy: doxycycline, 100 mg orally twice daily for 4 weeks; or tetracycline, 500 mg orally four times daily for 4 weeks
Tertiary (late) syphilis	Gummatous disease, cardiovascular disease	Nontreponemal tests (71% to 73%) Treponemal-specific tests (94% to 96%)	Same treatment as for late latent syphilis

Stage	Clinical mani-festations	Diagnosis (sensi-tivity)	Treatment
Neuro-syphilis	Seizures, ataxia, aphasia, paresis, hyperreflexia, personality changes, cog-nitive distur-bance, visual changes, hear-ing loss, neu-ropathy, loss of bowel or blad-der function, others	Cerebrospinal fluid examination	Aqueous crystalline penicillin G, 3 to 4 million units IV every 4 hours for 10 to 14 days; or penicillin G procaine, 2.4 million units IM once daily, plus probenecid, 500 mg orally four times daily, with both drugs given for 10 to 14 days

References, see page 372.

Gastrointestinal Disorders

Helicobacter Pylori Infection and Peptic Ulcer Disease

The spiral-shaped, gram-negative bacterium *Helicobacter pylori* is found in gastric mucosa or adherent to the lining of the stomach. Acute infection is most commonly asymptomatic but may be associated with epigastric burning, abdominal distention or bloating, belching, nausea, flatulence, and halitosis. *H. pylori* infection can lead to ulceration of the gastric mucosa and duodenum and is associated with malignancies of the stomach. The prevalence of *H. pylori* infection is as high as 52 percent.

I. Pathophysiology
   A. Helicobacter pylori (HP), a spiral-shaped, flagellated organism, is the most frequent cause of peptic ulcer disease (PUD). Nonsteroidal anti-inflammatory drugs (NSAIDs) and pathologically high acid-secreting states (Zollinger-Ellison syndrome) are less common causes. More than 90% of ulcers are associated with H. pylori. Eradication of the organism cures and prevents relapses of gastroduodenal ulcers.
   B. Complications of peptic ulcer disease include bleeding, duodenal or gastric perforation, and gastric outlet obstruction (due to inflammation or strictures).

II. Clinical evaluation
   A. Symptoms of PUD include recurrent upper abdominal pain and discomfort. The pain of duodenal ulceration is often relieved by food and antacids and worsened when the stomach is empty (eg, at nighttime). In gastric ulceration, the pain may be exacerbated by eating.
   B. Nausea and vomiting are common in PUD. Hematemesis ("coffee ground" emesis) or melena (black tarry stools) are indicative of bleeding.
   C. Physical examination. Tenderness to deep palpation is often present in the epigastrium, and the stool is often guaiac-positive.

Presentation of Uncomplicated Peptic Ulcer Disease

Epigastric pain (burning, vague abdominal discomfort, nausea)
   Often nocturnal
   Occurs with hunger or hours after meals
   Usually temporarily relieved by meals or antacids
   Persistence or recurrence over months to years
   History of self-medication and intermittent relief

   D. NSAID-related gastrointestinal complications. NSAID use and *H pylori* infection are independent risk factors for peptic ulcer disease. The risk is 5 to 20 times higher in persons who use NSAIDs than in the general population. Misoprostol (Cytotec) has been shown to prevent both NSAID ulcers and related complications. The minimum effective dosage is 200 micrograms twice daily; total daily doses of 600 micrograms or 800 micrograms are significantly more effective.

III. Indications for testing and treatment
   A. In the absence of alarm symptoms for cancer or complicated ulcer disease, the approach to testing in patients with dyspepsia can be divided into four clinical scenarios: (1) known peptic ulcer disease, currently or previously

documented; (2) known nonulcer dyspepsia; (3) undifferentiated dyspepsia, and (4) gastroesophageal reflux disease (GERD).

B. Peptic ulcer disease. Treatment of *H. pylori* infection in patients with ulcers almost always cures the disease and reduces the risk for perforation or bleeding.

C. Nonulcer disease. There is no convincing evidence that empiric eradication of *H. pylori* in patients with nonulcer dyspepsia improves symptoms.

D. Undifferentiated dyspepsia. A test-and-treat strategy is recommended in which patients with dyspepsia are tested for the presence of *H. pylori* with serology and treated with eradication therapy if the results are positive. Endoscopy is reserved for use in patients with alarm signs or those with persistent symptoms despite empiric therapy.

Alarm Signs for Risk of Gastric Cancer of Complicated Ulcer Disease

Older Than 45 years	Abdominal mass
Rectal bleeding or melena	Jaundice
Weight los of >10 percent of body weight	Family history of gastric cancer
Anemia	Previous history of peptic ulcer
Dysphagia	Anorexia/early satiety

Evaluation for Helicobacter pylori-Related Disease

Clinical scenario	Recommended test
Dyspepsia in patient with alarm symptoms for cancer or complicated ulcer (eg, bleeding, perforation)	Promptly refer to a gastroenterologist for endoscopy.
Known PUD, uncomplicated	Serology antibody test; treat if result is positive.
Dyspepsia in patient with previous history of PUD not previously treated with eradication therapy	Serology antibody test; treat if result is positive.
Dyspepsia in patient with PUD previously treated for *H. pylori*	Stool antigen or urea breath test; if positive, treat with regimen different from the one previously used; retest to confirm eradication. Consider endoscopy.
Undifferentiated dyspepsia (without endoscopy)	Serology antibody test; treat if result is positive.
Documented nonulcer dyspepsia (after endoscopy)	Unnecessary
GERD	Unnecessary
Asymptomatic with history of documented PUD not previously treated with eradication therapy	Serology antibody test; treat if result is positive.
Asymptomatic	Screening unnecessary

E. **Gastroesophageal Reflux Disease.** *H. pylori* infection does not increase the risk of GERD. Eradication therapy does not eliminate GERD symptoms (sensation of burning and regurgitation.

IV. *Helicobacter pylori* Tests

A. Once testing and eradication are chosen, several diagnostic tests are available. Unless endoscopy is planned, a practical approach is to use serology to identify initial infection, and use the stool antigen test or urea breath test to determine cure, if indicated.

Noninvasive Testing Options for Detecting Helicobacter pylori				
Test	What does it measure?	Sensitivity	Test of cure?	Comments
Serology: laboratory-based ELISA	IgG	90 to 93	No	Accurate; convenient for initial infection; titers may remain positive after one year
Whole blood: office-based ELISA	IgG	50 to 85	No	Less accurate but fast, convenient
Stool: HpSA	*H. pylori* antigens	95 to 98	Yes	Relatively convenient and available
Urea breath test	Urease activity	95 to 100	Yes	Sensitivity reduced by acid suppression

B. **Endoscopy and Biopsy.** Alarm symptoms for cancer or ulcer complication warrant prompt endoscopic evaluation. A gastric antral biopsy specimens is considered the gold standard for detecting the presence of *H. pylori*. Cultures of biopsy specimens obtained during endoscopy can be tested for antimicrobial resistance in cases of treatment failure.

C. **Serology/ELISA.** When endoscopy is not performed, the most commonly used diagnostic approach is the laboratory-based serologic antibody test. This enzyme-linked immunosorbent assay (ELISA) detects IgG antibodies to *H. pylori*, indicating current or past infection. A positive serologic test suggests active infection in patients who have not undergone eradication therapy. The serologic test results may not revert to negative once the organism is eradicated; therefore, the test is not used to identify persistent infection.

D. **Stool testing with enzyme-linked immunoassay** for *H. pylori* antigen in stool specimens is highly sensitive and specific, the stool antigen test reverts to negative from five days to a few months after eradication of the organism, with 90 percent specificity. This test is useful in confirming eradication, and, because it is office-based, is less costly and more convenient than the urea breath test. False-positive results may occur even four weeks following eradication therapy.

E. **Urea Breath Test.** The urea breath test is a reliable test for cure and can detect the presence or absence of active *H. pylori* infection with greater accuracy than the serologic test. It is usually administered in the hospital outpatient setting because it requires time and special equipment.

V. Treatment Regimens for Helicobacter Pylori

A. Initial treatment

1. The regimen of choice is triple therapy with a proton pump inhibitor (eg, lansoprazole 30 mg twice daily, omeprazole (Prilosec) 20 mg twice daily, pantoprazole (Protonix) 40 mg twice daily, rabeprazole (AcipHex) 20 mg twice daily, or esomeprazole (Nexium) 40 mg once daily), amoxicillin (1 g twice daily), and clarithromycin (500 mg twice daily) for two weeks (10 days may be adequate). The combination of lansoprazole, amoxicillin and clarithromycin is available in a daily-dose package, Prevpac.

2. Metronidazole (Flagyl [500 mg twice daily]) can be substituted for amoxicillin but only in penicillin-allergic individuals since metronidazole resistance is common.

3. A proton pump inhibitor (PPI) may be combined with bismuth (525 mg four times daily) and two antibiotics (eg, metronidazole 500 mg four times daily and tetracycline 500 mg four times daily) for two weeks. One week of bismuth based treatment may be sufficient as long as it is given with a PPI.

Triple Therapy Regimens for *Helicobacter pylori* Infection		
Treatment (10 to 14 days of therapy recommended)	Convenience factor	Tolerability
1. Omeprazole (Prilosec), 20 mg two times daily *or* Lansoprazole (Prevacid), 30 mg two times daily *plus* Metronidazole (Flagyl), 500 mg two times daily *or* Amoxicillin, 1 g two times daily *plus* Clarithromycin (Biaxin), 500 mg two times daily **Prepackaged triple-therapy(Prevpac)**: taken bid for 14 days; consists of 30 mg lansoprazole, 1 g amoxicillin, and 500 mg clarithromycin.	Twice-daily dosing	Fewer significant side effects, but more abnormal taste versus other regimens
2. Ranitidine bismuth citrate (Tritec), 400 mg twice daily *plus* Clarithromycin, 500 mg twice daily *or* Metronidazole, 500 mg twice daily *plus* Tetracycline, 500 mg twice daily *or* Amoxicillin, 1 g twice daily 92 (RMA)	Twice-daily dosing	Increased diarrhea versus other regimens

4. Dual therapy regimens using a PPI plus one antibiotic have eradication rates significantly lower (60 to 85 percent) than the standard regimens.

5. One-week treatment protocols have ulcer healing rates of 90 percent and H. pylori eradication rates of 77 to >85 percent.

B. Treatment failures.
Initial eradication of H. pylori fails in 5 to 12 percent of patients. For patients failing one course of H. pylori treatment, quadruple therapy consisting of a PPI twice daily and bismuth-based triple therapy (Pepto Bismol 2 tablets, tetracycline 500 mg, and high dose metronidazole 500 mg all four times daily) preferably given with meals for 14 days is recom-

mended. Two weeks should be the duration of subsequent courses of treatment.

C. **Side effects** are reported in up to 50 percent of patients taking one of the triple agent regimens:

1. The most common side effect is a metallic taste due to metronidazole or clarithromycin.
2. Metronidazole can cause peripheral neuropathy, seizures, and a disulfiram-like reaction when taken with alcohol.
3. Tetracycline can induce a photosensitivity reaction. It should not be administered to pregnant women.
4. Amoxicillin can cause diarrhea or an allergic reaction.
5. Bismuth side effects are rare. Proton pump inhibitors have no significant documented adverse effects.

D. **Treatment of NSAID-related ulcers**

1. When the ulcer is caused by NSAID use, healing of the ulcer is greatly facilitated by discontinuing the NSAID. Acid antisecretory therapy with an H2-blocker or proton pump inhibitor speeds ulcer healing. Proton pump inhibitors are more effective in inhibiting gastric acid production and are often used to heal ulcers in patients who require continuing NSAID treatment.
2. If serologic or endoscopic testing for H pylori is positive, antibiotic treatment is necessary.
3. **Acute H$_2$-blocker therapy**
   a. **Ranitidine (Zantac)**, 150 mg bid or 300 mg qhs.
   b. **Famotidine (Pepcid)**, 20 mg bid or 40 mg qhs.
   c. **Nizatidine (Axid Pulvules)**, 150 mg bid or 300 mg qhs.
   d. **Cimetidine (Tagamet)**, 400 mg bid or 800 mg qhs.
4. **Proton pump inhibitors**
   a. **Omeprazole (Prilosec)**, 20 mg qd.
   b. **Lansoprazole (Prevacid)**, 15 mg before breakfast qd.
   c. **Esomeprazole (Nexium)** 20-40 mg qd.
   d. **Pantoprazole (Protonix)** 40 mg PO, 20 minuted before the first meal of the day or IV once daily.
   e. **Rabeprazole (AcipHex)** 20 mg/day, 20 to 30 minutes before the first meal of the day.

VI. **Surgical treatment of peptic ulcer disease**

A. **Indications for surgery** include exsanguinating hemorrhage, >5 units transfusion in 24 hours, rebleeding during same hospitalization, intractability, perforation, gastric outlet obstruction, and endoscopic signs of rebleeding.

B. Unstable patients should receive a truncal vagotomy, oversewing of bleeding ulcer bed, and pyloroplasty.

References, see page 372.

Gastroesophageal Reflux Disease

Gastroesophageal reflux disease is caused by the combination of excess reflux of gastric juice and impaired clearance of this refluxate from the esophagus. GERD is defined as symptoms or tissue damage caused by reflux of gastric contents with or without esophageal inflammation.

I. Clinical manifestations

A. Typical symptoms of GERD are heartburn and regurgitation; atypical symptoms include odynophagia, dysphagia, chest pain, cough, and reactive airway disease. Up to half of the general population has monthly heartburn or regurgitation.

B. Heartburn, the most common symptom of GERD, is a substernal burning sensation that rises from the upper abdomen into the chest and neck. Dysphagia, the sensation that swallowed material is lodged in the chest, may be caused by esophageal inflammation or impaired motility. Esophageal cancer also is an important differential diagnostic consideration when dysphagia is the presenting complaint.

Symptoms of GERD

Heartburn (pyrosis)	Chronic cough
Regurgitation	Nocturnal cough
Dysphagia	Asthma
Water brash	Dyspepsia
Globus	Hiccups
Odynophagia	Chest pain
Hoarseness	Nausea

C. Chest pain due to GERD can mimic angina. Extraesophageal manifestations of GERD include asthma, chronic cough, sinusitis, pneumonitis, laryngitis, hoarseness, hiccups, and dental disease. Complications of long-standing GERD include esophageal stricture and Barrett's esophagus.

Differential diagnostic considerations in GERD

Esophageal neoplasm	Nonulcer dyspepsia
Infectious esophagitis	Coronary artery disease
Caustic esophagitis	Hepatobiliary disease
Pill esophagitis	Esophageal motility disorders
Gastritis	Cholelithiasis
Peptic ulcer disease	

II. Diagnosis

A. Diagnosis of GERD is often based on clinical findings and confirmed by the response to therapy. Diagnostic evaluation should be pursued if symptoms are chronic or refractory to therapy or if esophageal or extra-esophageal complications are suspected.

Indications for esophageal endoscopy in patients with GERD

Dysphagia or odynophagia
Persistent or progressive symptoms despite therapy
Esophageal symptoms in an immunocompromised patient
Mass, stricture, or ulcer on upper gastrointestinal barium study
Gastrointestinal bleeding or iron deficiency anemia
At least 10 years of GERD symptoms (screen for Barrett's esophagus)

B. Ambulatory esophageal pH monitoring is performed by placing a pH electrode just above the lower esophageal sphincter. This test has a sensitivity of 60-100%.

    C. Short PPI trials are useful for diagnosis of GERD and have a sensitivity of 70 to 90% and specificity of 55 to 85%.

III. **Treatment options**
  A. **Lifestyle modification.** Strategies include elevation of the head of the bed 6 to 8 in; reduced consumption of fatty foods, chocolate, alcohol, colas, red wine, citrus juices, and tomato products; avoidance of the supine position after meals; not eating within 3 hours of bedtime; avoidance of tight-fitting clothing; weight loss if obese; and smoking cessation.
  B. Although H_2-blockers are less expensive than PPIs, PPIs provide superior acid suppression, healing rates and symptom relief. Therefore, PPIs may be more cost-effective than H_2-blockers, especially in patients with more severe acid-peptic disorders, because of their lower and less frequent dosing requirements and their comparatively shorter duration of required therapy.
  C. **Histamine$_2$-blockers** are used extensively. The four available agents, cimetidine (Tagamet), famotidine (Pepcid), nizatidine (Axid), and ranitidine (Zantac), are equivalent. Dosage must be reduced in patients with renal failure. In general, doses of H_2 blockers required to control GERD symptoms and heal esophagitis are two to three times higher than those needed for treatment of peptic ulcer disease. Rates of symptom control and healing are about 50%.
    1. **Cimetidine (Tagamet)**, 800 mg twice daily; **ranitidine (Zantac)**, 150 mg four times daily; **famotidine (Pepcid)**, 40 mg twice daily; and **nizatidine (Axid)**, 150 mg twice daily.
  D. **Proton pump inhibitors (PPIs)** irreversibly bind and inhibit the proton pump.
    1. The five available PPIs, esomeprazole (Nexium), lansoprazole (Prevacid), omeprazole (Prilosec), pantoprazole (Protonix), and rabeprazole (AcipHex), have similar pharmacologic activities. PPIs should be taken 20 to 30 minutes before the first meal of the day. PPIs are more effective than are H2 blockers.
    2. In contrast to the other Proton Pump Inhibitors (PPIs), rabeprazole (AcipHex) forms a partially reversible bond with the proton pump. Therefore, it may have a more sustained acid-suppressing effect than the other PPIs. Rabeprazole and pantoprazole, seem to have fewer drug interactions. Pantoprazole is the least expensive.

Proton Pump Inhibitors	
Drug	**Dosage**
Esomeprazole - *Nexium*	20 mg or 40 mg, 20 to 30 minutes before the first meal of the day
Lansoprazole - *Prevacid*	30 mg, 20 to 30 minutes before the first meal of the day
Omeprazole - *Prilosec*, generic	20 mg/day, 20 to 30 minutes before the first meal of the day
Pantoprazole - *Protonix*	40 mg PO, 20 minuted before the first meal of the day or IV once daily
Rabeprazole - *AcipHex*	20 mg/day, 20 to 30 minutes before the first meal of the day

E. **Surgical treatment.** The most common of the antireflux procedures used to treat GERD is the Nissen fundoplication, which is a laparoscopic procedure. A portion of the stomach is wrapped around the distal esophagus. Indications include patient preference for surgical treatment over prolonged medical therapy, incomplete control despite medical therapy, and refractory manifestations of reflux (eg, pneumonia, laryngitis, asthma).

IV. **Management considerations**

A. Patients with frequent or unrelenting symptoms or esophagitis, or both, should be treated at the outset with a PPI once or twice daily as appropriate.

B. **Refractory GERD.** Increasing the dosage of PPIs often can control GERD in patients receiving a single daily dose. Sometimes switching to a different PPI can improve symptoms. Antireflux surgical treatment is an alternative.

Alternative diagnoses in patients with refractory GERD	
Esophageal hypersensitivity (visceral hyperalgesia)	Caustic exposure
Achalasia	Impaired gastric emptying
Distal esophageal cancer	Eosinophilic gastroenteritis
Stricture	Bile acid reflux
NSAID-induced symptoms	Nonulcer dyspepsia
Infection (eg, Candida, herpes, cytomegalovirus esophagitis)	Pill esophagitis

References, see page 372.

Abnormal Liver Function Tests

The most common liver function tests include the enzyme tests (serum aminotransferases, alkaline phosphatase, gamma glutamyl transpeptidase), tests of synthetic function (serum albumin concentration, prothrombin time), and serum bilirubin, which reflects hepatic transport capability.

I. Epidemiology

A. Abnormal liver function tests (LFTs) are frequently detected in asymptomatic patients. Serious underlying liver disease is uncommon. Abnormal serum aminotransferase levels are detected in 0.5 percent. A cause is found in only 12 percent (including chronic hepatitis B and C, autoimmune hepatitis, and cholelithiasis). No specific diagnosis can be established in 87 percent.

B. A diagnosis can be established noninvasively in most patients with abnormal LFTs. The majority of patients in whom the diagnosis remains unclear after obtaining a history and laboratory testing will have alcoholic liver disease, steatosis, or steatohepatitis.

C. **History.** Important considerations include exposure to any chemical or medication (including over-the-counter medications) which may be temporally related to the onset of LFT abnormalities.

1. The duration of LFT abnormalities.

2. The presence jaundice, arthralgias, myalgias, rash, anorexia, weight loss, abdominal pain, fever, pruritus, and changes in the urine and stool.

3. A history of arthralgias and myalgias predating jaundice suggests viral or drug-related hepatitis, while jaundice associated with the sudden onset of severe right upper quadrant pain and shaking chills suggests choledocholithiasis and ascending cholangitis.

    4. Transfusions, intravenous and intranasal drug use, tattoos, and sexual activity should be assessed. Recent travel history, exposure to people with jaundice, exposure to possibly contaminated foods, occupational exposure to hepatotoxins, and alcohol consumption should be assessed.

II. Physical examination

A. Temporal and proximal muscle wasting suggest longstanding diseases.

B. Stigmata of chronic liver disease include spider nevi, palmar erythema, gynecomastia, caput medusae.

C. Dupuytren's contractures, parotid gland enlargement, and testicular atrophy are commonly seen in advanced Laennec's cirrhosis and occasionally in other types of cirrhosis.

D. An enlarged left supraclavicular node (Virchow's node) or periumbilical nodule (Sister Mary Joseph's nodule) suggest an abdominal malignancy.

E. Jugular venous distension, a sign of right sided heart failure, suggests hepatic congestion

F. A right pleural effusion may be seen in advanced cirrhosis.

G. The abdominal examination should focus upon the size and consistency of the liver, the size of the spleen (a palpable spleen is enlarged), and should include an assessment for ascites (fluid wave or shifting dullness).

H. Patients with cirrhosis may have an enlarged left lobe of the liver (which can be felt below the xiphoid) and an enlarged spleen. A grossly enlarged nodular liver or an obvious abdominal mass suggests malignancy. An enlarged tender liver could be viral or alcoholic hepatitis or, less often, an acutely congested liver secondary to right-sided heart failure.

I. Severe right upper quadrant tenderness with respiratory arrest on inspiration (Murphy's sign) suggests cholecystitis or, occasionally, ascending cholangitis. Ascites in the presence of jaundice suggests either cirrhosis or malignancy with peritoneal spread.

III. Laboratory testing

A. A critical step in guiding the evaluation is determining the overall pattern of the abnormal LFTs, which can be broadly divided into two categories:

    1. Patterns predominantly reflecting hepatocellular injury.

    2. Patterns predominantly reflecting cholestasis.

B. aminotransferases compared with the alkaline phosphatase, while those with a cholestatic process have the opposite findings. The serum bilirubin can be prominently elevated in both hepatocellular and cholestatic conditions and therefore is not helpful in differentiating between the two.

C. The serum albumin and a prothrombin time should be obtained to assess liver function. A low albumin suggests a chronic process such as cirrhosis or cancer, while a normal albumin suggests a more acute process such as viral hepatitis or choledocholithiasis. An elevated prothrombin time indicates either vitamin K deficiency due to prolonged jaundice and malabsorption of vitamin K or significant hepatocellular dysfunction. The failure of the prothrombin time to correct with parenteral administration of vitamin K indicates severe hepatocellular injury.

D. The presence of bilirubin in the urine reflects direct hyperbilirubinemia and underlying hepatobiliary disease.

IV. Mild chronic elevation in serum aminotransferases. The laboratory evaluation of patients with chronic (≥six months), mild elevation (<250 U/L) of one or both of the aminotransferases is as follows:

A. Step one. Medication that can cause elevation of the serum aminotransferases, alcohol use, and testing viral hepatitis B and C, hemochromatosis, and fatty liver should be performed.

    1. Medications. Almost any medication can cause an elevation of liver enzymes. Common ones include nonsteroidal anti-inflammatory drugs, antibiotics, HMG-CoA reductase inhibitors, antiepileptic drugs, and antituberculous drugs. Herbal preparations and illicit drug use may also be the cause.

2. **Alcohol abuse** should be assessed by history. The diagnosis is supported by an AST to ALT ratio of 2:1 or greater. A twofold elevation of the gamma glutamyltransferase (GGT) in patients whose AST to ALT ratio is greater than 2:1 strongly suggests alcohol abuse. It is rare for the AST to be greater than eightfold elevated and even less common for the ALT to be greater than fivefold elevated.

3. **Hepatitis B.** Risk for hepatitis B is increased in patients with a history of parenteral exposures and in patients from southeast Asia, China, and sub-Saharan Africa.

   a. Initial testing for patients suspected of having chronic hepatitis B includes:
      (1) Hepatitis B surface antigen.
      (2) Hepatitis B surface antibody.
      (3) Hepatitis B core antibody.

   b. Patients who are surface antigen and core antibody positive are chronically infected and additional testing (hepatitis B "e" antigen and "e" antibody and a hepatitis B DNA) is indicated. A positive HBsAb and HBcAb indicates immunity to hepatitis B and another cause of aminotransferase elevation should be sought.

   c. The presence of a positive HBV DNA in the presence or absence of the "e" antigen indicates viral replication. A positive HBV DNA and a negative "e" antigen indicates that the patient has a precore mutant of hepatitis B. Both of these situations warrant further evaluation with a liver biopsy and possible treatment.

   d. A positive hepatitis B surface antigen with a negative HBV DNA and a negative "e" antigen suggests that the patient is a carrier of hepatitis B and in a non-replicative state. The presence of a carrier state does not explain elevated aminotransferases and another cause should be sought.

4. **Hepatitis C.** Chronic hepatitis C is very common in the United States. Approximately 3.9 million Americans are positive for the antibody to hepatitis C and an 2.7 million people are chronically infected. The risk is highest in individuals with a history of parenteral exposure (blood transfusions, intravenous drug use, occupational), cocaine use, tattoos, body piercing, and high risk sexual behavior.

   a. The initial test for hepatitis C is the hepatitis C antibody. It has a sensitivity of 92 to 97 percent. A positive hepatitis C antibody in a patient with risk factors for the infection is sufficient to make the diagnosis and a quantitative hepatitis C RNA, hepatitis C genotype, and liver biopsy should next be done to assess the need for treatment.

   b. A positive hepatitis C antibody in a low-risk patient should be verified with either a RIBA or a qualitative PCR test. A negative hepatitis C antibody in a patient with risk factors for hepatitis C should be verified with a qualitative PCR test.

5. **Hereditary hemochromatosis (HHC)** is a common genetic disorder. The frequency of heterozygotes is about 10 percent in Caucasians, with a frequency of about 0.5 percent for the homozygous state. Screening should begin with a serum iron and total iron binding capacity (TIBC), which permits the calculation of the iron or transferrin saturation (serum iron/TIBC). An iron saturation of greater than 45 percent warrants obtaining a serum ferritin. A serum ferritin concentration of greater than 400 ng/mL in men and 300 ng/mL in women further supports the diagnosis of HHC.

6. **Hepatic steatosis and non-steatohepatitis (NASH)** may present with mild elevations of the serum aminotransferases, which are usually less than

fourfold elevated. NASH is more common in women and associated with obesity and type 2 diabetes. In contrast to alcohol related liver disease, the ratio of AST to ALT is usually less than one. The initial evaluation to identify the presence of fatty infiltration of the liver is ultrasound, computed tomographic imaging, or magnetic resonance imaging.

B. Step two. The next set of tests should look for non-hepatic causes of elevated aminotransferases, which include principally muscle disorders and thyroid disease. Much less common causes are occult celiac disease and adrenal insufficiency.

  1. **Muscle disorders.** Elevated serum aminotransferases, especially AST, may be caused by disorders that affect striated muscle, such as inborn errors of muscle metabolism, polymyositis, and heavy exercise. If striated muscle is the source of increased aminotransferases, serum levels of creatine kinase and aldolase will be elevated.

  2. **Thyroid disorders** can produce elevated aminotransferases. TSH is a reasonable screening test for hypothyroidism while a set of thyroid function tests should be checked if hyperthyroidism is suspected.

  3. **Celiac disease.** The serum AST ranges from 29 to 80, and the serum ALT ranges from 60 to 130 with the ALT usually slightly greater than AST. Serum aminotransferases return to normal following a gluten-free diet. The diagnosis is suggested by antibody screening.

  4. **Adrenal insufficiency.** Aminotransferase elevation (1.5 to 3 times normal) has been described in patients with adrenal insufficiency (due to Addison's disease or secondary causes). Aminotransferases normalize within one week following treatment.

C. Step three. The next set of tests is aimed at identifying rarer liver conditions.

  1. **Autoimmune hepatitis (AIH)** is a condition found primarily in young to middle-aged women. The diagnosis is based upon elevated serum aminotransferases, the absence of other causes of chronic hepatitis, and serological evidence of AIH.

    a. A useful screening test for AIH is the serum protein electrophoresis (SPEP). Additional tests include antinuclear antibodies (ANA), anti-smooth muscle antibodies (SMA), and liver-kidney microsomal antibodies (LKMA).

  2. **Wilson's disease,** a genetic disorder of biliary copper excretion, may cause elevated aminotransferases in asymptomatic patients. The prevalence of Wilson's disease is very low.

    a. Patients usually present between ages 5 to 25, but the diagnosis should be considered in patients up to the age of 40. The initial screening test for Wilson's disease is a serum ceruloplasmin. If the ceruloplasmin is normal and Kayser-Fleischer rings are absent, but there is still a suspicion of Wilson's disease, the next test is a 24-hour urine collection for quantitative copper excretion.

  3. **Alpha-1-antitrypsin deficiency** is an uncommon cause of chronic liver disease in adults. Obtaining an alpha-1-antitrypsin phenotype is the most cost-effective test. In adults, alpha-1-antitrypsin deficiency should be suspected in patients who have a history of emphysema.

D. Step four. A liver biopsy is often considered in patients in whom all of the above testing has been unyielding. However, in some settings, the best course may be observation.

  1. **Who to observe.** Observation is recommended only in patients in whom the ALT and AST are less than twofold elevated and no chronic liver condition has been identified by the above noninvasive testing.

  2. **Who to biopsy.** A liver biopsy is recommended in patients in whom the ALT and AST are persistently greater than twofold elevated.

V. Isolated hyperbilirubinemia occurs principally in two settings:
  A. Overproduction of bilirubin.
  B. Impaired uptake, conjugation, or excretion of bilirubin.
  C. The initial step in evaluating an isolated elevated hyperbilirubinemia is to fractionate the bilirubin to determine whether the hyperbilirubinemia is predominantly conjugated or unconjugated.
    1. Unconjugated hyperbilirubinemia results from either overproduction, impairment of uptake, or impaired conjugation of bilirubin.
    2. Conjugated hyperbilirubinemia is caused by decreased excretion into the bile ductules or backward leakage of the pigment. It is characterized by mild hyperbilirubinemia (with a direct-reacting fraction of 50 percent) in the absence of other abnormalities of liver function tests. Normal levels of serum alkaline phosphatase and gamma-glutamyltranspepetidase help to distinguish these conditions from disorders associated with biliary obstruction.

Hepatocellular Conditions That Can Produce Jaundice
Viral hepatitis Hepatitis A, B, C, and E Epstein-Barr virus Cytomegalovirus
Alcohol
Drugs Predictable, dose-dependent (eg, acetaminophen) Unpredictable, idiosyncratic (many drugs)
Environment toxins Vinyl chloride Jamaica bush tea - Pyrrolizidine alkaloids
Autoimmune hepatitis
Wilson's disease

Classification of jaundice according to type of bile pigment and mechanism	
Unconjugated hyperbilirubinemia	**Conjugated hyperbilirubinemia**

Increased bilirubin production
    Extravascular hemolysis
    Extravasation of blood into tissues
    Dyserythropoiesis
Impaired hepatic bilirubin uptake
    Congestive hear failure
    Portosystemic shunts
    Some patients with Gilbert's syndrome
    Certain Drugs - rifampin, probenecid,
        flavaspidic acid, bunamiodyl
Impaired bilirubin conjugation
    Crigler-Najjar syndrome type I and II
    Gilbert's syndrome
    Neonates
    Hyperthyroidism
    Ethinyl estradiol
    Liver diseases - chronic persistent hepa-
        titis, advanced cirrhosis, Wilson's dis-
        ease
	Extrahepatic cholestasis (biliary obstruc-
	    tion)
	    Choledocholithiasis
	    Intrinsic and extrinsic tumors (eg,
	        cholangiocarcinoma)
	    Primary sclerosing cholangitis
	    AIDS cholangiopathy
	    Strictures after invasive procedures
	    Certain parasitic infections (eg, Ascaris
	        lumbricoides, liver flukes
	Intrahepatic cholestasis
	    Viral hepatitis
	    Nonalcoholic hepatitis
	    Primary biliary cirrhosis
	    Drugs and toxins (eg, alkylated steroids,
	        chlorpromazine, herbal medications
	        [eg, Jamaican bush tea], arsenic)
	    Sepsis and hypoperfusion states
	    Infiltrative diseases (eg, amyloidosis,
	        lymphoma, sarcoidosis, tuberculosis
	    Total parenteral nutrition
	    Postoperative patient
	    Following organ transplantation
	    Hepatic crisis in sickle cell disease
	    Pregnancy
	    End-stage liver disease
	Hepatocellular injury

D. **Isolated elevation of the alkaline phosphatase and/or gamma glutamyl transpeptidase.** Serum alkaline phosphatase is derived predominantly from the liver and bones. Individuals with blood types O and B can have elevated serum alkaline phosphatase after eating a fatty meal due to an influx of intestinal alkaline phosphatase.

E. **Determining the source of the alkaline phosphatase.** The first step in the evaluation of an elevated alkaline phosphatase is to identify its source. Electrophoretic separation is the most sensitive and specific method.

F. **Initial testing for alkaline phosphatase of hepatic origin.** Chronic cholestatic or infiltrative liver diseases should be considered in patients in whom the alkaline phosphatase is determined to be of liver origin and persists over time. The most common causes include partial bile duct obstruction, primary biliary cirrhosis (PBC), primary sclerosing cholangitis, adult bile ductopenia, and androgenic steroids and phenytoin. Infiltrative diseases include sarcoidosis, other granulomatous diseases, and cancer metastatic to the liver.

   1. Initial testing should include a right upper quadrant ultrasound (which can assess the hepatic parenchyma and bile ducts) and an antimitochondrial antibody (AMA), which is highly suggestive of PBC. The presence of biliary dilatation suggests obstruction of the biliary tree.

G. **Patients in whom initial testing is unrevealing.** A liver biopsy and either an ERCP or magnetic resonance cholangiopancreatogram (MRCP) are recommended if the AMA and ultrasound are both negative and the alkaline phosphatase is persistently more than 50 percent above normal for more than six months. If the alkaline phosphatase is less than 50 percent above normal, all of the other liver tests are normal, and the patient is asymptomatic, observation alone is suggested.

H. Gamma glutamyl transpeptidase. Gamma glutamyl transpeptidase (GGT) is found in hepatocytes and biliary epithelial cells. GGT is very sensitive for detecting hepatobiliary disease. Elevated levels of serum GGT have been reported in pancreatic disease, myocardial infarction, renal failure, chronic obstructive pulmonary disease, diabetes, and alcoholism. High serum GGT values are also found in patients taking phenytoin and barbiturates.

1. GGT is best used to evaluate elevations of other serum enzyme tests (eg, to confirm the liver origin of an elevated alkaline phosphatase or to support a suspicion of alcohol abuse in a patient with an elevated AST and an AST:ALT ratio of greater than 2:1). An elevated GGT with otherwise normal liver tests should not lead to an exhaustive work-up for liver disease.

VI. Evaluation of patients with simultaneous elevation of several LFTs. Patients should be divided into those with a predominantly hepatocellular process and those with a predominantly cholestatic process. Patients with a predominantly cholestatic pattern may be further divided into those with intra- or extrahepatic cholestasis.

A. While ALT and AST values less than eight times normal may be seen in either hepatocellular or cholestatic liver disease, values 25 times normal or higher are seen primarily in hepatocellular diseases.

B. Predominantly hepatocellular pattern with jaundice. Common hepatocellular diseases that can cause jaundice include viral and toxic hepatitis (including drugs, herbal therapies, alcohol) and end-stage cirrhosis from any cause. Wilson's disease should be considered in young adults.

1. **Autoimmune hepatitis** predominantly occurs in young to middle-aged women (although it may affect men and women of any age) and should particularly be considered in patients who have other autoimmune diseases.

2. **Alcoholic hepatitis** can be differentiated from viral and toxin related hepatitis by the pattern of the serum aminotransferases. Patients with alcoholic hepatitis typically have an AST:ALT ratio of at least 2:1. The AST rarely exceeds 300 U/L. In contrast, patients with acute viral hepatitis and toxin related injury severe enough to produce jaundice typically have aminotransferases greater than 500 U/L with the ALT greater than or equal to the AST.

3. **Viral hepatitis.** Patients with acute viral hepatitis can develop jaundice. Testing for acute viral hepatitis includes a:

4. Hepatitis A IgM antibody.

5. Hepatitis B surface antigen.

6. Hepatitis B core IgM antibody.

7. Hepatitis C viral RNA.

8. Patients with acute hepatitis C are usually asymptomatic. Testing for acute HCV should be performed by requesting an assay for serum hepatitis C viral RNA since hepatitis C antibody may take weeks to months to become detectable.

C. Toxic hepatitis. Drug-induced hepatocellular injury can be classified either as predictable or unpredictable. Predictable drug reactions are dose-dependent and affect all patients who ingest a toxic dose of the drug in question (eg, acetaminophen hepatotoxicity). Unpredictable, or idiosyncratic, drug reactions are not dose dependent and occur in a minority of patients. Virtually any drug can cause an idiosyncratic reaction. Environmental toxins are also an important cause of hepatocellular injury. Examples include industrial chemicals such as vinyl chloride, herbal preparations (Jamaica bush tea), and the mushrooms Amanita phalloides or verna containing highly hepatotoxic amatoxins.

D. **Shock liver (ischemic hepatitis).** Patients who have a prolonged period of systemic hypotension (cardiac arrest, severe heart failure) may develop ischemic injury to the liver. Aminotransferases levels may be exceeding high (1000 IU/L or 50 times the upper limit of normal) and lactic dehydrogenase may be seen. Patients may also develop jaundice, hypoglycemia, and hepatic synthetic dysfunction. The majority of patients have deterioration of renal function. Hepatic function usually returns to normal within several days of the acute episode.

E. **Wilson's disease** can occasionally present with acute and even fulminant hepatitis. The diagnosis should be considered in patients younger than 40, particularly those who have concomitant hemolytic anemia.

VII. **Predominantly cholestatic pattern.** The first step in evaluating patients whose LFT pattern predominantly reflects cholestasis is to determine whether the cholestasis is due to intra- or extrahepatic causes. The first step is to obtain a right upper quadrant ultrasound, which can detect dilation of the intra- and extrahepatic biliary tree with a high degree of sensitivity and specificity. The absence of biliary dilatation suggests intrahepatic cholestasis, while the presence of biliary dilatation indicates extrahepatic cholestasis.

References, see page 372.

Acute Pancreatitis

The incidence of acute pancreatitis ranges from 54 to 238 episodes per 1 million per year. Patients with mild pancreatitis respond well to conservative therapy, but those with severe pancreatitis may have a progressively downhill course to respiratory failure, sepsis, and death (less than 10%).

I. **Etiology**
   A. **Alcohol-induced pancreatitis.** Consumption of large quantities of alcohol may cause acute pancreatitis.
   B. **Cholelithiasis.** Common bile duct or pancreatic duct obstruction by a stone may cause acute pancreatitis. (90% of all cases of pancreatitis occur secondary to alcohol consumption or cholelithiasis).
   C. **Idiopathic pancreatitis.** The cause of pancreatitis cannot be determined in 10 percent of patients.
   D. **Hypertriglyceridemia.** Elevation of serum triglycerides (>l,000mg/dL) has been linked with acute pancreatitis.
   E. **Pancreatic duct disruption.** In younger patients, a malformation of the pancreatic ducts (eg, pancreatic divisum) with subsequent obstruction is often the cause of pancreatitis. In older patients without an apparent underlying etiology, cancerous lesions of the ampulla of Vater, pancreas or duodenum must be ruled out as possible causes of obstructive pancreatitis.
   F. **Iatrogenic pancreatitis.** Radiocontrast studies of the hepatobiliary system (eg, cholangiogram, ERCP) can cause acute pancreatitis in 2-3% of patients undergoing studies.
   G. **Trauma.** Blunt or penetrating trauma of any kind to the peri-pancreatic or perihepatic regions may induce acute pancreatitis. Extensive surgical manipulation can also induce pancreatitis during laparotomy.

Causes of Acute Pancreatitis	
Alcoholism	Infections
Cholelithiasis	Microlithiasis
Drugs	Pancreas divisum
Hypertriglyceridemia	Trauma
Idiopathic causes	

Medications Associated with Acute Pancreatitis	
Definitive Association:	**Probable Association:**
Azathioprine (Imuran)	Acetaminophen
Sulfonamides	Nitrofurantoin
Thiazide diuretics	Methyldopa
Furosemide (Lasix)	Erythromycin
Estrogens	Salicylates
Tetracyclines	Metronidazole
Valproic acid (Depakote)	NSAIDS
Pentamidine	ACE-inhibitors
Didanosine (Videx)	

II. **Pathophysiology.** Acute pancreatitis results when an initiating event causes the extrusion of zymogen granules, from pancreatic acinar cells, into the interstitium of the pancreas. Zymogen particles cause the activation of trypsinogen into trypsin. Trypsin causes auto-digestion of pancreatic tissues.

III. **Clinical presentation**
   A. **Signs and symptoms.** Pancreatitis usually presents with mid-epigastric pain that radiates to the back, associated with nausea and vomiting. The pain is sudden in onset, progressively increases in intensity, and becomes constant. The severity of pain often causes the patient to move continuously in search of a more comfortable position.
   B. **Physical examination**
      1. Patients with acute pancreatitis often appear very ill. Findings that suggest severe pancreatitis include hypotension and tachypnea with decreased basilar breath sounds. Flank ecchymoses (Grey Tuner's Sign) or periumbilical ecchymoses (Cullen's sign) may be indicative of hemorrhagic pancreatitis.
      2. Abdominal distension and tenderness in the epigastrium are common. Fever and tachycardia are often present. Guarding, rebound tenderness, and hypoactive or absent bowel sounds indicate peritoneal irritation. Deep palpation of abdominal organs should be avoided in the setting of suspected pancreatitis.

IV. **Laboratory testing**
   A. **Leukocytosis.** An elevated WBC with a left shift and elevated hematocrit (indicating hemoconcentration) and hyperglycemia are common. Pre-renal azotemia may result from dehydration. Hypoalbuminemia, hypertriglyceridemia, hypocalcemia, hyperbilirubinemia, and mild elevations of transaminases and alkaline phosphatase are common.
   B. **Elevated amylase.** An elevated amylase level often confirms the clinical diagnosis of pancreatitis.
   C. **Elevated lipase.** Lipase measurements are more specific for pancreatitis than amylase levels, but less sensitive. Hyperlipasemia may also occur in patients with renal failure, perforated ulcer disease, bowel infarction and bowel obstruction.

D. **Abdominal Radiographs** may reveal non-specific findings of pancreatitis, such as "sentinel loops" (dilated loops of small bowel in the vicinity of the pancreas), ileus and, pancreatic calcifications.

E. **Ultrasonography** demonstrates the entire pancreas in only 20 percent of patients with acute pancreatitis. Its greatest utility is in evaluation of patients with possible gallstone disease.

F. **Helical high resolution computed tomography** is the imaging modality of choice in acute pancreatitis. CT findings will be normal in 14-29% of patients with mild pancreatitis. Pancreatic necrosis, pseudocysts and abscesses are readily detected by CT.

Selected Conditions Other Than Pancreatitis Associated with Amylase Elevation

Carcinoma of the pancreas	Acute alcoholism
Common bile duct obstruction	Diabetic ketoacidosis
Post-ERCP	Lung cancer
Mesenteric infarction	Ovarian neoplasm
Pancreatic trauma	Renal failure
Perforated viscus	Ruptured ectopic pregnancy
Renal failure	Salivary gland infection
	Macroamylasemia

V. **Prognosis.** Ranson's criteria is used to determine prognosis in acute pancreatitis. Patients with two or fewer risk factors have a mortality rate of less than 1 percent, those with three or four risk-factors a mortality rate of 16 percent, five or six risk factors, a mortality rate of 40 percent, and seven or eight risk factors, a mortality rate approaching 100 percent.

Ranson's Criteria for Acute Pancreatitis

At admission	During initial 48 hours
1. Age >55 years	1. Hematocrit drop >10%
2. WBC >16,000/mm^3	2. BUN rise >5 mg/dL
3. Blood glucose >200 mg/dL	3. Arterial pO$_2$ <60 mm Hg
4. Serum LDH >350 IU/L	4. Base deficit >4 mEq/L
5. AST >250 U/L	5. Serum calcium <8.0 mg/dL
	6. Estimated fluid sequestration >6 L

VI. **Treatment of pancreatitis**

A. **Expectant management.** Most cases of acute pancreatitis will improve within three to seven days. Management consists of prevention of complications of severe pancreatitis.

B. **NPO and bowel rest.** Patients should take nothing by mouth. Total parenteral nutrition should be instituted for those patients fasting for more than five days. A nasogastric tube is warranted if vomiting or ileus.

C. **IV fluid resuscitation.** Vigorous intravenous hydration is necessary. A decrease in urine output to less than 30 mL per hour is an indication of inadequate fluid replacement.

D. **Pain control.** Morphine is discouraged because it may cause Oddi's sphincter spasm, which may exacerbate the pancreatitis. Meperidine (Demerol), 25-100 mg IV/IM q4-6h, is favored. Ketorolac (Toradol), 60 mg IM/IV, then 15-30 mg IM/IV q6h, is also used.

   E. Antibiotics. Routine use of antibiotics is not recommended in most cases of acute pancreatitis. In cases of infectious pancreatitis, treatment with cefoxitin (1-2 g IV q6h), cefotetan (1-2 g IV q12h), imipenem (1.0 gm IV q6h), or ampicillin/sulbactam (1.5-3.0 g IV q6h) may be appropriate.

   F. Alcohol withdrawal prophylaxis. Alcoholics may require alcohol withdrawal prophylaxis with lorazepam (Ativan) 1-2mg IM/IV q4-6h as needed x 3 days, thiamine 100mg IM/IV qd x 3 days, folic acid 1 mg IM/IV qd x 3 days, multivitamin qd.

   G. Octreotide. Somatostatin is also a potent inhibitor of pancreatic exocrine secretion. Octreotide is a somatostatin analogue, which has been effective in reducing mortality from bile-induced pancreatitis. Clinical trials, however, have failed to document a significant reduction in mortality

   H. Blood sugar monitoring and insulin administration. Serum glucose levels should be monitored.

VII. Complications
   A. Chronic pancreatitis
   B. Severe hemorrhagic pancreatitis
   C. Pancreatic pseudocysts
   D. Infectious pancreatitis with development of sepsis (occurs in up to 5% of all patients with pancreatitis)
   E. Portal vein thrombosis
References, see page 372.

Lower Gastrointestinal Bleeding

The spontaneous remission rates for lower gastrointestinal bleeding is 80 percent. No source of bleeding can be identified in 12 percent of patients, and bleeding is recurrent in 25 percent. Bleeding has usually ceased by the time the patient presents to the emergency room.

I. Clinical evaluation
   A. The severity of blood loss and hemodynamic status should be assessed immediately. Initial management consists of resuscitation with crystalloid solutions (lactated Ringers) and blood products if necessary.
   B. The duration and quantity of bleeding should be assessed; however, the duration of bleeding is often underestimated.
   C. Risk factors that may have contributed to the bleeding include nonsteroidal anti-inflammatory drugs, anticoagulants, colonic diverticulitis, renal failure, coagulopathy, colonic polyps, and hemorrhoids. Patients may have a prior history of hemorrhoids, diverticulosis, inflammatory bowel disease, peptic ulcer, gastritis, cirrhosis, or esophageal varices.
   D. Hematochezia. Bright red or maroon output per rectum suggests a lower GI source; however, 12 to 20% of patients with an upper GI bleed may have hematochezia as a result of rapid blood loss.
   E. Melena. Sticky, black, foul-smelling stools suggest a source proximal to the ligament of Treitz, but Melena can also result from bleeding in the small intestine or proximal colon.
   F. Clinical findings
      1. Abdominal pain may result from ischemic bowel, inflammatory bowel disease, or a ruptured aneurysm.
      2. Painless massive bleeding suggests vascular bleeding from diverticula, angiodysplasia, or hemorrhoids.
      3. Bloody diarrhea suggests inflammatory bowel disease or an infectious origin.

4. **Bleeding with rectal pain** is seen with anal fissures, hemorrhoids, and rectal ulcers.
5. **Chronic constipation** suggests hemorrhoidal bleeding. New onset of constipation or thin stools suggests a left sided colonic malignancy.
6. **Blood on the toilet paper** or dripping into the toilet water suggests a perianal source of bleeding, such as hemorrhoids or an anal fissure.
7. **Blood coating** the outside of stools suggests a lesion in the anal canal.
8. **Blood streaking** or mixed in with the stool may results from polyps or a malignancy in the descending colon.
9. **Maroon colored stools** often indicate small bowel and proximal colon bleeding.

II. Physical examination
   A. **Postural hypotension** indicates a 20% blood volume loss, whereas, overt signs of shock (pallor, hypotension, tachycardia) indicates a 30 to 40 percent blood loss.
   B. **The skin** may be cool and pale with delayed refill if bleeding has been significant.
   C. **Stigmata of liver disease**, including jaundice, caput medusae, gynecomastia and palmar erythema, should be sought because patients with these findings frequently have GI bleeding.

III. Differential diagnosis of lower GI bleeding
   A. **Angiodysplasia** and diverticular disease of the right colon accounts for the vast majority of episodes of acute lower GI bleeding. Most acute lower GI bleeding originates from the colon however 15 to 20 percent of episodes arise from the small intestine and the upper GI tract.
   B. **Elderly patients.** Diverticulosis and angiodysplasia are the most common causes of lower GI bleeding.
   C. **Younger patients.** Hemorrhoids, anal fissures and inflammatory bowel disease are most common causes of lower GI bleeding.

Clinical Indicators of Gastrointestinal Bleeding and Probable Source		
Clinical Indicator	**Probability of Upper Gastrointestinal source**	**Probability of Lower Gastrointestinal Source**
Hematemesis	Almost certain	Rare
Melena	Probable	Possible
Hematochezia	Possible	Probable
Blood-streaked stool	Rare	Almost certain
Occult blood in stool	Possible	Possible

IV. **Diagnosis and management of lower gastrointestinal bleeding**
   A. **Rapid clinical evaluation and resuscitation** should precede diagnostic studies. Intravenous fluids (1 to 2 liters) should be infused over 10- 20 minutes to restore intravascular volume, and blood should be transfused if there is rapid ongoing blood loss or if hypotension or tachycardia are present. Coagulopathy is corrected with fresh frozen plasma, platelets, and cryoprecipitate.
   B. When small amounts of bright red blood are passed per rectum, then lower GI tract can be assumed to be the source. In patients with large volume maroon

stools, nasogastric tube aspiration should be performed to exclude massive upper gastrointestinal hemorrhage.

C. If the nasogastric aspirate contains no blood then anoscopy and sigmoidoscopy should be performed to determine weather a colonic mucosal abnormality (ischemic or infectious colitis) or hemorrhoids might be the cause of bleeding.

D. **Colonoscopy** in a patient with massive lower GI bleeding is often nondiagnostic, but it can detect ulcerative colitis, antibiotic-associated colitis, or ischemic colon.

E. **Polyethylene glycol-electrolyte solution** (CoLyte or GoLytely) should be administered by means of a nasogastric tube (Four liters of solution is given over a 2-3 hour period), allowing for diagnostic and therapeutic colonoscopy.

V. **Definitive management of lower gastrointestinal bleeding**

A. **Colonoscopy**

1. Colonoscopy is the procedure of choice for diagnosing colonic causes of GI bleeding. It should be performed after adequate preparation of the bowel. If the bowel cannot be adequately prepared because of persistent, acute bleeding, a bleeding scan or angiography is preferable.

2. If colonoscopy fails to reveal the source of the bleeding, the patient should be observed because, in 80% of cases, bleeding ceases spontaneously.

B. **Radionuclide scan or bleeding scan.** Technetium- labeled (tagged) red blood cell bleeding scans can detect bleeding sites when bleeding is intermit-tent. Localization may not he a precise enough to allow segmental colon resection.

C. **Angiography**. Selective mesenteric angiography detects arterial bleeding that occurs at rates of 0.5 mL/per minute or faster. Diverticular bleeding causes pooling of contrast medium within a diverticulum. Bleeding angiodysplastic lesions appear as abnormal vasculature. When active bleeding is seen with diverticular disease or angiodysplasia, selective arterial infusion of vasopressin may be effective.

D. **Surgery**

1. If bleeding continues and no source can be found, surgical intervention is usually warranted. Surgical resection may be indicated for patients with recurrent diverticular bleeding, or for patients who have had persistent bleeding from colonic angiodysplasia and have required blood transfusions.

2. Surgical management of lower gastrointestinal bleeding is ideally under-taken with a secure knowledge of the location and cause of the bleeding lesion. A segmental bowel resection to include the lesion and followed by a primary anastomosis is usually safe and appropriate in all but the most unstable patients.

VI. **Diverticulosis**

A. Diverticulosis of the colon is present in more than 50% of the population by age 60 years. Bleeding from diverticula is relatively rare, affecting only 4% to 17% of patients at risk.

B. In most cases, bleeding ceases spontaneously, but in 10% to 20% of cases, the bleeding continues. The risk of rebleeding after an episode of bleeding is 25%. Right-sided colonic diverticula occur less frequently than left-sided or sigmoid diverticula but are responsible for a disproportionate incidence of diverticular bleeding.

C. Operative management of diverticular bleeding is indicated when bleeding continues and is not amenable to angiographic or endoscopic therapy. It also should be considered in patients with recurrent bleeding in the same colonic segment. The operation usually consists of a segmental bowel resection (usually a right colectomy or sigmoid colectomy) followed by a primary anasto-mosis.

VII. **Arteriovenous malformations**
   A. AVMs or angiodysplasias are vascular lesions that occur primarily in the distal ileum, cecum, and ascending colon of elderly patients. The arteriographic criteria for identification of an AVM include a cluster of small arteries, visualization of a vascular tuft, and early and prolonged filling of the draining vein.
   B. The typical pattern of bleeding of an AVM is recurrent and episodic, with most individual bleeding episodes being self-limited. Anemia is frequent, and continued massive bleeding is distinctly uncommon. After nondiagnostic colonoscopy, enteroscopy should be considered.
   C. Endoscopic therapy for AVMs may include heater probe, laser, bipolar electrocoagulation, or argon beam coagulation. Operative management is usually reserved for patients with continued bleeding, anemia, repetitive transfusion requirements, and failure of endoscopic management. Surgical management consists of segmental bowel resection with primary anastomosis.

VIII. **Inflammatory bowel disease**
   A. Ulcerative colitis and, less frequently, Crohn's colitis or enteritis may present with major or massive lower gastrointestinal bleeding. Infectious colitis can also manifest with bleeding, although it is rarely massive.
   B. When the bleeding is minor to moderate, therapy directed at the inflammatory condition is appropriate. When the bleeding is major and causes hemodynamic instability, surgical intervention is usually required. When operative intervention is indicated, the patient is explored through a midline laparotomy, and a total abdominal colectomy with end ileostomy and oversewing of the distal rectal stump is the preferred procedure.

IX. **Tumors of the colon and rectum**
   A. Colon and rectal tumors account for 5% to 10% of all hospitalizations for lower gastrointestinal bleeding. Visible bleeding from a benign colonic or rectal polyp is distinctly unusual. Major or massive hemorrhage rarely is caused by a colorectal neoplasm; however, chronic bleeding is common. When the neoplasm is in the right colon, bleeding is often occult and manifests as weakness or anemia.
   B. More distal neoplasms are often initially confused with hemorrhoidal bleeding. For this reason, the treatment of hemorrhoids should always be preceded by flexible sigmoidoscopy in patients older than age 40 or 50 years. In younger patients, treatment of hemorrhoids without further investigation may be appropriate if there are no risk factors for neoplasm, there is a consistent clinical history, and there is anoscopic evidence of recent bleeding from enlarged internal hemorrhoids.

X. **Anorectal disease**
   A. When bleeding occurs only with bowel movements and is visible on the toilet tissue or the surface of the stool, it is designated *outlet bleeding*. Outlet bleeding is most often associated with internal hemorrhoids or anal fissures.
   B. Anal fissures are most commonly seen in young patients and are associated with severe pain during and after defecation. Other benign anorectal bleeding sources are proctitis secondary to inflammatory bowel disease, infection, or radiation injury. Additionally, stercoral ulcers can develop in patients with chronic constipation.
   C. Surgery for anorectal problems is typically undertaken only after failure of conservative medical therapy with high-fiber diets, stool softeners, and/or hemorrhoidectomy.

XI. **Ischemic colitis**
   A. Ischemic colitis is seen in elderly patients with known vascular disease. The abdomen pain may be postprandial and associated with bloody diarrhea or rectal bleeding. Severe blood loss is unusual but can occur.

B. Abdominal films may reveal "thumb-printing" caused by submucosal edema. Colonoscopy reveals a well-demarcated area of hyperemia, edema and mucosal ulcerations. The splenic flexure and descending colon are the most common sites. Most episodes resolve spontaneously, however, vascular bypass or resection may be required.

References, see page 372.

Acute Diarrhea

Acute diarrhea is defined as diarrheal disease of rapid onset, often with nausea, vomiting, fever, and abdominal pain. Most episodes of acute gastroenteritis will resolve within 3 to 7 days.

I. Clinical evaluation of acute diarrhea
   A. The nature of onset, duration, frequency, and timing of the diarrheal episodes should be assessed. The appearance of the stool, buoyancy, presence of blood or mucus, vomiting, or pain should be determined.
   B. Contact with a potential source of infectious diarrhea should be sought.
   C. Drugs that may cause diarrhea include laxatives, magnesium-containing compounds, sulfa-drugs, and antibiotics.

II. Physical examination
   A. Assessment of volume status. Dehydration is suggested by dry mucous membranes, orthostatic hypotension, tachycardia, mental status changes, and acute weight loss.
   B. Abdominal tenderness, mild distention and hyperactive bowel sounds are common in acute infectious diarrhea. The presence of rebound tenderness or rigidity suggests toxic megacolon or perforation.
   C. Evidence of systemic atherosclerosis suggests ischemia. Lower extremity edema suggests malabsorption or protein loss.

III. Acute infectious diarrhea
   A. Infectious diarrhea is classified as noninflammatory or inflammatory, depending on whether the infectious organism has invaded the intestinal mucosa.
   B. Noninflammatory infectious diarrhea is caused by organisms that produce a toxin (enterotoxigenic E coli strains, Vibrio cholerae). Noninflammatory, infectious diarrhea is usually self-limiting and lasts less than 3 days.
   C. Blood or mucus in the stool suggests inflammatory disease, usually caused by bacterial invasion of the mucosa (enteroinvasive E coli, Shigella, Salmonella, Campylobacter). Patients usually have a septic appearance and fever; some have abdominal rigidity and severe abdominal pain.
   D. Vomiting out of proportion to diarrhea is usually related to a neuroenterotoxin-mediated food poisoning from Staphylococcus aureus or Bacillus cereus, or rotavirus (in an infant), or Norwalk virus (in older children or adults). The incubation period for neuroenterotoxin food poisoning is less than 4 hours, while that of a viral agent is more than 8 hours.
   E. Traveler's diarrhea is a common acute diarrhea. Three or four unformed stools are passed/per 24 hours, usually starting on the third day of travel and lasting 2-3 days. Anorexia, nausea, vomiting, abdominal cramps, abdominal bloating, and flatulence may also be present.
   F. Antibiotic-related diarrhea
      1. Antibiotic-related diarrhea ranges from mild illness to life-threatening pseudomembranous colitis. Overgrowth of Clostridium difficile causes pseudomembranous colitis. Amoxicillin, cephalosporins and clindamycin have been implicated most often, but any antibiotic can be the cause.

2. Patients with pseudomembranous colitis have high fever, cramping, leukocytosis, and severe, watery diarrhea. Latex agglutination testing for C difficile toxin can provide results in 30 minutes.

3. **Enterotoxigenic E coli**

   a. The enterotoxigenic E coli include the E coli serotype 0157:H7. Grossly bloody diarrhea is most often caused by E. coli 0157:H7, causing 8% of grossly bloody stools.

   b. Enterotoxigenic E coli can cause hemolytic uremic syndrome, thrombotic thrombocytopenic purpura, intestinal perforation, sepsis, and rectal prolapse.

IV. **Diagnostic approach to acute infectious diarrhea**

   A. An attempt should be made to obtain a pathologic diagnosis in patients who give a history of recent ingestion of seafood (Vibrio parahaemolyticus), travel or camping, antibiotic use, homosexual activity, or who complain of fever and abdominal pain.

   B. Blood or mucus in the stools indicates the presence of Shigella, Salmonella, Campylobacter jejuni, enteroinvasive E. coli, C. difficile, or Yersinia entero-colitica.

   C. Most cases of mild diarrheal disease do not require laboratory studies to determine the etiology. In moderate to severe diarrhea with fever or pus, a stool culture for bacterial pathogens (Salmonella, Shigella, Campylobacter) is submitted. If antibiotics were used recently, stool should be sent for Clostridium difficile toxin.

V. **Laboratory evaluation of acute diarrhea**

   A. **Fecal leukocytes** is a screening test which should be obtained if moderate to severe diarrhea is present. Numerous leukocytes indicate Shigella, Salmonella, or Campylobacter jejuni.

   B. **Stool cultures for bacterial pathogens** should be obtained if high fever, severe or persistent (>14 d) diarrhea, bloody stools, or leukocytes is present.

   C. **Examination for ova and parasites** is indicated for persistent diarrhea (>14 d), travel to a high-risk region, gay males, infants in day care, or dysentery.

   D. **Blood cultures** should be obtained prior to starting antibiotics if severe diarrhea and high fever is present.

   E. **E coli 0157:H7 cultures.** Enterotoxigenic E coli should be suspected if there are bloody stools with minimal fever, when diarrhea follows hamburger con-sumption, or when hemolytic uremic syndrome is diagnosed.

   F. **Clostridium difficile cytotoxin** should be obtained if diarrhea follows use of an antimicrobial agent.

   G. **Rotavirus antigen test (Rotazyme)** is indicated for hospitalized children <2 years old with gastroenteritis. The finding of rotavirus eliminates the need for antibiotics.

VI. **Treatment of acute diarrhea**

   A. **Fluid and electrolyte resuscitation**

   1. **Oral rehydration.** For cases of mild to moderate diarrhea in children, Pedialyte or Ricelyte should be administered. For adults with diarrhea, flavored soft drinks with saltine crackers are usually adequate.

   2. **Intravenous hydration** should be used if oral rehydration is not possible.

   B. **Diet.** Fatty foods should be avoided. Well-tolerated foods include complex carbohydrates (rice, wheat, potatoes, bread, and cereals), lean meats, yogurt, fruits, and vegetables. Diarrhea often is associated with a reduction in intesti-nal lactase. A lactose-free milk preparation may be substituted if lactose intolerance becomes apparent.

VII. **Empiric antimicrobial treatment of acute diarrhea**
  A. **Febrile dysenteric syndrome**
    1. If diarrhea is associated with high fever and stools containing mucus and blood, empiric antibacterial therapy should be given for Shigella or Campylobacter jejuni.
    2. Norfloxacin (Noroxin) 400 mg bid **OR**
    3. Ciprofloxacin (Cipro) 500 mg bid.
  B. **Travelers' diarrhea**. Adults are treated with norfloxacin 400 mg bid, ciprofloxacin (Cipro) 500 mg bid, or ofloxacin (Floxin) 300 mg bid for 3 days.
References, see page 372.

Chronic Diarrhea

Diarrhea is considered chronic if it lasts longer than 2 weeks.

I. **Clinical evaluation of chronic diarrhea**
  A. Initial evaluation should determine the characteristics of the diarrhea, including volume, mucus, blood, flatus, cramps, tenesmus, duration, frequency, effect of fasting, stress, and the effect of specific foods (eg, dairy products, wheat, laxatives, fruits).
  B. **Secretory diarrhea**
    1. Secretory diarrhea is characterized by large stool volumes (>1 L/day), no decrease with fasting, and a fecal osmotic gap <40.
    2. **Evaluation of secretory diarrhea** consists of a giardia antigen, Entamoeba histolytica antibody, Yersinia culture, fasting serum glucose, thyroid function tests, and a cholestyramine (Cholybar, Questran) trial.
  C. **Osmotic diarrhea**
    1. Osmotic diarrhea is characterized by small stool volumes, a decrease with fasting, and a fecal osmotic gap >40. Postprandial diarrhea with bloating or flatus also suggests osmotic diarrhea. Ingestion of an osmotically active laxative may be inadvertent (sugarless gum containing sorbitol) or covert (with eating disorders).
    2. **Evaluation of osmotic diarrhea**
      a. Trial of lactose withdrawal.
      b. Trial of an antibiotic (metronidazole) for small-bowel bacterial over-growth.
      c. Screening for celiac disease (anti-endomysial antibody, antigliadin antibody).
      d. Fecal fat measurement (72 hr) for pancreatic insufficiency.
      e. Trial of fructose avoidance.
      f. Stool test for phenolphthalein and magnesium if laxative abuse is sus-pected.
      g. Hydrogen breath analysis to identify disaccharidase deficiency or bacte-rial overgrowth.
  D. **Exudative diarrhea**
    1. Exudative diarrhea is characterized by bloody stools, tenesmus, urgency, cramping pain, and nocturnal occurrence. It is most often caused by inflam-matory bowel disease, which may be suggested by anemia, hypoalbuminemia, and an increased sedimentation rate.
    2. **Evaluation of exudative diarrhea** consists of a complete blood cell count, serum albumin, total protein, erythrocyte sedimentation rate, electrolyte measurement, Entamoeba histolytica antibody titers, stool culture, Clostridium difficile antigen test, ova and parasite testing, and flexible sigmoidoscopy and biopsies.

References, see page 372.

Inflammatory Bowel Disease

Ulcerative colitis is limited to the rectum and colon. Crohn's disease may involve both the small and the large bowel, but 15% to 25% of cases are isolated to the colon. Both Crohn's disease and ulcerative colitis can follow an active and remitting course and have a highly variable response to therapy.

I. Clinical presentation

A. Crohn's disease is a chronic, transmural, granulomatous disorder that can involve any segment of gastrointestinal tract from the mouth to the anus. In the bowel it may affect multiple distinct segments, with normal intervening bowel. Crohn's disease also may be complicated by intestinal strictures, fistulas, and perianal fistulas. The clinical presentation of Crohn's disease ranges from intestinal obstruction, to bloody or nonbloody diarrhea, to malabsorption.

B. Ulcerative colitis is a nongranulomatous inflammatory condition that always starts in the rectum and extends proximally throughout the colon in a continuous and confluent fashion, never involving the small bowel. The clinical presentation of ulcerative colitis is more uniform than that of Crohn's disease and includes rectal bleeding or bloody diarrhea. In addition to gastrointestinal symptoms, extraintestinal manifestations can occur and may involve the skin (eg, erythema nodosum, pyoderma gangrenosum), joints (sacroiliitis, ankylosing spondylitis, and peripheral arthritis), eyes (iritis and uveitis), and liver (sclerosing cholangitis). Extraintestinal manifestations are due to the release of bacterial antigens from the colonic lumen.

C. Differential diagnosis. In patients with new-onset bloody diarrhea and abdominal cramps, an infectious cause must first be ruled out. In addition to routine cultures, cultures for *Clostridium difficile,* ova and parasites, and hemorrhagic *Escherichia coli* should be done. Colonic ischemia presents with symptoms similar to those of IBD--abdominal cramps, rectal bleeding, and diarrhea--and should be a consideration in older patients. Nonsteroidal anti-inflammatory drugs can also cause colonic ulcerations that mimic colonic Crohn's disease.

II. Induction therapy

A. Mild-to-moderate Crohn's disease

1. Patients with mild to moderate colonic Crohn's disease may be managed successfully with 5-ASA products, such as sulfasalazine (Azulfidine), 1 g two to four times daily, which produces remission in about 50%.

2. Sulfasalazine is composed of a sulfapyridine moiety attached to 5-ASA. It is activated in the colon by colonic bacteria that releases sulfapyridine, which is then absorbed. The 5-ASA remains in the colon. Side effects include nausea, gastrointestinal upset, rash, headache, and reversible male infertility. Rare hypersensitivity reactions include hemolytic anemia, neutropenia, and hepatitis.

3. For patients with colonic Crohn's disease who are unable to tolerate sulfasalazine or who are allergic to sulfa drugs, sulfa-free 5-ASA products have been developed. Olsalazine (Dipentum), 500 mg two or three times daily, and balsalazide (Colazal), 2.25 g three times daily, work exclusively in the colon, whereas the mesalamine preparations--Asacol, 800 to 1,600 mg three or four times daily, and Pentasa, 1 g four times daily--are released in the small bowel and the colon.

4. Antibiotics also have been used in the treatment of colonic Crohn's disease. Metronidazole (Flagyl), 250 to 500 mg three times daily, has been shown to be beneficial in colonic Crohn's disease as well as in Crohn's in patients with

perianal abscesses and fistulas. Ciprofloxacin (Cipro) has been used as an alternative to metronidazole for both colonic and perianal Crohn's disease.

B. Mild-to-moderate ulcerative colitis

1. **Ulcerative colitis** with fewer than six loose bowel movements per day, with or without blood, and without significant weight loss or anemia is considered to be mild-to-moderate disease. In this setting, 5-ASA drugs such as sulfasalazine or Asacol are often used as primary therapy. Onset of action is usually within 1 week, but peak effect is not reached for 3 to 6 weeks.

2. For patients with isolated proctitis, corticosteroid (Anusol) or mesalamine (Canasa) suppository given once or twice a day is usually sufficient therapy. When ulcerative colitis extends beyond the rectum, corticosteroid foam (Cortifoam, ProctoFoam) or enema (Cortenema) or mesalamine enema (Rowasa) may be used nightly.

C. Moderate-to-severe Crohn's disease

1. Patients with moderate to severe Crohn's disease often present with severe abdominal pain, diarrhea, weight loss, fever, and symptoms of obstruction.

2. Budesonide (Entocort), 9 mg once daily, is approved for the treatment of ileal and ileocecal Crohn's disease. Although prednisone and budesonide are equally efficacious, budesonide's extensive first-pass metabolism through the liver and high affinity for the glucocorticoid receptor in the small bowel.

3. Another novel therapy for Crohn's disease is infliximab (Remicade), which is approved for induction of remission. Infliximab is a monoclonal antibody to tumor necrosis factor alpha and is given intravenously. A single outpatient infusion of infliximab yielded a clinical response in up to 80%.

4. Methotrexate, 25 mg intramuscularly, has been shown to be efficacious in a subgroup of steroid-dependent patients.

D. Moderate-to-severe ulcerative colitis

1. Patients presenting with moderate to severe ulcerative colitis usually have more than six loose to watery bowel movements per day, often containing blood, along with abdominal cramps, weight loss, and anemia. Patients with ulcerative colitis may be treated with oral prednisone or intravenous therapy. If a severely ill patient fails to respond within 7 to 10 days, intravenous cyclosporine or colectomy should be considered.

2. **Cyclosporine.** In a trial of patients with ulcerative colitis refractory to corticosteroids, 83% responded to cyclosporine. Cyclosporine should be used as a transitional agent or bridge to longer-term therapy with an immunomodulating drug or to elective colectomy.

III. Maintenance therapy

A. Most of the drugs used for induction of remission also may be used for maintenance therapy. Treatments include 5-ASA products, immunomodulators (6-mercaptopurine [Purinethol] and azathioprine [Imuran]), and infliximab. Corticosteroids, however, should almost never be used for long-term therapy.

B. For patients with Crohn's disease or ulcerative colitis refractory to prednisone therapy or who become prednisone-dependent, use of immunomodulating agents such as 6-mercaptopurine, 1.5 to 2 mg/kg per day, and its prodrug azathioprine, 2 to 2.5 mg/kg per day, has proved beneficial. Infliximab has recently been shown to be efficacious in the maintenance of remission for Crohn's disease.

References, see page 372.

Neurologic Disorders

Acute Ischemic Stroke

I. **Initial general assessment.** Sudden loss of focal brain function is the core feature of the onset of ischemic stroke. The goals in this initial phase include:
   A. Medically stabilize the patient.
   B. Reverse any conditions that are contributing to the patient's problem.
   C. Assess the pathophysiologic basis of the neurologic symptoms.
   D. Screen for potential contraindications to thrombolysis in acute ischemic stroke patients.
   E. Diagnosing an intracerebral hemorrhage (ICH) or subarachnoid hemorrhage (SAH) as soon as possible can be lifesaving. The presence of onset headache and vomiting favor the diagnosis of ICH or SAH compared with a thromboembolic stroke, while the abrupt onset of impaired cerebral function without focal symptoms favors the diagnosis of SAH.
   F. **History and physical examination** should distinguish between seizures, syncope, migraine, and hypoglycemia, which can mimic acute ischemia. In patients with focal signs and altered level of consciousness, it is important to determine whether the patient takes insulin or oral hypoglycemic agents, has a history of a seizure disorder or drug overdose or abuse, medications on admission, or recent trauma.

Acute stroke differential diagnosis

Migraine
Intracerebral hemorrhage
Head trauma
Brain tumor
Todd's palsy (paresis, aphasia, neglect, etc., after a seizure episode)
Functional deficit (conversion reaction)
Systemic infection
Toxic-metabolic disturbances (hypoglycemia, acute renal failure, hepatic insufficiency, exogenous drug
   intoxication)

   G. **Physical examination** should evaluate the neck and retroorbital regions for vascular bruits, and palpate of pulses in the neck, arms, and legs to assess for their absence, asymmetry, or irregular rate.
   1. The heart should be auscultated for murmurs. Fluctuations in blood pressure occasionally precede fluctuations in clinical signs.
   2. The skin should be examined for signs of endocarditis, cholesterol emboli, purpura, or ecchymoses. The funduscopic examination may reveal cholesterol emboli or papilledema. The head should be examined for signs of trauma. A tongue laceration may occur during a seizure.
   3. The neck should be immobilized until evaluated radiographically for evidence of serious trauma if there is a suspicion of a fall. The chest x-ray is helpful if it shows cardiomegaly, metastases, or a widened mediastinum suggesting aortic dissection. Examination of the extremities is important to detect deep vein thrombosis.

4. **Breathing.** Patients with increased ICP due to hemorrhage, vertebrobasilar ischemia, or bihemispheric ischemia can present with a decreased respiratory drive or muscular airway obstruction. Intubation may be necessary to restore adequate ventilation. Patients with adequate ventilation should have the oxygen saturation monitored. Patients who are hypoxic should receive supplemental oxygen.

H. Immediate laboratory studies

1. All patients with acute neurologic deterioration or acute stroke should have an electrocardiogram. Chest radiography is indicated if lung or heart disease is suspected. Oxygen saturation or arterial blood gas tests are indicated if hypoxia is suspected.

2. **Blood studies include:**
   a. Complete blood count including platelets, and erythrocyte sedimentation rate.
   b. Electrolytes, urea nitrogen, creatinine.
   c. Serum glucose. Finger stick for faster glucose measurement if diabetic, taking insulin or oral hypoglycemic agents, or if there is clinical suspicion for hypoglycemia.
   d. Liver function tests.
   e. Prothrombin time and partial thromboplastin time.
   f. Toxicology screen and blood alcohol level in selected patients.
   g. Blood for type and cross match in case fresh frozen is needed to reverse a coagulopathy if ICH is suspected.
   h. Urine human chorionic gonadotropin in women of child-bearing potential.
   i. Consider evaluation for hypercoagulable state in young patients without apparent stroke risk factors.

Laboratory studies

Complete blood count and erythrocyte sedimentation rate
Electrolytes, urea nitrogen, creatinine, glucose
Liver function tests
Prothrombin time and partial thromboplastin time
Toxicology screen
Blood for type and cross match
Urine human chorionic gonadotropin in women of child-bearing potential
Consider evaluation for hypercoagulable state in young patients without apparent stroke risk factors

---

3. Anticoagulant use is a common cause of intracerebral hemorrhage. Thus, the prothrombin and partial thromboplastin time and the platelet count should be checked. The effects of warfarin are corrected with intravenous vitamin K and fresh-frozen plasma (typically 4 units) in patients with intracerebral hemorrhage.

4. A drug overdose can mimic an acute stroke. In addition, cocaine, intravenous drug abuse, and amphetamines can cause an ischemic stroke or intracranial hemorrhage. Hyponatremia and thrombotic thrombocytopenic purpura (TTP) can present with focal neurologic deficits, suggesting the need for measurement of serum electrolytes and a complete blood count with platelet count.

5. **Hyperglycemia,** defined as a blood glucose level >108 mg/dL, is associated with poor functional outcome from acute stroke at presentation. Stress hyperglycemia is common in stroke patients, although newly diagnosed diabetes may be detected. Treatment with fluids and insulin to reduce serum glucose to less than 300 mg/dL is recommended.

6. **Hypoglycemia** can cause focal neurologic deficits mimicking stroke. The blood sugar should be checked and rapidly corrected if low. Glucose should be administered immediately after drawing a blood sample in "stroke" patients known to take insulin or oral hypoglycemic agents.

7. **Fever.** Primary central nervous system infection, such as meningitis, subdural empyema, brain abscess, and infective endocarditis, need to be excluded as the etiology of fever. Common etiologies of fever include aspiration pneumonia and urinary tract infection. Fever may contribute to brain injury in patients with an acute stroke. Maintaining normothermia is recommended after an acute stroke. Prophylactic administration of acetaminophen (1 g four times daily) is more effective in preventing fever than placebo (5 versus 36 percent).

8. **Blood pressure management.** Acute management of blood pressure (BP) may vary according to the type of stroke.

   a. **Ischemic stroke.** Blood pressure should not be treated acutely in the patient with ischemic stroke unless the hypertension is extreme (diastolic BP above 120 mm Hg and/or systolic BP above 220 mm Hg), or the patient has active ischemic coronary disease, heart failure, or aortic dissection. If pharmacologic therapy is given, intravenous labetalol is the drug of choice.

   b. **Intracranial hemorrhage.** With ICH, intravenous labetalol, nitroprusside, or nicardipine, should be given if the systolic pressure is above 170 mm Hg. The goal is to maintain the systolic pressure between 140 and 160 mm Hg. Intravenous labetalol is the first drug of choice in the acute phase since it allows rapid titration.

I. **Neurologic evaluation.** The history should focus upon the time of symptom onset, the course of symptoms over time, possible embolic sources, items in the differential diagnosis, and concomitant diseases. The neurologic examination should attempt to confirm the findings from the history and provide a quantifiable examination for further assessment over time.

J. **Neuroimaging** studies are used to exclude hemorrhage as a cause of the deficit, to assess the degree of brain injury, and to identify the vascular lesion responsible for the ischemic deficit.

1. **Computed tomography.** In the hyperacute phase, a non-contrast CT (NCCT) scan is usually ordered to exclude or confirm hemorrhage. A NCCT scan should be obtained as soon as the patient is medically stable.

   a. **Noncontrast CT.** Early signs of infarction include: Subtle parenchymal hypodensity, which can be detected in 45 to 85 percent of cases. Early focal brain swelling is present in up to 40 percent of patients with early infarction and also has been adversely related to outcome. A hyperdense middle cerebral artery (MCA) can be visualized in 30 to 40 percent of patients with an MCA distribution stroke, indicating the presence of thrombus inside the artery lumen (bright artery sign).

2. **Transcranial Doppler ultrasound (TCD)** visualizes intracranial vessels of the circle of Willis. It is a noninvasive means of assessing the patency of intracranial vessels.

3. **Carotid duplex ultrasound** is as a noninvasive examination to evaluate extracranial atherosclerotic disease. It may help to establish the source of an embolic stroke, but is not used acutely.

Initial management of acute stroke

Determine whether stroke is ischemic or hemorrhagic by computed tomography
Consider administration of t-PA if less than three hours from stroke onset
General management:
- Blood pressure (avoid hypotension)
- Assure adequate oxygenation
- Administer intravenous glucose
- Take dysphagia/aspiration precautions
- Consider prophylaxis for venous thrombosis if the patient is unable to walk
- Suppress fever, if present
- Assess stroke mechanism (eg, atrial fibrillation, hypertension)
- Consider aspirin or clopidogrel (Plavix) therapy if ischemic stroke and no contraindications (begin 24 hours after t-PA).

Antiplatelet Agents for Prevention of Ischemic Stoke

- Enteric-coated aspirin (Ecotrin) 325 mg PO qd
- Clopidogrel (Plavix) 75 mg PO qd
- Extended-release aspirin 25 mg with dipyridamole 200 mg (Aggrenox) one tab PO qd

Eligibility criteria for the treatment of acute ischemic stroke with recombinant tissue plasminogen activator (rt-PA)

Inclusion criteria
Clinical diagnosis of ischemic stroke, with the onset of symptoms within three hours of the initiation of treatment (if the exact time of stroke onset is not know, it is defined as the last time the patient was known to be normal), and with a measurable neurologic deficit.

Exclusion criteria
Historical
    Stroke or head trauma within the prior 3 months
    Any prior history of intracranial hemorrhage
    Major surgery within 14 days
    Gastrointestinal or genitourinary bleeding within the previous 21 days

Clinical
Rapid improving stroke symptoms
Only minor and isolated neurologic signs
Seizure at the onset of stroke with postictal residual neurologic impairments
Symptoms suggestive of subarachnoid hemorrhage, even if the CT is normal
Clinical presentation consistent with acute MI or post-MI pericarditis
Persistent systolic BP >185 diastolic >110 mm Hg, or requiring aggressive therapy to control BP
Pregnancy or lactation
Active bleeding or acute trauma (fracture)

Laboratory
Platelets <100,000/mm^3
Serum glucose <50 mg/dL or >400 mg/dL
INR >1.5 if on warfarin
Elevated partial thromboplastin time if on heparin

Head CT scan
Evidence of hemorrhage
Evidence major early infarct signs, such as diffuse swelling of the affected hemisphere,
parenchymal hypodensity, and /or effacement of >35 percent of the middle cerebral artery
territory

  K. Thrombolytic therapy. Patients presenting within three hours of symptom
     onset may be given IV alteplase (Activase) (0.9 mg/kg up to 90 mg; 10 percent
     as a bolus, then a 60 minute infusion).
References, see page 372.

Transient Cerebral Ischemia

Transient ischemic attack (transient cerebral ischemia, TIA) is a temporary focal
neurologic deficit caused by the brief interruption of local cerebral blood flow. The
prevalence of TIAs 1.6-4.1 percent. Stroke occurs in one-third of patients who have
a TIA. The duration of a focal neurologic deficit that leads to cerebral infarction is 24
hours or greater. Transient ischemic attacks (TIA) are divided into three subtypes:
Large artery low flow TIA (true TIA), embolic TIA, and lacunar or small penetrating
vessel TIA.

I. **Pathophysiology.** The most frequent mechanism of TIA is embolization by a
   thrombus from an atherosclerotic plaque in a large vessel (stenotic carotid
   artery). TIAs may also occur as manifestations of intracranial atherosclerotic
   disease (lacunar TIAs) or large-vessel occlusion. In addition, they can be
   associated with atrial fibrillation or mitral valve prolapse, carotid or vertebral dissection, and hypercoagulable states (antiphospholipid antibody syndrome).
II. **Evaluation of TIA symptoms**
   A. The primary objective when evaluating a patient with a transient ischemic
       attack (TIA) is to determine whether the ischemic insult has occurred in the
       anterior or posterior circulation.
   B. Anterior circulation ischemia causes motor or sensory deficits of the
       extremities or face, amaurosis fugax, aphasia, and/or homonymous
       hemianopia.
   C. Posterior circulation ischemia causes motor or sensory dysfunction in
       association with diplopia, dysphasia, dysarthria, ataxia, and/or vertigo.
   D. Assessment should determine the activity in which the patient was engaged
       and the patient's physical position at the onset of the attack. A description of
       the specific symptoms of the attack should be obtained, including the speed
       with which they developed, whether they were bilateral or unilateral, and their
       duration.
   E. History of hypertension, diabetes, cardiac disease, previous TIA or stroke,
       cigarette smoking, or use of street drugs should be sought.
   F. Differentiating TIAs from other entities
       1. Seizures almost always involve a change in the level of consciousness or
           awareness, excessive motor activity and confusion, none of which charac-
           terizes a TIA.
       2. Syncope. Changes in cardiac output produce generalized, rather than
           focal, cerebral ischemia, characterized by loss of consciousness and a
           rapid heartbeat (often due to an arrhythmia).
       3. Benign positional vertigo. Recurrent waves of dizziness, which last 2-10
           seconds and are related to movement (standing up or sitting down), are
           characteristic.

G. Physical examination

1. Heart rate and rhythm and the blood pressure in both arms, peripheral pulses, skin lesions (petechiae of embolic origin), and skin manifestations of connective tissue disease should be assessed.
2. Carotid bruits may suggest carotid stenosis. Ophthalmoscopic examination can detect arterial or venous occlusion and emboli.
3. **Neurologic examination**
   a. The neurologic examination should be normal in TIA patients unless the patient has had a previous stroke or is currently experiencing a TIA or stroke.
   b. Evaluation should include the level of consciousness, orientation, ability to speak and understand language; cranial nerve function, especially eye movements and pupil reflexes and facial paresis. Neglect, gaze preference, arm and leg strength, sensation, and walking ability should be assessed.

Common Clinical Findings Associated with Ischemia in Various Arterial Distributions

Anterior cerebral artery	**Lenticulostriate arteries**
Weakness in contralateral leg	Pure motor hemiparesis (lacunar syndrome)
Sensory loss in contralateral leg, with or without weakness or numbness in proximal contralateral arm	**Posterior cerebral artery**
Middle cerebral artery	Visual field disturbance
Contralateral hemiparesis	Contralateral sensory loss
Deviation of head and eyes toward side of lesion	Amnesia
Contralateral hemianesthesia	**Vertebrobasilar arteries**
Contralateral hemianopia	Vertigo
Aphasia (if dominant hemisphere is affected)	Nausea and vomiting
Unawareness of stroke (if nondominant hemisphere is affected)	Ataxia
	Nystagmus

H. Laboratory testing
is helpful in ruling out metabolic and hematologic causes of neurologic symptoms, including hypoglycemia, hyponatremia, and thrombocytosis.

1. **Electrocardiogram** may reveal unsuspected cases of atrial fibrillation or a recent myocardial infarction.

Initial Evaluation of a Patient with Transient Ischemic Attack

Complete blood cell count with platelet count
Chemistry profile (including cholesterol and glucose levels)
Prothrombin time and activated partial thromboplastin time
Erythrocyte sedimentation rate
Syphilis serology
Electrocardiography
Cranial computed tomography (particularly with hemispheric transient ischemic attack)
Noninvasive arterial imaging (ultrasonography, magnetic resonance angiography)

I. Imaging studies.
Brain imaging with CT or MRI is indicated in all patients with suspected TIA to search for an obstructive lesion in a larger artery supplying the affected territory. The presence of a brain infarct on CT or MRI scan, particularly in an area suggested by the anatomy of the TIA or stroke.

Infarction is more likely to be identified acutely on MRI than on CT. However, CT scanners are more widely available emergently than MRI.

J. **Cardiac evaluation.** All patients with TIA should have the following tests:
1. Standard 12 lead electrocardiogram (ECG)
2. Chest radiography
3. **Echocardiography** is indicated for patients who are candidates for anticoagulation or for patients who have suspected endocarditis.
   a. Transesophageal echocardiography (TEE) is the test of choice for evaluation of aortic atherosclerosis.
   b. Transthoracic echocardiography (TTE) with agitated saline contrast is usually a first test because it is noninvasive and better tolerated. It is also less sensitive than TEE. Transesophageal echocardiography (TEE) should be performed if the TTE is negative and treatment decisions hinge on identifying one of the possible TEE findings.
4. **Cardiac monitoring** is an essential part of this evaluation to exclude atrial fibrillation. Holter monitoring or continuous telemetry may be most useful in patients with a history of palpitations, paroxysmal atrial fibrillation, evidence of spontaneous echo contrast on TEE, and cryptogenic TIA.
K. **Other tests.** Blood cultures, an erythrocyte sedimentation rate, or antinuclear antibody testing are indicated if bacterial or nonbacterial endocarditis is suspected.
L. **Neurovascular evaluation.** Noninvasive options for evaluation of large vessel occlusive disease include magnetic resonance angiography (MRA), computed tomography angiography (CTA), carotid duplex ultrasonography (CDUS), and transcranial Doppler ultrasonography (TCD).
1. **Anterior circulation.** Patients with symptoms referable to the anterior circulation require extracranial carotid artery evaluation.
2. **Posterior circulation.** Patients with symptoms referable to the posterior circulation should have MRA or CTA of the neck to detect dissection and vertebral origin atherosclerosis.
3. **Intracranial large vessels.** In most cases, cardiac and extracranial evaluations should be performed prior to intracranial evaluation. Evaluation of intracranial vessels with CTA, MRA, or TCD should be performed routinely, especially for the following higher prevalence situations:
   a. Age less than 50 without clear cardiac or extracranial source
   b. Patients with recurrent stereotyped TIAs
   c. Patients with posterior circulation event and no clear cardiac source
   d. Patients with preoperative evaluation of collateral circulation before carotid endarterectomy
4. **Small vessels** are not directly visible with any of the currently available imaging techniques. However, evaluation of the extracranial carotid artery is recommended for patients with lacunar infarction or suspected small vessel TIA referable to the anterior circulation.
M. **Blood tests**
1. In patients with TIA, the following tests should be considered:
   a. Complete blood count (CBC)
   b. Partial thromboplastin time (aPTT)
   c. Erythrocyte sedimentation rate (ESR)
2. Suspicion for blood disorders as potential sources of cerebral ischemia should be raised in the following settings:
   a. Cryptogenic stroke
   b. Age 45 or younger
   c. History of clotting dysfunction
   d. Multiple venous and arterial occlusions
   e. Suspected or confirmed cancer

      f. Family history of thrombotic events

III. Treatment of transient cerebral ischemia and minor stroke

A. Large vessel disease

1. **Antiplatelet therapy.** Patients with large vessel atherothrombotic disease in anterior and posterior cerebral circulation sites other than the internal carotid artery and patients with the latter lesions who cannot undergo carotid endarterectomy benefit from antiplatelet therapy.

2. **Anticoagulation (eg, with warfarin).** Virtually all patients with atrial fibrillation who have a history of stroke or TIA should be treated with warfarin in the absence of contraindications since long-term anticoagulation reduces the risk of recurrent stroke. In contrast, warfarin has not been found to be superior to antiplatelet agents as secondary prevention in patients without atrial fibrillation.

3. **Carotid revascularization.** Carotid endarterectomy (CEA) should be considered for patients with large vessel atherothrombotic disease in the internal carotid artery that causes low flow or embolic TIAs.

4. **Amaurosis fugax** refers to transient monocular blindness caused by a small embolus to the ophthalmic artery. It accounts for one-quarter of TIAs involving the anterior cerebral circulation. Amaurosis fugax frequently occurs as a result of carotid stenosis. Amaurosis fugax is more typical of carotid stenosis than atrial fibrillation. Carotid endarterectomy may improve outcomes in those with additional risk factors for stroke.

5. **Risk factor management** is appropriate for all patients with less than 50 percent carotid stenosis or for those who are at high risk of developing complications from surgery. Risk factor management includes treatment of hypertension, diabetes mellitus, smoking, dyslipidemia, and hyperhomocysteinemia.

6. **Carotid occlusion.** Surgical revascularization is a viable option only when residual flow can be demonstrated in the carotid artery. Carotid artery occlusion can be associated with TIA and stroke. Short-term (three to six months) anticoagulation may be administered for acute symptomatic occlusion.

7. **Vertebral revascularization.** Large artery lesions at the origin of the vertebral artery have been treated with angioplasty, stenting, and vertebral artery transposition to the common carotid artery. These procedures are considered when maximal medical therapy has failed to prevent embolism or low-flow ischemic events.

8. **Intracranial large vessel disease**

    a. There is no clear difference in effectiveness for either aspirin or anticoagulation for large vessel intracranial disease. Therefore, aspirin or other antiplatelet therapy is recommended, since warfarin is potentially more hazardous.

    b. Antiplatelet therapy (eg, aspirin 75 to 325 mg/day) and risk factor management should be initiated for patients with large vessel intracranial disease. However, warfarin may still benefit selected patients with large artery lesions who have recurrent embolic or low-flow TIAs despite maximal antiplatelet therapy. Use of warfarin (goal INR 2 to 3) may be considered for such patients if there is thrombus in the basilar artery, middle cerebral artery stem, or the siphon portion of the internal carotid artery.

9. **Dissection.** Patients who experience acute ischemic symptoms due to carotid or vertebral dissection should be treated with intravenous heparin followed by warfarin therapy until the carotid or vertebral artery is occluded and healed, or is resolved back to a clonic state of circulation. This usually involves treatment for six months to one year.

B. Small vessel disease. Small vessel disease that causes transient ischemia is a diagnosis of exclusion. The efficacy of aspirin versus warfarin in preventing further TIAs or stroke in the setting of a small vessel TIA is uncertain. Attention to serum lipids, homocysteine metabolism, hypertension, and other modifiable risk factors are additional means of preventing lacunar strokes in patients with small vessel disease.

C. Cardiogenic embolism. Approximately 60 percent of all strokes are caused by embolism (eg, heart, aorta, or an unknown source).

1. The distinction between artery-to-artery and non-artery-to-artery sources of embolism can be difficult. Suspicion of the former typically arises once vascular pathology in a large vessel has been identified (eg, with noninvasive testing). Repetitive spells within a single vascular territory are also suggestive of an artery-to-artery source, as is a normal echocardiogram. Transesophageal echocardiography (TEE) is better for identifying these lesions. TTE with agitated saline contrast should be performed as a first test, and proceeding to TEE if there is a strong suspicion of a cardioembolic source. Cardiac monitoring is also an essential part of this evaluation to exclude atrial fibrillation.

2. Definite cardiac sources of embolism for which antithrombotic therapy has proven effective include:
   a. Atrial fibrillation.
   b. Left ventricular thrombus.
   c. Left atrial thrombus.
   d. Rheumatic valve disease.
   e. Mechanical prosthetic heart valve.
   f. Bioprosthetic heart valve.
   g. Cardiomyopathy with an ejection fraction less than 30 percent.
   h. Recent myocardial infarction in high-risk patients, with risk factors including anterior wall MI, coexisting left ventricular dysfunction, hypertension before MI, and history of systemic or pulmonary embolism.

3. **Atrial fibrillation** is a major risk factor for ischemic stroke. Anticoagulation is the most effective treatment to reduce stroke risk.
   a. **Acute heparin therapy.** It is reasonable to follow the guidelines for acute heparin therapy after stroke.
   b. **Warfarin.** Virtually all patients with atrial fibrillation who have a history of embolic stroke or TIA should be treated with warfarin in the absence of contraindications. Warfarin treatment can reduce the risk of stroke by 70 percent. An INR between 2.0 and 3.0 is recommended for most patients with AF who receive warfarin anticoagulation.

4. **Infective endocarditis.** An important cause of embolic TIA for which anticoagulation is hazardous is infective endocarditis. Emboli from vegetations can cause focal neurologic signs which are fleeting. Thus, endocarditis must be excluded in any patient with a TIA and other suggestive findings such as fever and a heart murmur. Treatment consists of antibiotic therapy for the infection.

5. **Minor causes of cardiogenic embolism.** Minor potential sources of cardiogenic embolism include left ventricular regional wall motion abnormalities, severe mitral annular calcification, mitral valve prolapse, and mitral valve strands. The risk of stroke associated with these sources is uncertain, as is the efficacy of and need for treatment.

D. Antiplatelet agents for stroke prevention

1. The Sixth American College of Chest Physicians (ACCP) Consensus Conference on Antithrombotic Therapy recommended that every patient with an atherothrombotic stroke or TIA and no contraindication should receive an antiplatelet agent to reduce the risk of recurrent stroke and

other vascular events. Fewer gastrointestinal side effects and bleeding occur with lower doses (75 to 150 mg/day). Aspirin, clopidogrel (75 mg/day), and the combination of aspirin and dipyridamole are all acceptable options. However, initial therapy with aspirin (50 to 325 mg/day) is recommended; doses less than 150 mg/day are associated with less gastrointestinal toxicity.

2. Clopidogrel is an alternative for patients who cannot tolerate aspirin. Combination therapy with aspirin and dipyridamole can be considered in patients who have an event while on aspirin alone. Ticlopidine should be reserved for patients intolerant of both aspirin and clopidogrel.

References, see page 372.

Dementia

Dementia is characterized by a general decrease in the level of cognition (especially memory), behavioral disturbances, and interference with daily function and independence. Alzheimer's disease (AD) is the most common form of dementia, accounting for 60 to 80 percent of cases.

I. Identification of dementia

A. The normal cognitive decline associated with aging consists of mild changes in memory and the rate of information processing, which are not progressive and do not affect daily function.

B. Patients with dementia may have difficulty with one or more of the following:
   1. Learning and retaining new information (eg, trouble remembering events).
   2. Handling complex tasks (eg, balancing a checkbook).
   3. Reasoning (eg, unable to cope with unexpected events).
   4. Spatial ability and orientation (eg, getting lost in familiar places).
   5. Language (eg, word finding).
   6. Behavior.

C. The date of onset of dementia can often be identified when the patient stopped driving or managing finances. Useful questions are, "When did you first notice the memory loss?" and "How has the memory loss progressed since then?"

D. The diagnosis of dementia must be distinguished from delirium and depression. Delirium is usually acute in onset with a clouding of the sensorium. Patients with delirium may have fluctuations in their level of consciousness and have difficulty with attention and concentration.

E. Patients with depression are more likely to complain about memory loss than those with dementia. Patients with depression may have psychomotor slowing and poor effort on testing.

F. **Mild cognitive impairment (MCI)** is defined by the following features:
   1. Memory complaint, corroborated by an informant.
   2. Objective memory impairment.
   3. Normal general cognitive function.
   4. Intact activities of daily living.
   5. Not demented.

G. Patients with MCI are at increased risk of dementia. The prevalence of MCI was estimated at 3 to 4 percent.

H. **Dementia syndromes.** The major dementia syndromes include:
   1. Alzheimer's disease.
   2. Vascular ("multi-infarct") dementia.
   3. Parkinson's disease and related dementias (including Lewy body dementia and progressive supranuclear palsy).
   4. Frontal lobe dementia.
   5. Reversible dementias.

6. Most elderly patients with chronic dementia have Alzheimer's disease (60 to 80 percent). The vascular dementias account for 10 to 20 percent, and Parkinson's disease 5 percent. Alcohol-related dementia, medication side effects, depression, normal pressure hydrocephalus, and other central nervous system illnesses are responsible for the remainder of the chronic dementias.

DSM-IV Criteria for Dementia

1. Memory impairment
2. At least one of the following:
   - Aphasia
   - Apraxia
   - Agnosia
   - Disturbance in executive functioning
3. The disturbance in 1 and 2 significantly interferes with work, social activities, or relationships
4. Disturbance does not occur exclusively during delirium

Additional criteria for dementia type
Dementia of the Alzheimer's type:
   Gradual onset and continuing cognitive decline
   Not caused by identifiable medical, psychiatric, or neurologic condition

---

Vascular dementia
Focal from history, physical exam, or laboratory findings of a specific medical condition

---

Dementia due to other medical conditions
Evidence from history, physical exam, or laboratory findings of a specific medical condition causing cognitive deficits (HIV disease, head trauma, Parkinson's disease, Huntington's disease, Pick's disease, Creutzfeldt-Jacob)

I. **Alzheimer's disease** is a progressive neurologic disorder that results in memory loss, personality changes, global cognitive dysfunction, and functional impairments. Loss of short-term memory is most prominent early. In the late stages of disease, patients are totally dependent upon others for basic activities of daily living, such as feeding and toileting.

1. Alzheimer's disease is characterized by cerebral extracellular deposition of amyloid-beta protein, intracellular neurofibrillary tangles, and loss of neurons. The DSM-IV criteria for the diagnosis of Alzheimer's dementia include the following:

   a. The gradual onset and continuing decline of cognitive function from a previously higher level, resulting in impairment in social or occupational function.

   b. Impairment of recent memory (inability to learn new information) and at least one of the following: disturbance of language; inability to execute skilled motor activities in the absence of weakness; disturbances of visual processing; or disturbances of executive function (including abstract reasoning and concentration).

   c. The cognitive deficits are not due to other psychiatric, neurologic, or systemic diseases.

   d. The deficits do not occur exclusively in the setting of delirium.

    2. Behavioral problems are common in Alzheimer's disease; personality changes (progressive passivity to open hostility) may precede the cognitive impairments. Delusions (particularly paranoid) and hallucinations contribute to the behavioral difficulties.

J. Vascular dementia. Features that suggest the diagnosis include:
   1. The onset of cognitive deficits associated with a stroke.
   2. Abrupt onset of symptoms followed by stepwise deterioration.
   3. Findings on neurologic examination consistent with prior stroke(s).
   4. Infarcts on cerebral imaging.

K. Poststroke dementia develops in 19.3 percent of subjects with stroke. Subjects with stroke have a twofold higher risk of dementia at 10 years.

L. Mixed dementia. Many individuals have mixed features of vascular and Alzheimer's dementia.

M. **Reversible dementia.** The potentially reversible dementias include the following:
   1. **Medication-induced** (eg, analgesics, anticholinergics, psychotropic medications, and sedative-hypnotics).
   2. **Alcohol-related** (eg, intoxication, withdrawal).
   3. **Metabolic disorders** (eg, thyroid disease, vitamin B12 deficiency, hyponatremia, hypercalcemia, hepatic and renal dysfunction).
   4. **Depression.**
   5. **Central nervous system neoplasms,** chronic subdural hematomas, chronic meningitis.
   6. **Normal pressure hydrocephalus.**
   7. **Bismuth exposure** can cause a myoclonic encephalopathy that can be confused with CJD.
   8. **Hashimoto's thyroiditis** can cause encephalopathy with myoclonus or choreoathetosis and seizures.
   9. **Whipple's disease** is characterized by dementia, supranuclear gaze palsy, oculomasticatory myorhythmia, and myoclonus.

N. Normal pressure hydrocephalus is often considered in patients who present with the triad of gait disturbance, urinary incontinence, and cognitive dysfunction.
   1. The Miller Fisher test, consisting of objective gait assessment before and after the removal of 30 mL of spinal fluid, is useful to confirm the diagnosis of normal pressure hydrocephalus. Radioisotope diffusion studies in the cerebrospinal fluid also confirm the diagnosis.

O. Other disorders
   1. **Creutzfeldt-Jakob disease** is a rare neurodegenerative disease caused by prions. It presents with a rapidly progressive dementia that is usually fatal within one year. The diagnosis may be suspected on the basis of the rapid onset of cognitive impairment, motor deficits, and seizures. The disease is not treatable, but the disease is potentially transmissible.
   2. Other more common infectious disorders that may be associated with dementia include tertiary syphilis and HIV infection.

II. Diagnostic approach

A. History of cognitive and behavioral changes should be assessed. Drugs that impair cognition (eg, analgesics, anticholinergics, psychotropic medications, and sedative-hypnotics) should be sought.

B. Physical examination, including neurologic examination. The work-up may include laboratory and imaging studies should be completed.

C. Mini-Mental State Examination (MMSE) is the most widely used cognitive test for dementia. It tests a broad range of cognitive functions, including orientation, recall, attention, calculation, language manipulation, and constructional praxis. The MMSE includes the following tasks:

1. **Orientation**
   a. What is the date: (year, season, date, day, month) - 5 points
   b. Where are we: (state)(county)(town)(hospital)(floor) - 5 points

2. **Registration**
   a. Name three objects. Ask the patient all three after you have said them. Give one point for each correct answer. Then repeat them until he learns all three. Maximum score - 3 points.

3. **Attention and calculation**
   a. Serial 7s, beginning with 100 and counting backward. One point for each correct, stop after 5 answers. Alternatively, spell WORLD backwards (one point for each letter that is in correct order). Maximum score - 5 points.
   b. Ask for the three objects repeated above. One point for each correct. Maximum score - 3 points.
   c. Show and ask patient to name a pencil and wrist watch - 2 points.
   d. Repeat the following, "No ifs ands or buts." Allow only one trial - 1 point.
   e. Follow a three stage command, "Take a paper in your right hand, fold it in half, and put it on the floor." Score one point for each task executed. Maximum score - 3 points.
   f. On a blank piece of paper write "close your eyes" and ask the patient to read and do what it says - 1 point.
   g. Give the patient a blank piece of paper and ask him to write a sentence. The sentence must contain a noun and verb and be sensible - 1 point.
   h. Ask the patient to copy intersecting pentagons. All ten angles must be present and two must intersect - 1 point.

4. A total maximal score on the MMSE is 30 points. A score of less than 24 points is suggestive of dementia or delirium. The MMSE has a sensitivity of 87 percent and a specificity of 82 percent. However, the test is not sensitive in cases of mild dementia, and scores are spuriously low in individuals with a low education level, poor motor function, black or Latino ethnicity, poor language skills, or impaired vision.

D. **Physical examination and a neurologic examination** should seek for focal neurologic deficits that may be consistent with prior strokes, signs of Parkinson's disease (eg, cogwheel rigidity and tremors), gait, and eye movements.

E. **Laboratory testing**
   1. Screening for B12 deficiency and hypothyroidism is recommended. Routine laboratory studies may include a complete blood count, electrolytes, calcium, glucose, blood urea nitrogen, creatinine, and liver function tests. Screening for neurosyphilis (RPR) is not recommended unless there is a high clinical suspicion of neurosyphilis.
   2. Red blood cell folate should be obtained in ethanol dependence. Ionized serum calcium should be measured in multiple myeloma, prostate cancer, or breast cancer.

F. **Neuroimaging.** A noncontrast head CT or MRI is recommended for all patients with dementia.

III. **Treatment of dementia**

A. **Cholinesterase inhibitors**
   1. Patients with AD have reduced cerebral production of choline acetyl transferase, which leads to a decrease in acetylcholine synthesis and impaired cortical cholinergic function. Cholinesterase inhibitors increase cholinergic transmission by inhibiting cholinesterase at the synaptic cleft.
   2. Four cholinesterase inhibitors, tacrine, donepezil, rivastigmine, and galantamine are currently approved. Tacrine was can cause hepatotoxicity

and is rarely used. The choice between the other three agents is based upon cost and patient tolerability because efficacy is similar.

3. **Donepezil (Aricept)** has relatively little peripheral anticholinesterase activity and is generally well-tolerated. This combined with its once-daily dosing has made it a popular drug in patients with AD. The recommended dose for donepezil is 5 mg per day for 4 weeks, then increasing to 10 mg per day.

   a. Cognition, as measured by the Alzheimer's Disease Assessment Scale (ADAS-cog), and the Clinician's global ratings significantly improved.

   b. There was a small but significant beneficial effect of donepezil for cognition compared with placebo, with a 0.8 point difference in the Mini Mental Status Exam (MMSE) score (95% CI 0.5-1.2).

   c. Donepezil may have some symptomatic benefit in patients with mild cognitive impairment (MCI) who are likely to convert to AD, delaying the clinical diagnosis but not changing the underlying course of the disease.

   d. Prolonged treatment with donepezil appears to be safe and effective. Cholinergic side effects (primarily diarrhea, nausea, and vomiting) are transient and generally mild, occurring in about 20 percent of patients.

4. **Rivastigmine (Exelon)** appears to be beneficial for patients with mild-to-moderate AD. Its side-effect profile is related to cholinergic effects, with significant nausea, vomiting, anorexia, and headaches. It should be given with food to minimize nausea. One case of esophageal rupture do to severe vomiting has been reported. Therapy is initiated at 1.5 mg BID with titration every two weeks up to 6 mg BID and, if treatment is interrupted for longer than several days, it should be restarted at the lowest daily dose and then titrated again. Its efficacy appears similar although it may have more gastrointestinal side-effects.

5. **Galantamine (Reminyl)** and appears to be effective in patients with mild-to-moderate AD. Treatment with galantamine (maintenance dose 24 or 32 mg/day) slows the decline in both cognition and activities of daily living compared with placebo in patients with early Alzheimer's disease.

   a. Gastrointestinal symptoms (nausea, vomiting, diarrhea, anorexia, weight loss) are the most common adverse effects of galantamine. Like rivastigmine, galantamine appears to have similar efficacy to donepezil in patients with AD, but may have more gastrointestinal side-effects.

6. **Degree of benefit.** Cholinesterase inhibitors can improve cognitive function in patients with AD, vascular dementia, and diffuse Lewy body disease. However, the average benefit is a small improvement in cognition and activities of daily living.

7. **Administration.** Cholinesterase inhibitors are a symptomatic treatment and not disease-modifying; therefore, the drugs should be given for eight weeks and the patient's response should be reviewed. Treatment is continued if improvement is noted. The medication should be discontinued when a patient progresses to advanced dementia

Cholinesterase Inhibitors for the Treatment of Mild-to-Moderate Alzheimer's Disease

Drug	Dosage	Side effects	Specific cautions
Donepezil (Aricept)	Initial dosage is 5 mg once daily; if necessary, dosage can be increased to 10 mg once daily after 4 to 6 weeks.	Mild side effects, nausea, vomiting, and diarrhea; effects can be reduced by taking with food. Initial agitation in some subsides after a few weeks.	Possible interactions with cimetidine (Tagamet), theophylline, warfarin (Coumadin), and digoxin (Lanoxin)
Rivastigmine (Exelon)	Initial dosage of 1.5 mg bid (3 mg per day) is well tolerated; dosage can be increased as tolerated to maximum of 6 mg twice daily (12 mg per day).	Nausea, vomiting, diarrhea, headaches, dizziness, abdominal pain, fatigue, malaise, anxiety, and agitation; these effects can be reduced by taking rivastigmine with food.	Weight loss Interacting drugs include aminoglycosides and procainamide (Procanbid).
Galantamine (Reminyl)	Initial dosage is 4 mg bid (8 mg per day) for 4 weeks; dosage is then increased to 8 mg twice daily (16 mg per day) for at least 4 weeks. An increase to 12 mg twice daily (24 mg per day) should be considered.	Mild side effects, including nausea, vomiting, and diarrhea; these effects can be reduced by taking galantamine with food No apparent association with sleep disturbances (which can occur with other cholinergic treatments)	Contraindicated for use in patients with hepatic or renal impairment
Tacrine (Cognex)	Initial dosage is 10 mg four times daily (40 mg per day) for 4 weeks.	High incidence of side effects, including gastrointestinal problems.	Hepatotoxicity is a problem; hence, liver tests should be performed.

IV. **Disease-modifying agents**

   A. **Memantine** (Namenda) is an N-methyl-D-aspartate (NMDA) receptor antagonist. Glutamate is the principle excitatory amino acid neurotransmitter in cortical and hippocampal neurons. One of the receptors activated by glutamate is the NMDA receptor, which is involved in learning and memory. Excessive NMDA stimulation can be induced by ischemia and lead to excitotoxicity, suggesting that agents that block pathologic stimulation of NMDA receptors may protect against further damage in patients with vascular dementia.

   1. Memantine results in a small but statistically significant improvement in ADAS-cog scores compared with placebo (difference between the groups 2 points on a 70 point scale.

   2. Memantine appears to be effective in patients with moderate to severe Alzheimer's disease. A 28-week randomized trial in 252 patients with MMSE scores of 3 to 14 (mean approximately 8) at study entry found that memantine significantly reduced deterioration on multiple scales of clinical efficacy.

3. The mechanism of action of memantine is distinct from that of the cholinergic agents; it appears to be neuroprotective. Memantine also appears to have fewer side effects than the cholinergic agents.

4. **Memantine plus cholinesterase inhibitors.** Treatment with memantine plus donepezil results in significantly better outcomes than placebo plus donepezil on measures of cognition, activities of daily living, global outcome, and behavior. Memantine is used in combination with a cholinesterase inhibitor in patients with advanced disease. Since it may be disease-modifying. Memantine should be continued even when there is no clinical improvement.

B. Recommendations

1. Start patients with mild-to-moderate dementia on a cholinesterase inhibitor. Tacrine should not be used. The choice between donepezil, rivastigmine, and galantamine can be based upon cost, individual patient tolerance, and physician experience, as efficacy appears to be similar.

2. In patients with moderate to advanced dementia, add memantine to a cholinesterase inhibitor, or use memantine alone in patients who do not tolerate or benefit from a cholinesterase inhibitor.

3. In patients with severe dementia, cholinesterase inhibitors can be discontinued, but they should be restarted if the patient worsens without the medication. Memantine should be continued even in severe dementia, given the possibility that memantine may be disease modifying. However, in some patients with advanced dementia medications should be discontinued to maximize quality of life and patient comfort.

4. For delusions and hallucinations, the atypical neuroleptics olanzapine (starting at a dose of 2.5 mg daily, titrating up to a maximum of 5 mg twice a day) or quetiapine (starting at a dose of 25 mg at bedtime, titrating up to a maximum of 75 mg twice a day) are recommended at the lowest effective doses.

5. For depression, avoid tricyclic antidepressants. SSRIs are preferred, but fluoxetine should be avoided because of its long half-life and drug interactions, and avoid paroxetine because it is more anticholinergic than other SSRIs.

6. For agitation and aggression, look for triggers and try to treat those first. Most behavioral symptoms have precipitants (constipation, urinary retention, fear of unrecognized caregivers, etc). Frightening delusions respond to atypical neuroleptics, and agitation may be due to unrecognized depression and responds to SSRIs. If a treatable etiology cannot be found, treat with trazodone starting with 25 mg at bedtime or twice daily and titrating the dose up to 50 to 100 mg twice daily. If this is unsuccessful, an atypical neuroleptic should be used.

References, see page 372.

Seizures

A seizure is a sudden change in behavior that is the result brain dysfunction. Epileptic seizures result from electrical hypersynchronization of the cerebral cortex. Epilepsy is characterized by recurrent epileptic seizures caused by a brain disorder. Approximately 0.5 to 1 percent of the population has epilepsy.

I. Etiology

A. Epileptic seizures

1. An identifiable cause can be determined in less than one-half of epilepsy cases. Epilepsy in most of these other patients is genetically determined. In causes of epileptic seizures include congenital brain malformations, inborn errors of metabolism, high fevers, head trauma, brain tumors, stroke, intracranial infection, cerebral degeneration, withdrawal states, and iatrogenic drug reactions.

2. In the elderly, vascular, degenerative, and neoplastic etiologies are more common than in younger adults and children. A higher proportion of epilepsy in children is due to congenital brain malformations. Head injury accounts for a relatively small proportion of epilepsy overall.

B. Physiological nonepileptic seizures

1. Hyperthyroidism can cause seizures and can exacerbate seizures in patients with epilepsy.

2. Hypoglycemic seizures are most common in diabetic patients who take excessive amounts of insulin or oral hypoglycemics.

3. Nonketotic hyperglycemia most commonly occurs in elderly diabetics and can cause focal motor seizures.

4. Precipitous falls in serum sodium concentrations can trigger generalized tonic-clonic seizures.

5. Hypocalcemia is a rare cause of seizures and most often occurs in neonates. In adults, hypocalcemia may occur after thyroid or parathyroid surgery or with renal failure, hypoparathyroidism, or pancreatitis. Magnesium levels below 0.8 mEq/L may result in irritability, agitation, confusion, myoclonus, tetany, and convulsions. Renal failure and uremia are often associated with seizures.

6. Cerebral anoxia as a complication of cardiac or respiratory arrest, carbon monoxide poisoning, drowning, or anesthetic complication can cause myoclonic and generalized tonic-clonic seizures. Cerebral anoxia due to syncope can result in very brief tonic and/or clonic movements without a prolonged postictal state.

Nonepileptic paroxysmal disorders that can mimic epileptic seizure

Syncope
Reflex (vasovagal, carotid sinus, glossopharyngeal, cough)
Decreased cardiac output
Decreased left ventricular filling (hypovolemia, orthostatic hypotension, pulmonary embolism)
Cardiac arrhythmia
Migraine with auras, basilar migraine, confusional migraine
Transient ischemic attack
Periodic paralysis
Sleep disorders (parasomnias, daytime amnestic episodes)
Gastrointestinal disorders (reflux, motility disorders)
Movement disorders (tics, Tourette's syndrome, nonepileptic myoclonus, paroxysmal choreoathetosis, shuddering attacks)
Psychiatric disorders (panic, somatization, dissociation, conversion [nonepileptic psychogenic seizures])
Drug toxicity and substance abuse
Breath-holding spells

Classification of epileptic seizures	
Generalized	**Partial**
Absence Myoclonic Tonic Atonic Clonic Tonic-clonic (grand mal seizure)	Simple partial (consciousness not impaired) Complex partial (consciousness impaired) Partial with secondary generalization (can be tonic-clonic, tonic, or clonic)

A. Differential diagnosis

1. **REM behavior disorder** is a parasomnia that consists of sudden arousals from REM sleep immediately followed by complicated, often aggressive, behaviors for which the patient is amnestic. Diagnosis is clarified by sleep testing (polysomnography).

2. **Transient ischemic attacks (TIAs)** may last seconds to minutes. They are generally characterized by "negative" symptoms and signs (such as weakness or visual loss rather than jerking movements, stiffening, that accompany seizures.

3. **Transient global amnesia** is a condition of possibly vascular or migrainous etiology, that typically occurs after the age of 50. Affected patients have a deficit of short-term memory that begins abruptly and persists for minutes to hours.

4. **Migraine** auras such as visual illusions and altered consciousness can mimic complex partial seizures.

II. Clinical evaluation

A. Seizure precipitants or triggers.
Environmental or physiological precipitants or triggers immediately preceding the seizure should be assessed. Triggers of seizures include strong emotions, intense exercise, flashing lights, and loud music. Fever, the menstrual period, lack of sleep, and stress can also cause seizures. However, the majority of patients with epilepsy have no identifiable or consistent trigger to their seizures.

B. Seizure symptoms and signs

1. **Auras.** The symptoms that a patient experiences at the beginning of the seizure are referred to as the aura. Auras are seizures that cause symptoms, but not enough to interfere with consciousness. Auras are called simple partial seizures; "simple" means that consciousness is not impaired and "partial" means that only part of the cortex is disrupted by the seizure. A seizure that begins in the occipital cortex may result in flashing lights, while a seizure that affects the motor cortex will result in rhythmic jerking movements of the face, arm, or leg on the side of the body opposite to the involved cortex (Jacksonian seizure).

2. **Complex partial seizures** are characterized by an abrupt loss of consciousness. Complex partial seizures are the most common type of seizure in adults. Patients appear to be awake but are not in contact with others. They often seem to stare into space and either remain motionless or engage in repetitive behaviors, called automatisms, such as facial grimacing, gesturing, chewing, lip smacking, snapping fingers, repeating words or phrases, walking, running, or undressing. Complex partial seizures typically last less than three minutes and may be preceded by a simple partial seizure. The postictal phase is characterized by somnolence, confusion, and headache. The patient has no memory of the seizure.

3. **Generalized seizures** originate in all the regions of the cortex. Absence seizures and generalized tonic-clonic seizures are types of generalized

seizures. Other subtypes of generalized seizures are clonic, myoclonic, tonic, and atonic seizures.

a. **Absence seizures** usually occur during childhood and typically last between 5 and 10 seconds. Absence seizures cause sudden staring with impaired consciousness.

b. **Generalized tonic-clonic seizure** begins with an abrupt loss of consciousness. Muscles of the arms and legs as well as the chest and back then become stiff. The patient may begin to appear cyanotic. After one minute, the muscles begin to jerk and twitch for one to two minutes. The tongue can be bitten. The postictal phase begins once the twitching movements end. The patient is initially in a deep sleep, breathing deeply, and then gradually wakes up, often complaining of a headache.

c. **Clonic seizures** cause rhythmical jerking muscle contractions that usually involve the arms, neck, and face.

d. **Myoclonic seizures** consist of sudden, brief muscle contractions that may occur singly or in clusters and that can affect any group of muscles, although typically the arms are affected. Consciousness is not impaired.

e. **Tonic seizures** cause sudden muscle stiffening, often associated with impaired consciousness and falling to the ground.

f. **Atonic seizures** produce a sudden loss of control of the muscles, particularly of the legs, that results in collapsing to the ground and possible injuries.

Phases of Tonic-clonic Seizures	
Aura	**None**
Tonic Phase	10 to 20 seconds
Sudden loss of consciousness Loss of posture with high risk of self injury depending on activity Brief flexion of arms, eyes deviated upward Extension of back, neck, arms, and legs Involuntary crying out from contraction of respiratory muscles Shallow respiration, cyanosis may occur Ends with tremors, which gradually slow and merge with clonic phase	
Clonic phase	30 to 90 seconds
Brief, violent, generalized flexor contractions alternating with progressively longer muscle relaxation Cyanosis Possible cheek or tongue biting Foamy salivation Possible loss of bowel or bladder control Ends with deep inspiration, sustained muscle relaxation	
Postictal phase	Minutes to several hours
Headache, mild confusion Muscles sore Fatigue, patient may sleep and awake refreshed	
Other features	

Aura	None
Fast heart rate Elevated blood pressure Respiratory and metabolic acidosis Dilated pupils Risk of vertebral fracture, pneumonia	

- **C. Other aspects of the patient history**
  1. **Medication history.** Some medications have been associated with iatrogenic seizures. Partial-onset seizures are less likely to be drug-induced than generalized tonic-clonic seizures.
  2. **Past medical history.** Risk factors for epileptic seizures include head injury, stroke, Alzheimer's disease, history of intracranial infection, and alcohol or drug abuse.
  3. **Family history** of seizures is highly suggestive of epilepsy. Absence seizures and myoclonic seizures may be inherited.
- **D. Physical and neurologic examination** is generally unrevealing in patients with epileptic seizures, but is important to exclude meningitis or intracerebral hemorrhage. Weakness, hyperreflexia, or a positive Babinski sign may point to a contralateral structural brain lesion.

History of a suspected seizure

Before the event
Unusual stress (eg, severe emotional trauma)
Sleep deprivation
Recent illness
Unusual stimuli (eg, flickering lights)Use of medications and drugs
Activity immediately before event (eg, change in posture, exercise)

During the event
Symptoms at onset (eg, aura)
Temporal mode of onset: gradual versus sudden
Duration: brief (ictal phase <5 min) versus prolonged
Stereotypy: duration and features of episodes nearly identical versus frequently changing
Time of day: related to sleep or occurring on awakening
Ability to talk and respond appropriately
Ability to comprehend
Ability to recall events during the seizure
Abnormal movements of the eyes, mouth, face, head, arms, and legs
Bowel or bladder incontinence
Bodily injury

After the event
Confusion
Lethargy
Abnormal speech
Focal weakness or sensory loss (ie, Todd's paralysis)
Headache, muscle soreness, or physical injury

III. Diagnostic studies
- **A. Laboratory screening** includes glucose, calcium, magnesium, hematology studies, renal function tests, and toxicology screens.
- **B. Lumbar puncture** is essential if an acute infectious process involving the central nervous system is possible or the patient has a history of cancer that is

known to metastasize to the meninges. Lumbar puncture should only be performed after a space occupying brain lesion has been excluded by neuroimaging studies.

C. **Electroencephalography (EEG)** is an essential study. If abnormal, the EEG may substantiate the diagnosis of epileptic seizures. Obtaining the EEG in the sleep-deprived state and using provocative measures, such as hyperventilation and intermittent photic stimulation, increase the yield. A normal EEG does not rule out epilepsy.

D. **Neuroimaging** study should be done to exclude a structural brain abnormality. Brain magnetic resonance imaging (MRI) is preferred over computed tomography (CT) to identify cortical dysplasias, infarcts, or tumors.

IV. **Management of epilepsy**

A. Chronic drug therapy is not necessary if a first seizure is provoked by factors that resolve. Antiepileptic drug therapy should be started if a patient appears to be at increased risk for recurrent seizures. The overall risk of recurrence following a first seizure in adults is 14% at one year. The worst prognosis is in patients with a history of a neurologic insult and provoked seizures in the past; these individuals have an 80% recurrence rate at five years.

B. **Factors contributing to the risk of recurrent seizures include:**
1. A history of brain insult (eg, head injury with loss of consciousness).
2. A lesion on brain CT or MRI studies.
3. Focal abnormalities detected during the neurologic examination.
4. Cognitive impairment.
5. A partial seizure as the first seizure.
6. An abnormal EEG (particularly epileptiform abnormalities).

C. AED therapy should be initiated after the first incident if the patient is considered at high risk for recurrence. Antiepileptic drug treatment is generally started after the second seizure. The risk of another seizure after two unprovoked seizures is greater than 65 percent.

Initial treatment for partial and generalized epilepsies		
Type of epilepsy	First-line agents	Second-line agents
Partial	Carbamazepine, oxcarbazepine (Trileptal), phenytoin (Dilantin)	Divalproex (Depakote), felbamate (Felbatol), gabapentin (Neurontin), lamotrigine (Lamictal), levetiracetam (Keppra), tiagabine (Gabitril Filmtabs), topiramate (Topamax), valproate (Depakene), zonisamide (Zonegran)
Generalized		
Absence seizures	Ethosuximide (Zarontin), valproate	Lamotrigine, levetiracetam
Idiopathic	Lamotrigine, valproate	Topiramate, zonisamide
Symptomatic	Lamotrigine, topiramate, valproate, zonisamide	Barbiturates, benzodiazepines

Dosing of Antiepileptic Drugs		
Drug	**Intravenous dose**	**Oral dose**
Barbiturates, Mysoline	Phenobarbital: 90 to 120 mg every 10 to 15 min as needed to maximum of 100 mg	1 to 5 mg/kg/day
Carbamazepine (Tegretol; Tegretol-XR; Carbatrol)	Not applicable	Start at 2 to 3mg/kg/day; increase dose every 5 days to 10 mg/kg/day; dose may need to be increased to 15 to 20 mg/kg/day after 2 to 3 months because of hepatic autoinduction
Ethosuximide (Zarontin)	Not applicable	20 to 40 mg/day in 1 to 3 divided doses
Felbamate (Felbatol)	Not applicable	12 mg/day in 3 divided doses; increase by 600 to 1200 mg/day every 2 weeks to recommended maximum of 3600 mg/day
Gabapentin (Neurontin)	Not applicable	300 mg on the first day, 300 mg twice daily on the second day, 300 mg three times daily on the third day; increase as needed to 1800 mg/day in 3 divided doses; lower doses recommended in patients with renal insufficiency
Lamotrigine (Lamictal)	Not applicable	For patients taking an enzyme-inducing antiepileptic drug: 25 mg BID, titrated upward by 5 mg increments every 1 to 2 weeks as needed. For patients taking valproate: 25 mg every other day, with increases of 25 to 50 mg every 2 weeks as needed to a maximum of 300 to 500 mg/day.

Drug	Intravenous dose	Oral dose
Levetiracetam (Keppra)	Not applicable	Start at 500 mg twice daily; increase as needed by 100 mg/day every two weeks to a maximum total dose of 400 mg per day in two divided doses; lower doses recommended in patients with renal insufficiency
Oxcarbazepine (Trileptal)	Not applicable	Start at 300 to 600 mg/day in two or three divided doses; increase by 600 mg/day weekly to a total dose of 900 to 3000 mg per day in two or three divided doses

D. Choosing an antiepileptic drug. Treatment should be started with a single drug (monotherapy) with gradual increase in dosage as needed to produce optimal seizure control. Combination therapy should be attempted only when at least two sequential trials of single agents have failed. With the exception of felbamate, second-generation AEDs (eg, gabapentin, lamotrigine, topiramate, tiagabine, levetiracetam, oxcarbazepine, zonisamide) have significant advantages over older AEDs (eg, phenobarbital, phenytoin, carbamazepine, valproate) with generally lower side effect rates, little or no need for serum monitoring, and fewer drug interactions.

Pharmacokinetics of Antiepileptic Drugs			
Drug	Frequency of dosing	Frequency of initial laboratory monitoring	Therapeutic level (µg/mL)
Carbamazepine	BID, TID, or QID	3, 6, or 9 weeks	4 to 12
Ethosuximide	QD, BID, or TID	2 to 3 weeks	40 to 100
Felbamate	BID or TID	Every 2 weeks for other antiepileptic drugs until felbamate dose stabilized. Blood count and liver function weekly to monthly	Not established
Gabapentin	TID	None	Not established
Lamotrigine	BID	None	Not established
Levetiracetam	BID	None	Not established
Oxcarbazepine	BID or TID	None	Not established

Drug	Frequency of dosing	Frequency of initial laboratory monitoring	Therapeutic level (µg/mL)
Phenobarbital	QD or BID	3 to 4 weeks	10 to 40
Phenytoin	QD or BID	2 to 3 weeks	10 to 20
Tiagabine	BID, TID, QID	None	Not established
Topiramate	BID	None	Not established
Valproate	BID or TID	1 to 2 weeks (obtain platelet count if level >100)	50 to 150
Zonisamide	QD or BID	None	Not established

Side Effects of Antiepileptic Drugs

Drug	Systemic side effects	Neurotoxic side effects
Carbamazepine	Nausea, vomiting, diarrhea, hyponatremia, rash, pruritus	Drowsiness, dizziness, blurred or double vision, lethargy, headache
Ethosuximide	Nausea, vomiting	Sleep disturbance, drowsiness, hyperactivity
Felbamate	Nausea, vomiting, anorexia, weight loss	Insomnia, dizziness, headache, ataxia
Gabapentin	None	Somnolence, dizziness, ataxia
Lamotrigine	Rash, nausea	Dizziness, somnolence
Levetiracetam	Infection	Fatigue, somnolence, dizziness, agitation, anxiety
Oxcarbazepine	Nausea, rash, hyponatremia	Sedation, headache, dizziness, vertigo, ataxia, diplopia
Phenytoin	Gingival hypertrophy, body hair increase, rash, lymphadenopathy	Confusion, slurred speech, double vision, ataxia, neuropathy
Primidone, phenobarbital	Nausea, rash	Alteration of sleep cycles, sedation, lethargy, behavioral changes, hyperactivity, ataxia, tolerance, dependence

Drug	Systemic side effects	Neurotoxic side effects
Tiagabine	None known	Dizziness, lack of energy, somnolence, nausea, nervousness, tremor, difficulty concentrating, abdominal pain
Topiramate	Weight loss, renal stones, paresthesias	Fatigue, nervousness, difficulty concentrating, confusion, depression, anorexia, language problems, anxiety, mood problems, tremor
Valproate	Weight gain, nausea, vomiting, hair loss, easy bruising	Tremor
Zonisamide	Nausea, anorexia	Somnolence, dizziness, ataxia, confusion, difficulty concentrating

Rare side effects of antiepileptic drugs	
Drug	Side effects
Carbamazepine	Agranulocytosis, Stevens-Johnson syndrome, aplastic anemia, hepatic failure, dermatitis/rash, serum sickness, pancreatitis
Ethosuximide	Agranulocytosis, Stevens-Johnson syndrome, aplastic anemia, hepatic failure, dermatitis/rash, serum sickness
Felbamate	Aplastic anemia, liver failure
Gabapentin	Unknown
Lamotrigine	Stevens-Johnson syndrome, hypersensitivity
Levetiracetam	Unknown
Oxcarbazepine	Unknown
Phenytoin	Agranulocytosis, Stevens-Johnson syndrome, aplastic anemia, hepatic failure, dermatitis/rash, serum sickness
Primidone, phenobarbital	Agranulocytosis, Stevens-Johnson syndrome, hepatic failure, dermatitis/rash, serum sickness
Tiagabine	Unknown
Topiramate	Acute myopia and glaucoma; oligohidrosis and hyperthermia, which primarily occur in children

Drug	Side effects
Valproate	Agranulocytosis, Stevens-Johnson syndrome, aplastic anemia, hepatic failure, dermatitis/rash, serum sickness, pancreatitis
Zonisamide	Rash, Stevens-Johnson syndrome, toxic epidermal necrolysis, aplastic anemia, agranulocytosis, nephrolithiasis; in children, fever and hyperhidrosis

   E. Oral contraceptive therapy. The expected contraceptive failure rate of 0.7 per 100 woman-years with oral contraceptive therapy is increased to 3.1 per 100 woman-years in patients who are receiving a first-generation antiepileptic drug (AED [carbamazepine, phenobarbital, or phenytoin]). Valproate and benzodiazepines are exceptions.

F. Surgical procedures for refractory epilepsy include surgical resection of epileptogenic tissue, surgical removal of the cortex of a grossly diseased hemisphere, multiple subpial transection, callosotomy, and implantation of the vagus nerve stimulator. Patients with poorly controlled epileptic seizures that are interfering with daily activities, education, employment, or family and social activities should be considered for surgical therapy.

   G. Vagal nerve stimulation. Many patients who fail AED therapy are not candidates for standard epilepsy surgery. Others may undergo resective surgery and still have excessive numbers of seizures. These patients may be candidates for vagal nerve stimulation (VNS). VNS reduces seizure frequency by about 50 percent in 50 percent of patients.

References, see page 372.

Migraine Headache

Migraine is an episodic headache that may occur in up to 17 percent of women and 6 percent of men. Migraine is three times more common in women than men. It tends to run in families, and typically it is a disorder of young, healthy women. Migraine without aura is the most common type, accounting for 80 percent of all migraine sufferers.

I. Pathophysiology
   A. Primary neuronal dysfunction leads to a sequence of changes intracranially and extracranially that account for migraine.
   B. Serotonin (released from brainstem serotonergic nuclei) plays an important role in the pathogenesis of migraine; this is probably mediated via its direct action upon the cranial vasculature, through its role in central pain control pathways and through cerebral cortical projections of brainstem serotonergic nuclei.

II. Clinical manifestations
   A. Migraine often begins early in the morning but can occur at any time. Nocturnal headaches, which awaken the patient from sleep, are common with cluster headaches, but migraine can also awaken patients.
   B. The headache is lateralized during severe migraine attacks in 60 to 70 percent of patients; bifrontal or global headache occurs in up to 30 percent. Occasionally, other locations are described, including biocccipital headaches. The pain is usually gradual in onset, following a crescendo pattern with gradual but complete resolution. The headache is usually dull, deep, and steady when mild to moderate; it becomes throbbing or pulsatile when severe.

C. Migraine headaches are often worsened by rapid head motion, sneezing, straining, motion, or physical exertion. Many individuals report photophobia or phonophobia during attacks.

D. Premonitory symptoms precede a migraine attack by several hours to one or two days. Typical symptoms include fatigue, concentration difficulty, neck stiffness, sensitivity to light or sound, nausea, blurred vision, yawning, or pallor.

E. Migraine aura is the complex of neurologic symptoms that accompanies migraine headache. An aura presents as a progressive neurologic deficit or disturbance with subsequent complete recovery. Auras are caused by cortical spreading depression occurring in regions of the cortex.

F. Auras typically occur before the onset of migraine headache, and the headache usually begins simultaneously with or just after the end of the aura phase.

G. Typical auras may involve any of the following manifestations:
   1. Visual disturbances
   2. Sensory symptoms
   3. Motor weakness
   4. Speech disturbances

H. Visual disturbances are the most common type of aura, accounting for the majority of the neurologic symptoms associated with migraine. Numbness and tingling of the lips, lower face, and fingers of one hand (cheio-oral) is the second most common type of aura.
   1. The typical visual aura starts with a flickering uncolored zig-zag line in the center of the visual field and gradually progressed toward the periphery of one hemifield, often leaving a scotoma.

I. Autonomic and sinus symptoms characteristically occur in cluster headaches but are also commonly associated with migraine headache. These symptoms may include nasal congestion, rhinorrhea, tearing, color and temperature change, and changes in pupil size.

J. Cutaneous allodynia is the perception of pain produced by innocuous stimulation of normal skin. Brushing hair, touching the scalp, shaving, or wearing tight clothes may trigger allodynic symptoms of pain during migraine.

K. **Complications of migraine:**
   1. Chronic migraine
   2. Status migrainosus
   3. Persistent aura without infarction
   4. Migrainous infarction
   5. Migraine-triggered seizure

L. **Precipitating factors**. Migraine headaches may be precipitated by stress, worry, menstruation, oral contraceptives, exertion, fatigue, lack of sleep, hunger, head trauma, and certain foods and beverages containing nitrites, glutamate, aspartate, and tyramine.

M. **Menstrual migraine** is defined as migraine headache that occurs in close temporal relationship to the onset of menstruation; this time period usually encompasses two days before through three days after the onset of menstrual bleeding.

N. **Migraine with aura** is a recurrent disorder manifesting in attacks of reversible focal neurologic symptoms that usually develop gradually over 5 to 20 minutes and last for less than 60 minutes. A headache begins during the aura or follows aura within 60 minutes.

Features of Migraine Headache and Headache Caused by Underlying Disease	
Migraine headache	**Headache caused by serious underlying disease**
History	
• Chronic headache pattern similar from attack to attack • Gastrointestinal symptoms • Aura, especially visual • Prodrome	• Onset before puberty or after age 50 (tumor) • "Worst headache ever" (subarachnoid hemorrhage) • Headache occurring after exertion, sex, or bowel movement (subarachnoid hemorrhage) • Headache on rising in the morning (increased intracranial pressure, tumor) • Personality changes, seizures, alteration of consciousness (tumor) • Pain localized to temporal arteries or sudden loss of vision (giant cell arteritis) • Very localized headache (tumor, subarachnoid hemorrhage, giant cell arteritis)
Physical examination	
• No signs of toxicity • Normal vital signs • Normal neurologic examination	• Signs of toxicity (infection, hemorrhage) • Fever (sinusitis, meningitis, or other infection) • Meningismus (meningitis) • Tenderness of temporal arteries (giant cell arteritis) • Focal neurologic deficits (tumor, meningitis, hemorrhage) • Papilledema (tumor)
Laboratory tests and neuroimaging	
• Normal results	• Erythrocyte sedimentation rate >50 mm/hr (giant cell arteritis) • Abnormalities on lumbar puncture (meningitis, hemorrhage) • Abnormalities on CT or MRI (tumor, hemorrhage, aneurysm)

III. Diagnostic testing

A. Neuroimaging is not necessary for most patients with migraine. Neuroimaging is recommended in the following patients with nonacute headache:

1. Patients with an unexplained abnormal finding on neurologic examination.
2. Patients with atypical headache features or headaches that do not fulfill the strict definition of migraine or other primary headache disorder (or have some additional risk factor, such as immune deficiency).
3. Patients with sudden severe headache also need neuroimaging because of the suspicion of subarachnoid hemorrhage.

B. Symptoms which increase the odds of finding an abnormality on neuroimaging:

1. Rapidly increasing headache frequency
2. History of lack of coordination
3. History of localized neurologic signs or numbness or tingling
4. History of headache causing awakening from sleep

C. A head CT scan (without and with contrast) is sufficient in many patients when neuroimaging is deemed necessary. An MRI is indicated when posterior fossa lesions or cerebrospinal fluid (CSF) leak are suspected. Magnetic resonance angiography (MRA) and mMagnetic resonance venography (MRV) are indicated when arterial or venous lesions are suspected.

IV. Acute treatment of migraine in adults

A. Mild analgesics

1. Some patients with migraine have an optimal response with nonsteroidal antiinflammatory drugs (NSAIDs) or acetaminophen. Acetaminophen and many other analgesics are not advisable, in the patient who requires frequent medication, since they have been associated with rebound headaches.

2. **Nonsteroidal anti-inflammatory drugs** (NSAIDs) with efficacy in migraine therapy include ibuprofen (Advil, 400 to 1200 mg), naproxen (Naprosyn, 750 to 1250 mg), diclofenac (Voltaren, 50 to 100 mg), tolfenamic acid (Clotam Rapid, 200 mg), and aspirin (650 to 1000 mg).

3. Indomethacin (Indocin) is a potent NSAID that is also available in suppository form, which may be helpful for nauseated patients. Indomethacin suppositories contain 50 mg of the drug; the suppositories may be cut into halves or thirds.

4. Acetaminophen is an effective abortive agent in some patients. Acetaminophen can be used in combination with NSAIDs. The combination of acetaminophen, aspirin, and caffeine (Excedrin, 2 extra strength tablets) alleviates headaches.

B. Triptans

1. Triptans inhibit the release of vasoactive peptides, promote vasoconstriction, and block pain pathways in the brainstem. Triptans inhibit transmission in the trigeminal nucleus caudalis. Triptans may also activate 5-HT 1b/1d receptors in descending brainstem pain modulating pathways.

2. Preparations and efficacy. Sumatriptan can be given as a subcutaneous injection, as a nasal spray, or orally. Zolmitriptan is also available for both nasal and oral use. The others are available for oral use only.

3. **Side effects of subcutaneous sumatriptan** include an injection site reaction, chest pressure, flushing, weakness, drowsiness, dizziness, malaise, warmth, and paresthesias. Most of these reactions resolve spontaneously within 30 minutes. There have been rare reports of myocardial infarction and sudden death. The most common side effect of intranasal sumatriptan is an unpleasant taste.

4. **Choice of triptan.** All of the available oral serotonin agonists are effective and well tolerated. The highest likelihood of consistent success was found with rizatriptan (10 mg), eletriptan (80 mg), and almotriptan (12.5 mg). Sumatriptan (Imitrex) offers the most options for drug delivery.

5. Rizatriptan has the fastest onset of action; the dose must be adjusted downward in patients who take propranolol since propranolol increases rizatriptan levels by 70 percent. Almotriptan has fewer side effects than sumatriptan. Patients who do not respond well to one triptan may respond to another.

6. Triptans should be avoided in patients with familial hemiplegic migraine, basilar migraine, ischemic stroke, ischemic heart disease, Prinzmetal's angina, uncontrolled hypertension, and pregnancy.

7. Combination with monoamine oxidase inhibitors is contraindicated with triptans other than eletriptan, frovatriptan (Frova), and naratriptan. Triptans should not be used within 24 hours of the use of ergotamine preparations.
8. Eletriptan is metabolized by cytochrome P-450 enzyme CYP3A4. Therefore, eletriptan should not be used within at least 72 hours of treatment with other drugs that are potent CYP3A4 inhibitors, such as ketoconazole, itraconazole, nefazodone, troleandomycin, clarithromycin, ritonavir, and nelfinavir.

Drugs for Treatment of Migraine and Tension Headache	
Drug	**Dosage**
5-HT₁ Receptor Agonists ("Triptans")	
Rizatriptan (Maxalt)	5- or 10-mg tablet or wafer (MLT); can be repeated in 2 hours; max 30 mg/day, 15 mg/day in patients on propranolol
Almotriptan (Axert)	12.5 mg at the onset of a migraine. Patients with hepatic or renal impairment should start with 6.25 mg. Max 2 doses per day.
Sumatriptan (Imitrex)	6 mg SC; can be repeated in 1 hour; max 2 injections/day 50 mg PO; can be repeated in 2 hours; max 100 mg 20 mg intranasally; can be repeated after 2 hours; max 40 mg/day Max in combination: two injections or sprays; or one of either plus two tablets
Naratriptan (Amerge)	2.5-mg tablet, can be repeated 4 hours later; max 5 mg/day
Zolmitriptan (Zomig, Zomig-ZMT, Zomig nasal spray)	2.5-5 mg PO; can be repeated in 2 hours. Tablets and orally disintegrating tablets, 2.5, 5 mg. Intranasally 5 mg; can be repeated after 2 hours; max 10 mg/day
Frovatriptan (Frova)	2.5 mg PO, repeat after 2 hours if the headache recurs; max 3 tabs in 24 hours. Longest half-life, slow onset, less effective
Eletriptan (Relpax)	20 or 40 mg, repeated after 2 hours if headache recurs; max 80 mg in 24 hours.
NSAIDs	
Ibuprofen (Motrin)	400-800 mg, repeat as needed in 4 hr
Naproxen sodium (Anaprox DS)	550-825 mg, repeat as needed in 4 hr

Drug	Dosage
Ergot Alkaloids	
Dihydroergotamine DHE 45 Migranal Nasal Spray	1 mg IM; can be repeated twice at 1-hour intervals (max 3 mg/attack) 1 spray (0.5 mg)/nostril, repeated 15 minutes later (2 mg/dose; max 3 mg/24 hours)
Ergotamine 1 mg/caffeine 100 mg (Ercaf, Gotamine, Wigraine)	2 tablets PO, then 1 q30min, x 4 PRN (max 6 tabs/attack)
Butalbital combinations	
Aspirin 325 mg, caffeine 40 mg, butalbital 50 mg (Fiorinal)	2 tablets, followed by 1 tablet q4-6h as needed
Isometheptene combination	
Isometheptene 65 mg, acetaminophen 325 mg, dichloral-phenazone 100 mg (Midrin)	2 tablets, followed by 1 tablet as needed q4-6h prn
Opioid Analgesics	
Butorphanol (Stadol NS)	One spray in one nostril; can be repeated in the other nostril in 60-90 minutes; the same two-dose sequence can be repeated in 3 to 5 hours

  C. **Ergots**
     1. Ergotamine preparations, alone and in combination with caffeine and other analgesics, have been used for the abortive treatment of migraine. Both ergotamine and dihydroergotamine (DHE 45) bind to 5HT 1b/d receptors.
     2. Ergotamine
        a. Ergotamine may worsen the nausea and vomiting associated with migraine. Vascular occlusion and rebound headaches have been reported with oral doses. Years of use also may be associated with valvular heart disease.
        b. Ergots should be avoided in patients with coronary artery disease because they cause sustained coronary artery constriction, peripheral vascular disease, hypertension, and hepatic or renal disease. In addition, ergotamine overuse has been associated with an increased risk of cerebrovascular, cardiovascular, and peripheral ischemic complications. Ergotamine should not be used in patients who have migraine with prolonged aura because they may reduce cerebral blood flow.
        c. Ergotamine is the drug of choice in relatively few patients with migraine.
  D. **Antiemetic**
     1. Chlorpromazine IV appears to be more effective than placebo in the acute treatment of migraine. IV prochlorperazine also appears to be as effective or more effective than placebo in the acute treatment of migraine.
     2. Metoclopramide should be considered a primary agent for acute migraine treatment in emergency departments. In addition, parenteral metoclopramide may be effective when combined with other treatments.
V. **Drug choice and sequence**
  A. Migraine therapy should begin with a triptan for outpatients.

    B. Intravenous (IV) metoclopramide (10 mg) or prochlorperazine (10 mg) are suggested for initial treatment of patients who present to the hospital emergency department with severe migraine

VI. Preventive treatment of migraine in adults

A. Indications for prophylactic headache treatment:

1. Recurring migraines that significantly interfere with daily routine, despite acute treatment
2. Contraindication to or failure or overuse of acute therapies
3. Adverse events with acute therapies
4. Patient preference
5. Hemiplegic migraine
6. Basilar type migraine
7. Migraine with prolonged aura
8. Migrainous infarction

B. Antihypertensives

1. **Beta blockers.** Chronic therapy with propranolol reduces the frequency and severity of migraine in 60 to 80 percent of patients. Propranolol is more effective than placebo in the short-term treatment of migraine. Only propranolol and timolol have been approved for migraine prophylaxis, but metoprolol, nadolol, and atenolol are commonly used.
2. The use of beta blockers may be limited in patients with erectile dysfunction, peripheral vascular disease, Raynaud's syndrome or disease, and in patients with baseline bradycardia or low blood pressure. They must be used cautiously as well asthma, diabetes mellitus, and those with cardiac conduction disturbances or sinus node dysfunction.
3. **Calcium channel blockers** are widely used for migraine prophylaxis. These agents may relieve aura symptoms as well as prevent migraines. Verapamil is frequently a first choice for prophylactic therapy because of a favorable side effect profile.
4. **Antidepressants** are useful for migraine prophylaxis. The tricyclic antidepressants (eg, amitriptyline and clomipramine) and serotonin blockers (eg, pizotifen, mirtazapine) are effective in preventing chronic migraines.
5. The tricyclic antidepressants most commonly used for migraine prophylaxis include amitriptyline, nortriptyline, doxepin, and protriptyline. Amitriptyline is the only tricyclic that has proven efficacy for migraine.
6. Side effects are common with tricyclic antidepressants. Most are sedating, particularly with amitriptyline and doxepin. Therefore, these drugs are usually used at bedtime and started at a low dose. Additional side effects of tricyclics include dry mouth, constipation, tachycardia, palpitations, orthostatic hypotension, weight gain, blurred vision, and urinary retention. Confusion can occur, particularly in the elderly.

C. Anticonvulsants.
The anticonvulsants sodium valproate, gabapentin, and topiramate are more effective than placebo for reducing the frequency of migraine attacks. Both valproate and topiramate are approved for migraine prophylaxis.

D. Valproate (Depakote)
decreases headache frequency by approximately 50 percent. Divalproex (valporate and valproic acid)is at least as effective as beta blockers and may be better tolerated. It can cause weight gain and hair loss and is contraindicated in pregnancy.

E. Gabapentin (Neurontin)
has been found to reduce migraine headache frequency.

F. Topiramate (Topamax)
is an effective prophylactic therapy.

1. Significant reductions in migraine frequency occur within the first month at topiramate doses of 100 and 200 mg/day.

Prophylactic treatment of migraine and tension type headache			
Drug	Starting dose	Maximum dose	Special precautions
Calcium channel blockers			
Verapamil	120 mg/day	720 mg/day	3 to 4 weeks required until effective; contraindicated in heart block, hypotension, congestive heart failure, atrial flutter and fibrillation
Nifedipine	30 mg/day	180 mg/day	
Diltiazem	60 mg/day	360 mg/day	
Flunarizine (not approved in U.S.)			
Tricyclic antidepressants			
Nortriptyline	10 mg/day	125 mg/day	Contraindicated in urinary retention, glaucoma, bundle branch block; severe anticholinergic effects and weight gain
Amitriptyline	10 mg/day	250 mg/day	
SSRIs			
Fluoxetine (Prozac)	10 mg/day	80 mg/day	Less anticholinergic side effects; generally better tolerated
Paroxetine (Paxil)	10 mg/day	40 mg/day	
Sertraline (Zoloft)	25 mg/day	200 mg/day	
Beta blockers			
Propranolol	60 mg/day	320 mg/day	3 to 4 weeks before effective; contraindicated in asthma, diabetes mellitus, congestive heart failure, heart block; depression, impotence, or hypotension
Nadolol	40 mg/day	240 mg/day	
Timolol	10 mg/day	40 mg/day	
Atenolol	50 mg/day	150 mg/day	
Metoprolol	50 mg/day	300 mg/day	
Anticonvulsants			
Carbamazepine (Tegretol)	100 mg/day	200-600 mg TID	Monitor CBC, LFTs
Valproate (Depakote)	250 mg BID	500 mg TID/QID	Teratogenic
Gabapentin (Neurontin)	100 mg TID or 300 mg QHS	300-800 mg TID	No blood monitoring required
Topiramate (Topamax)	25 mg/day	100 mg BID	Slow titration minimizes adverse events Weight loss common

VII. **Menstrual migraine**
   A. NSAIDs are often used for prophylaxis. Naproxen sodium 550 mg twice daily during the perimenstrual period is one commonly used regimen.

B. For patients who fail NSAID treatment or have contraindications to NSAIDs, frovatriptan (Frova, 2.5 mg daily or 2.5 mg twice daily) for six days is an alternative.

References, see page 372.

Vertigo

The clinical evaluation of vertigo begins with the patient's description of symptoms and the circumstances in which they occur. Many drugs can cause dizziness. Common nonvestibular causes (eg, hyperventilation, orthostatic hypotension, panic disorder) are often diagnosed.

I. History and physical examination
   A. Patients may use the term "dizziness" to describe one or more different sensations. These sensations include vertigo (spinning), light-headedness, unsteadiness and motion intolerance. The onset of symptoms, whether the sensation is constant or episodic, how often episodes occur and the duration of episodes should be assessed. Activities or movements that provoke or worsen a patient's dizziness should be sought as well as activities that minimize symptoms. Rotational vertigo when rolling over in bed is highly suggestive of BPPV.
   B. Vertigo is a sensation of movement of the self or of one's surroundings. Patients may describe vertigo as a sensation of floating, giddiness or disorientation. The duration of vertiginous symptoms and whether head movement provokes symptoms (positional vertigo) or if attacks occur without provocation (spontaneous vertigo) should be assessed.
   C. Hearing loss, tinnitus and aural fullness should be sought. Vision, strength and sensation, coordination, speech and swallowing should be evaluated. Double vision or hemiplegia strongly suggest a central nervous system lesion rather than a peripheral vestibular disorder. History for cardiac disease, migraine, cerebrovascular disease, thyroid disease and diabetes should be sought.

Drugs Associated with Dizziness		
Class of drug	**Type of dizziness**	**Mechanism**
Alcohol	Positional vertigo	Specific-gravity difference in endolymph vs cupula
Intoxication	CNS depression	Disequilibrium Cerebellar dysfunction
Tranquilizers	Intoxication	CNS depression
Anticonvulsants	Intoxication Disequilibrium	CNS depression Cerebellar dysfunction
Antihypertensives	Near faint	Postural hypotension
Aminoglycosides	Vertigo Disequilibrium Oscillopsia	Asymmetric hair-cell loss Vestibulospinal reflex loss Vestibulo-ocular reflex loss

D. Physical examination should evaluate orthostatic blood pressure changes followed by a complete head and neck examination as well as otologic and neurologic examinations. A pneumatic otoscope should be used to confirm normal tympanic membrane mobility. Balance, gait, cerebellar and cranial nerve function, and nystagmus should be evaluated.

E. Nystagmus consists of involuntary eye movements caused by asymmetry of signals from the right and left vestibular systems. Nystagmus of peripheral vestibular origin is usually horizontal with a slight or dramatic rotary component. Nystagmus of central origin is usually predominantly vertical.

F. The Dix-Hallpike test is particularly helpful to elicit nystagmus associated with BPPV. This maneuver stimulates the posterior semicircular canal, which is the semicircular canal most commonly involved in BPPV.

G. An audiogram should be performed if a specific cause of dizziness cannot be found after a thorough history and physical examination. Additional testing may include electronystagmography, auditory evoked brainstem response testing, radiologic imaging of the brain, brainstem and temporal bone and selected blood tests. Auditory evoked brainstem response testing measures the integrity of the auditory system and is useful to screen for acoustic tumors. Magnetic resonance imaging (MRI) should be reserved for patients with unilateral otologic symptoms or neurologic symptoms or those in whom dizziness persists despite appropriate treatment.

II. Benign paroxysmal positional vertigo

A. The most common cause of peripheral vestibular vertigo is BPPV. This condition is characterized by sudden, brief and sometimes violent vertigo after a change in head position. The sensation of vertigo usually lasts for only a few seconds. This form of vertigo is often noticed when a patient lies down, arises or turns over in bed. BPPV does not cause hearing loss, ear fullness or tinnitus. BPPV can occur at any age but is most commonly seen in elderly persons. Although usually unilateral, bilateral BPPV occurs in up to 15 percent of patients. Nystagmus is characteristic of BPPV.

B. BPPV is caused by displacement of otoconia from the utricle or saccule into the posterior semicircular canal. Therefore, when a patient moves the head into a provocative position, the otoconia provoke movement of the endolymphatic fluid inside the semicircular canal, creating a sensation of vertigo.

C. Treatment of BPPV. In-office physical therapy, known as repositioning maneuvers, redirects displaced otoconia into the utricle. This form of treatment is effective in 85 to 90 percent of patients.

D. During these exercises, the patient initially sits upright on the edge of a bed or couch. Then the patient rapidly lies down on his side with the affected ear down. Vertigo usually occurs. After the vertigo subsides (or after one minute if no vertigo occurs), the patient rapidly turns in a smooth arc to the opposite side. After vertigo associated with this movement subsides (or after one minute if no vertigo occurs), the patient slowly sits upright. Surgical treatment is reserved for the 2 to 5 percent of cases that fail to respond to nonsurgical treatment.

III. Vestibular neuronitis

A. Vestibular neuronitis is characterized by acute onset of intense vertigo associated with nausea and vomiting that is unaccompanied by any neurologic or audiologic symptoms. The symptoms usually reach their peak within 24 hours and then gradually subside. During the first 24 to 48 hours of a vertiginous episode, severe truncal unsteadiness and imbalance are present.

B. Vestibular neuronitis is presumed to have a viral etiology because it is often associated with a recent history of a flu-like illness. Management of the initial stage of vestibular neuronitis includes bed rest and the use of antiemetics (eg, promethazine [Phenergan]) and vestibular suppressants (eg, diazepam [Valium]). After the patient is able to stand, the brain begins compensating for the acute loss of unilateral vestibular function. The compensation process may be enhanced by performance of vestibular exercises twice per day for eight to 10 weeks.

IV. **Ménière's disease**
   A. Ménière's disease is characterized by fluctuating hearing loss, tinnitus, episodic vertigo and, occasionally, a sensation of fullness or pressure in the ear. Vertigo rapidly follows and is typically severe, with episodes occurring abruptly and without warning. The duration of vertigo is usually several minutes to hours. Unsteadiness and dizziness may persist for days after the episode of vertigo.
   B. Diseases with similar symptoms include syphilis, acoustic neuroma and migraine. Isolated episodes of hearing loss or vertigo may precede the characteristic combination of symptoms by months or years.
   C. Ménière's disease results from excessive accumulation of endolymphatic fluid (endolymphatic hydrops). As inner-ear fluid pressure increases, symptoms of Ménière's disease develop.
   D. Diuretics (eg, triamterene-hydrochlorothiazide [Dyazide, Maxzide]) and a low-salt diet are the mainstays of treatment. This combined regimen reduces endolymphatic fluid pressure. Other preventive measures include use of vasodilators and avoidance of caffeine and nicotine. Acute vertiginous episodes may be treated with oral or intravenous diazepam. Promethazine or glycopyrrolate (Robinul) is effective in the treatment of nausea.
   E. Surgical treatments are an option when appropriate prophylactic measures fail to prevent recurrent episodes of vertigo. Surgical procedures used in the treatment of Ménière's disease range from draining excess endolymphatic fluid from the inner ear (endolymphatic shunt) to severing the vestibular nerve (with hearing preservation). In selected cases, a chemical labyrinthectomy may be performed. Chemical labyrinthectomy involves the injection of a vestibulotoxic gentamicin (Garamycin) solution into the middle ear.

Antivertiginous and Antiemetic Drugs		
Classes and agents	**Dosage**	**Comments**
Antihistamines		
Dimenhydrinate (Benadryl)	50 mg PO q4-6h or 100-mg supp. q8h	Available without prescription, mild sedation, minimal side effects
Meclizine (Antivert)	25-50 mg PO q4-6h	Mild sedation, minimal side effects
Promethazine (Phenergan)	25-50 mg PO, IM, or suppository q4-6h	Good for nausea, vertigo, more sedation, extrapyramidal effects
Monoaminergic agents		
Amphetamine	5 or 10 mg PO q4-6h	Stimulant, can counteract sedation of antihistamines, anxiety
Ephedrine	25 mg PO q4-6h	Available without prescription
Benzodiazepine		
Diazepam (Valium)	5 or 10 mg PO q6-8h	Sedation, little effect on nausea

Classes and agents	Dosage	Comments
Phenothiazine		
Prochlorperazine (Compazine)	5-25 mg PO, IM, or suppository q4-6h	Good antiemetic; extrapyramidal side effects, particularly in young patients

References, see page 372.

Chronic Fatigue Syndrome

Chronic fatigue syndrome is characterized by clinically evaluated, unexplained, persistent or relapsing fatigue plus four or more specifically defined associated symptoms. Many people can have unexplained chronic fatigue and not fit the case criteria for CFS. Such individuals are defined as having idiopathic chronic fatigue. Twenty-four percent of patients complain of fatigue for more than one month. CFS is primarily a disorder of young to middle aged adults, but cases in children have been recognized.

I. Clinical presentation
A. Relatively sudden onset of fatigue is common, often associated with a typical infection, such as an upper respiratory infection or mononucleosis. After resolution of the initial infection, the patient is left with overwhelming fatigue and a number of additional symptoms, especially altered sleep and cognition. Excessive physical activity exacerbates the symptoms. There is often, however, a history of psychiatric disorders in the past.
B. Physical examination is usually normal.
1. Patients commonly feel febrile; however, few ever demonstrate elevated temperatures (greater than 37.4°C).
2. Joints ache, but there is no erythema, effusion, or limitation of motion.
3. Although the muscles are easily fatigued, strength is normal, as are biopsies and electromyograms.
4. Mild lymphadenitis is occasionally noted, and painful lymph nodes (lymphadynia) is a frequent complaint, but not true lymphadenopathy.
5. Many patients with chronic fatigue syndrome are partially or totally disabled by the fatigue.

Symptoms in Patients with Chronic Fatigue Syndrome	
Symptom	**Percent of patients**
Easy fatigability	100
Difficulty concentrating	90
Headache	90
Sore throat	85
Tender lymph nodes	80
Muscle aches	80
Joint aches	75
Feverishness	75
Difficulty sleeping	70
Psychiatric problems	65
Allergies	55
Abdominal cramps	40
Weight loss	20
Rash	10
Rapid pulse	10
Weight gain	5
Chest pain	5
Night sweats	5

Diagnostic criteria for the chronic fatigue syndrome

Major criteria

New onset of fatigue lasting six months, severe enough to reduce daily activity to less than 50 percent of the patient's premorbid activity level
The exclusion of other conditions that can produce fatigue

Minor criteria

Symptom criteria
  Low-grade fever: temperature 37.5 to 38.6°C orally or chills
  Sore throat
  Painful cervical or axillary lymph nodes
  Generalized muscle weakness
  Muscle pain
  Postexertional fatigue lasting more than 24 hours
  Generalized headaches
  Migratory arthralgia
  Neuropsychological complaints (photophobia, transient visual scotomata, forgetfulness, excessive
    irritability, confusion, difficulty thinking, inability to concentrate, or depression)
  Sleep disturbance
  Acute onset of symptoms over a few hours to a few days

Physical criteria. Determined by the physician on two occasions at least two months apart
  Low-grade fever
  Nonexudative pharyngitis
  Palpable cervical or axillary lymph nodes up to 2 cm in diameter

Common causes of fatigue		
Diagnosis	**Frequency in primary care**	**Fatigued patients (%)**
Depression	Very common	18
Environment (lifestyle)	Very common	17
Anxiety, anemia, asthma	Very common	14
Diabetes	Very common	11
Infections	Common	10
Thyroid, tumors	Common	7
Rheumatologic	Common	5
Endocarditis, cardiovascular	Common	8
Drugs	Common	5

II. **Diagnosis.** The diagnosis of CFS is made by exclusion. Patients with CFS must have clinically evaluated, unexplained, persistent or relapsing fatigue plus four or more associated symptoms. Under 10 percent of patients with chronic fatigue have CFS.

 A. Recommended testing in the patients suspected of CFS including complete blood count with differential, erythrocyte sedimentation rate, standard chemistries including plasma calcium concentration, thyroid function tests, antinuclear antibody titer, urinalysis, tuberculin skin test, and screening questionnaires for psychiatric disorders. Other tests may include plasma cortisol, rheumatoid factor, immunoglobulin levels, Lyme serology in endemic areas, and tests for HIV antibody.

Laboratory evaluation of chronic fatigue

For all patients
    Complete blood cell count with differential
    Erythrocyte sedimentation rate
    Urinalysis
Other tests based on findings
    Thyroid stimulating hormone
    Blood Chemistry levels:
        Alanine aminotransferase
        Aspartate aminotransferase
        Blood urea nitrogen
        Electrolytes
        Glucose
    Heterophil antibody test (Monospot)
    Serologic studies for Lyme or HIV antibody titers

 B. Serologies for EBV, CMV, or Lyme disease or antinuclear antibodies are recommended only in specific cases.

    C. The diagnosis of CFS is generally made if the patient has a typical history and no abnormality can be detected on physical examination or in the screening tests.

III. Management of the fatigued patient

A. Regular exercise will improve functional capacity, mood, and sleep. Regular sleep habits should be advised. In those complaining of depressive symptoms or sleep disturbance, an antidepressant or sleep hypnotic is indicated. A sedating antidepressant, such as amitriptyline (Elavil) 25 mg qhs, may be helpful for complaints of insomnia or restlessness. If the primary complaints are hypersomnia and psychomotor retardation, a selective serotonin reuptake inhibitor is indicated.

B. For physical symptoms such as headaches, myalgias, or arthralgias, nonsteroidal anti-inflammatory agents may be helpful. Therapies for which no effectiveness has been demonstrated in CFS include vitamins, acyclovir, gamma globulin, folic acid, cyanocobalamin, and magnesium.

C. Antidepressants

    1. Selective serotonin reuptake inhibitors (SSRIs) are the drugs of choice. Fluoxetine (Prozac), paroxetine (Paxil), sertraline (Zoloft), and fluvoxamine (LuVox) are effective in reducing fatigue, myalgia, sleep disturbance, and depression.

    2. For the patient who has significant difficulty with insomnia or with pain, paroxetine at bedtime is recommended because it is mildly sedating. Fluoxetine is useful in patients who complain of lack of energy because it has activating properties. Fluoxetine often improves cognitive functioning, especially concentrating ability.

    3. Initial dosage should be low because many CFS patients are sensitive to side effects.

        a. Fluoxetine (Prozac) 20 mg PO qAM; 20-40 mg/d [20 mg].

        b. Paroxetine (Paxil) 10 mg qAM; increase as needed to max of 40 mg/d. [10, 20, 30, 40 mg].

        c. Fluvoxamine (LuVox) 50-100 mg qhs; max 300 mg/d [50, 100 mg]

        d. Sertraline (Zoloft) 50-100 mg PO qAM [50, 100 mg].

IV. Prognosis.
CFS is a chronic illness, but 40-60% of patients improve within 1-3 years after diagnosis. The mean duration of illness prior to diagnosis is 52.6 months.

References, see page 372.

Dermatologic and Allergic Disorders

Herpes Simplex Virus Type 1 Infection

Herpes simplex virus type 1 (HSV-1) is the etiologic agent of vesicular lesions of the oral mucosa commonly referred to as "cold sores." HSV-1 can also cause clinical disease in the genitalia, liver, lung, eye, and central nervous system.

I. **Primary infection**
  A. Inoculation of HSV-1 at mucosal surfaces or skin sites permits entry of the virus into the epidermis, the dermis, and eventually to sensory and autonomic nerve endings. Disease is characterized by sudden appearance of multiple vesicular lesions on an inflammatory, erythematous base. Primary infection may also be associated with systemic symptoms, such as fever and malaise. The severity of symptoms and the number of lesions is considerably less with reactivation.
  B. The lesions can be painful and last for 10 to 14 days. Vesicles are usually grouped in a single anatomic site.
  C. Although the symptoms can be severe, most primary HSV-1 infections are asymptomatic. Only 20 to 25 percent of patients with HSV-1 antibodies and 10 to 20 percent of those with HSV-2 antibodies have a history of oral-labial or genital infections.

II. **Recurrent infection**
  A. Once HSV infection has occurred, the virus lives in a latent state in nerve cell bodies in ganglion neurons and can reactivate.
  B. In contrast to primary HSV-1, recurrent HSV-1 is rarely associated with systemic signs or symptoms except for local lymphadenopathy. Prodromal symptoms may herald the onset of a reactivation episode, such as pain, burning, tingling, and pruritus. These symptoms may last from 6 to 53 hours prior to the appearance of the first vesicles.
  C. Subclinical shedding is common in both immunocompetent and immunocompromised patients.
  D. **Immunocompetent hosts.** Recurrent episodes are usually of shorter duration than the primary episode. The median time from onset of prodromal symptoms to healing of the lesion is five days.
  E. **Precipitating factors** for HSV-1 recurrence include exposure to sunlight, fever, menstruation, emotional stress, and trauma to the area of primary infection.
  F. **Recurrences** occur as frequently as once per month (24 percent) or as infrequently as twice per year (19 percent).
  G. **Immunocompromised hosts.** The initial containment of HSV infection requires intact cellular immunity. Thus, immunocompromised hosts are at risk for increased frequency and severity of recurrent HSV infections. They are also at risk for dissemination of infection, which may include the lungs or gastrointestinal tract.
  H. **HIV infection.** Patients with advanced HIV infection (CD4 count <200 cells/μL) are at increased risk for recurrent and extensive HSV infections. HSV infections can occur anywhere on the skin, often presenting as extensive oral or perianal ulcers. HIV-infected patients can also develop esophagitis, colitis, chorioretinitis, acute retinal necrosis, tracheobronchitis, and pneumonia.

III. Oral infections

A. **Gingivostomatitis and pharyngitis** are the most frequent clinical manifestations of first-episode HSV-1 infection. Herpes labialis is the most frequent sign of reactivation disease.

B. **Children.** Primary HSV-1 oral infection usually presents as gingivostomatitis in children. After a brief incubation period (median 6 to 8 days, range 1 to 26 days), fever, pharyngitis and painful vesicular lesions develop suddenly. Lesions can occur anywhere on the pharyngeal and oral mucosa and progress over several days, eventually involving the soft palate, buccal mucosa, tongue, and the floor of the mouth. Gingivitis and extensions to lips and cheeks can be seen.

C. Common systemic symptoms and signs include fever, malaise, myalgias, irritability, and cervical lymphadenopathy. Transmission can occur through close contact with oral lesions.

D. Adults. Primary oral HSV-1 infection in adults can present as severe pharyngitis, fever, malaise, myalgia and cervical lymphadenopathy. Severe mouth pain and fever usually persist for two to eight days, during which time vesicles crust over and heal; cervical lymphadenopathy may persist for weeks.

E. Recurrences involving the oral cavity and lips are common. Lesions progress from vesicle to crust in about eight days, with significant diminution of pain after the first 24 hours.

F. Differential diagnosis. Recurrent aphthous ulcers, which are most often confused with HSV infection, are never preceded by vesicles and occur exclusively on mucosal surfaces such as the inner surfaces of lips, buccal mucosa, ventral tongue, and mucobuccal fold in the anterior part of the oral cavity. In contrast, recurrent oral HSV-1 lesions ("cold sores") occur at the border of the vermillion (ie, the colored portion of the lips).

G. Other diseases that present with oral lesions and/or severe pharyngitis include aphthous stomatitis, syphilis, bacterial pharyngitis, enteroviruses (eg, herpangina), Epstein-Barr virus, and Stevens-Johnson syndrome.

IV. Skin infections

A. HSV-1 can cause primary infection anywhere on the skin, especially if there is disruption of skin integrity. Primary infections begin with a typical prodrome of pruritus and pain, followed by the development of vesicular lesions. Associated symptoms include neuralgia and lymphadenopathy.

B. There are also a variety of syndromes associated with HSV-1 infection of the skin: HSV infection of the finger, known as herpetic whitlow, can occur as a complication of primary oral or genital herpes by inoculation of the virus through a break in the skin barrier.

V. Genital HSV-1 infections . The majority of genital HSV infections are due to HSV-2. Genital HSV-1 infection is transmitted through oral-genital contact.

VI. Ocular infections. Primary ocular HSV infections occur in less than 5 percent of patients, but can cause significant morbidity due to keratitis and acute retinal necrosis.

A. **Keratitis.** Recurrent HSV-1 keratitis continues to be a leading cause of corneal blindness. HSV keratitis has an acute onset with symptoms of pain, visual blurring, and discharge. Physical examination is notable for chemosis, conjunctivitis, and characteristic dendritic lesions of the cornea.

B. Use of topical steroid drops can exacerbate the infection and lead to blindness.

C. **Recurrent infection.** The acute disease is usually self-limited. Recurrences are common. Recurrent superficial keratitis heals without affecting vision. In comparison, recurrent attacks involving stromal tissue may lead to blindness.

D. Acute retinal necrosis (ARN) is a rare, potentially blinding retinal disease resulting from ocular infection with HSV or varicella-zoster virus (VZV).

VII. **Neurologic syndromes.** HSV-1 causes sporadic cases of encephalitis, characterized by the rapid onset of fever, headache, seizures, focal neurologic signs, and impaired consciousness. Other neurologic syndromes include aseptic meningitis, autonomic dysfunction, transverse myelitis, benign recurrent lymphocytic meningitis, and Bell's palsy.

VIII. **Diagnosis**
   A. **Viral culture.** The diagnosis of HSV infection is generally based upon tissue culture identification. Recovery of virus from secretions is possible in only 7 to 25 percent of patients with active lesions.
   B. **Polymerase chain reaction.** While viral culture has remained the standard diagnostic method for isolating HSV, real-time HSV PCR assays have emerged as a more sensitive method to confirm HSV infection in clinical specimens obtained from genital ulcers, mucocutaneous sites, and cerebrospinal fluid.

IX. **Treatment and prevention of herpes simplex virus type 1 infection**
   A. Children with gingivostomatitis often require either topical or oral analgesics and, in severe cases, intravenous rehydration. Short-term relief can be achieved with viscous lidocaine. Zilactin, a nonprescription topical medication may be used to protect lesions. Ziladent, a similar agent with benzocaine can provide pain relief for up to six hours. In more severe cases, oral opiate elixirs may be required.
   B. Acyclovir may be beneficial if begun early during primary (or recurrent) infections (400 mg PO three times per day or 200 mg PO five times per day or 15 mg/kg up to a dose of 200 mg PO, with each dose taken five times daily for seven days).
   C. Topical acyclovir 5 percent is minimally effective in the treatment of primary oral lesions since it has poor penetration.
   D. Recurrent herpes labialis is usually not treated with antivirals unless a prodromal stage before the appearance of lesions can be identified. In these cases oral acyclovir or penciclovir cream can be prescribed for four days duration.

Dosage Regimens for Primary Genital Herpes Infection	
Drug	**Dosage**
Acyclovir (Zovirax)	200-400 mg three times daily for 10 days
Famciclovir (Famvir)	250 mg three times daily for 10 days
Valacyclovir (Valtrex)	1 g twice daily for 10 days

   E. **Suppressive therapy to prevent recurrences**
      1. Chronic suppression has proven helpful in preventing HSV recurrences, decreasing in occurrence of new lesions by 50 to 78 percent in immunocompetent patients on prophylactic regimens of oral acyclovir. The number of recurrences per four months is lower with acyclovir (0.85 versus 1.80 with placebo). A daily suppressive regimen (Zovirax, 200 mg three to five times daily) has been shown to be safe and effective when used continuously for up to one year.
      2. Valacyclovir (Valtrex, 500 mg once daily) helps prevent recurrences (60 versus 38 percent), and the time to first recurrence is significantly longer (13 versus 9.6 weeks).

3. Short-term antiviral prophylaxis can also be considered in UV light-induced HSV recurrences.

References: See page 372.

Genital Herpes Simplex Virus Infection

The seroprevalence of herpes simplex virus type-2 (HSV-2) is 17 percent. HSV-2 remains the causative agent for most genital herpes infections. Recurrences are common following primary genital herpes. About 89 percent have one recurrence. And 38 percent of patients have six recurrences and 20 percent have more than ten.

I. **Types of infection**
   A. **Primary infection** refers to infection in a patient without preexisting antibodies to HSV-1 or HSV-2.
   B. **Nonprimary first episode infection** refers to the acquisition of genital HSV-1 in a patient with preexisting antibodies to HSV-2 or the acquisition of genital HSV-2 in a patient with preexisting antibodies to HSV-1.
   C. **Recurrent infection** refers to reactivation of genital HSV in which the HSV type recovered in the lesion is the same type as antibodies in the serum
   D. Each of these types can be either symptomatic or asymptomatic (also called subclinical).

II. **Clinical features**
   A. **Acute primary and recurrent infection.** The initial presentation can be severe with painful genital ulcers, dysuria, fever, tender local inguinal lymphadenopathy, and headache. In other patients, however, the infection is mild, subclinical, or entirely asymptomatic.
   B. Recurrent infection is typically less severe than primary or nonprimary first episode infection.
   C. **Primary infection.** The average incubation period after exposure is four days (range two to twelve days). Patients with primary infections usually have multiple, bilateral, ulcerating, pustular lesions which resolve after a mean of 19 days.
   D. **Other symptoms and signs in these first episode infections:**
      1. Systemic symptoms, including fever, headache, malaise, and myalgias — 67 percent
      2. Local pain and itching — 98 percent
      3. Dysuria — 63 percent
      4. Tender lymphadenopathy — 80 percent
   E. **Recurrent infection** is more common with HSV-2 than HSV-1 (60 versus 14 percent with HSV-1). The frequency of recurrences may correlate with the severity of the initial primary infection.
   F. **Subclinical infection** (asymptomatic viral shedding). After resolution of the primary genital HSV infection, intermittent viral shedding in the absence of genital lesions has been documented in both men and women
   G. **Diagnosis.** Among patients with genital herpes who present with a genital ulcer, the primary differential diagnosis includes syphilis chancroid, and drug eruptions, and Behcet's disease.
      1. The clinical diagnosis of genital herpes should be confirmed by laboratory testing.
      2. **Viral culture.** If active genital lesions are present, the vesicle should be unroofed for sampling of vesicular fluid for culture. However, the overall sensitivity of viral culture of genital lesions is only 50 percent.

3. Polymerase chain reaction. While viral culture is the standard diagnostic method for isolating HSV, real-time HSV PCR assays have emerged as a more sensitive method to confirm HSV infection.

4. Direct fluorescent antibody. Many diagnostic laboratories provide a rapid type-specific direct fluorescent antibody (DFA) test to detect HSV in clinical specimens. This test is specific, reproducible, and less expensive than current real-time HSV PCR assays.

III. **Treatment**

A. **Acyclovir, famciclovir, and valacyclovir,** which is a prodrug that is converted acyclovir, appear to have equivalent efficacy for the treatment of genital herpes and for the suppression of recurrent infection. Famciclovir and valacyclovir have greater oral availability than acyclovir.

B. Pain control with topical agents or opioid medications should be administered.

C. Although there is no difference in efficacy, acyclovir is substantially less expensive than famcicovir and valacyclovir.

D. **Acyclovir (Zovirax)** dose is 400 mg PO three times per day or 200 mg PO five times per day for 7 to 10 days There is no clinical benefit from higher doses.

E. Patients with primary genital herpes infections accompanied by more severe clinical manifestations, such as aseptic meningitis, may be treated with intravenous **acyclovir** (5 to 10 mg/kg every eight hours for five to seven days).

   1. **Famciclovir (Famvir)** dose is 250 mg PO three times daily for seven to ten days.

   2. **Valacyclovir (Valtrex)** dose is 1000 mg PO twice daily for seven to ten days.

Dosage Regimens for Primary Genital Herpes Infection	
Drug	**Dosage**
Acyclovir (Zovirax)	400 mg three times daily for 7-10 days
Famciclovir (Famvir)	250 mg three times daily for 7-10 days
Valacyclovir (Valtrex)	1 g twice daily for 7-10 days

F. **Recurrent episodes.** When compared to primary infection, recurrent genital HSV is typically less severe, with fewer lesions that are often in a unilateral, rather than bilateral distribution. In addition, treatment of the primary infection does not appear to reduce the frequency of subsequent recurrences.

G. **Recommendations.** Antiviral therapy of recurrent episodes is most likely to be effective if started within the first 24 hours.

   1. Although there is no difference in efficacy, acyclovir is substantially less expensive.

   2. The recommended dose of acyclovir is 800 mg PO three times daily for two days or 400 mg PO three times daily for three to five days.

   3. The recommended dose of famciclovir is 125 mg PO two times daily for three to five days.

   4. The recommended dose of valacyclovir is 500 mg PO twice daily for three days.

Dosages of Antiviral Agents for Treatment of Episodic Genital Herpes	
Drug	Dosage
Acyclovir (Zovirax)	400 mg three times daily daily for 3-5 days 800 mg twice daily for 2 days
Famciclovir (Famvir)	125 mg twice daily for 3-5 days
Valacyclovir (Valtrex)	500 mg twice daily for 3 days

  H. Suppression of recurrence and asymptomatic shedding. Suppressive therapy
     diminishes the frequency of viral shedding, reduces the rates of reactivation,
     and decreases transmission to uninfected partners.
     1. Suppressive therapy can diminish viral shedding and the rate of clinical
        recurrence.
     2. The recommended dose regimens for the prevention of recurrent infection
        are as follows. Although there is no difference in efficacy, acyclovir is
        substantially less expensive.
        a. Acyclovir. 400 mg twice daily.
        b. Famciclovir. 250 mg PO two times daily.
        c. Valacyclovir. 500 mg once daily; a higher dose of 500 mg twice daily or
           1000 mg once daily is recommended in patients with >10 recurrences
           per year.

Dosages and Characteristics of Chronic Suppressive Treatment Regimens for Recurrent Genital Herpes Infection			
Drug	Dosage	Decrease in recurrence rate (percentage)	Use in patients with >6 recurrences per year
Acyclovir (Zovirax)	400 mg twice daily	78 to 79	Yes
Famciclovir (Famvir)	250 mg twice daily	79	Yes
Valacyclovir (Valtrex)	1 g once daily	78 to 79	Yes
	250 mg twice daily	78 to 79	Yes
	500 mg once daily	71	No

  I. STD screening. Patients with genital herpes should be screened for other
     sexually transmitted diseases.
  J. Prevention. Behavioral changes, including condom use, may prevent the
     spread of genital HSV.
IV. Counseling
  A. Patients should be counseled that the acquisition of HSV can be asymptom-
     atic and only serologic testing can determine if their infection was recently
     acquired. They should be educated about the probability of recurrence
     (60%).
  B. All persons with genital HSV infection should be encouraged to inform their
     current and future sex partners that they have genital herpes. Serologic

testing should be considered for those who are asymptomatic to determine the risk of HSV acquisition.
  C. Couples who are serologically discordant should be advised to use condoms to decrease the risk of transmission and to abstain from intercourse when active lesions or prodromal symptoms are present. Patients may also be counseled that suppressive therapy may decrease the risk of transmission to the sexual partner.

References, see page 372.

Herpes Zoster and Postherpetic Neuralgia

Following primary infection with varicella-zoster virus (VZV), which causes chickenpox, latent infection is established in the sensory dorsal root ganglia. Reactivation of endogenous latent VZV infection within the sensory ganglia results in herpes zoster or "shingles", characterized by a painful, unilateral vesicular eruption in a restricted dermatomal distribution.

I. **Epidemiology**
  A. Cumulative lifetime incidence is 10 to 20 percent of the population. Older age groups have the highest incidence of zoster, because of the decline in VZV-specific cell mediated immunity. Approximately 4 percent of individuals will experience a second episode of herpes zoster.
  B. Herpes zoster cases has the highest incidence (5 to 10 cases per 1,000 persons) after the sixth decade.
  C. The incidence of shingles is significantly lower in black subjects versus white (5 versus 16 percent).
  D. HIV-infected patients. Herpes zoster preferentially occurs in immunosuppressed patients, including transplant recipients and HIV-infected patients. The development of herpes zoster suggests the need for assessment of HIV-1 seropositivity in populations at risk for HIV-1 infection.

II. **Natural history and infectivity**
  A. Approximately 75 percent of patients patients have prodromal pain in the dermatome where the rash subsequently appears. The rash appears as grouped vesicles or bullae which evolve into pustular or occasionally hemorrhagic lesions within three to four days. In immunocompetent hosts, the lesions crust by day 7 to 10 and are no longer infectious; crusting of the rash occurs within three to four weeks. Recurrence of clinical zoster in the immunocompetent host is rare.
  B. Pain is the most common symptom of zoster and can precede the rash by days to weeks; prodromal pain may be constant or intermittent. The pain is a deep "burning", "throbbing" or "stabbing" sensation.
  C. Zoster is generally limited to one dermatome in normal hosts, but can occasionally affect two or three neighboring dermatomes.
  D. The thoracic and lumbar dermatomes are the most commonly involved sites of herpes zoster. Zoster keratitis or zoster ophthalmicus can result from involvement of the ophthalmic branch of the trigeminal cranial nerve. These can be sight-threatening infections.
  E. Fewer than 20 percent of patients have significant systemic symptoms, such as headache, fever, malaise, or fatigue.

III. **Complications in immunocompetent patients.**
  A. Complications of herpes zoster include ocular, neurologic, bacterial superinfection of the skin and postherpetic neuralgia. Herpes zoster may also extend centrally which can result in meningeal inflammation and clinical

meningitis. Occasionally VZV reactivation affects motor neurons in the spinal cord and brain stem resulting in motor neuropathies.

B. Postherpetic neuralgia. Approximately 10 to 15 percent of all patients with herpes zoster will develop postherpetic neuralgia (PHN); individuals older than 60 years account for 50 percent of these cases. PHN has been generally defined as the persistence of sensory symptoms (pain, numbness, dysesthesias, allodynia, which is pain precipitated by movement) in the affected dermatome for >30 days after the onset of zoster.

  1. Prodromal sensory symptoms were associated with a twofold higher prevalence of PHN.
  2. Immunosuppressed individuals (HIV, transplant, connective tissue disease) had higher PHN prevalence.
  3. Treatment of herpes zoster with steroids does not reduce the prevalence of PHN.
  4. Acyclovir therapy does not reduce the prevalence of PHN.
  5. The current standard therapeutic approach has employed tricyclic antidepressants (amitriptyline, desipramine) alone or in combination with carbamazepine or opioids. Tricyclic antidepressants may be contraindicated in elderly patients with cardiovascular disease. Intrathecal corticosteroids were effective in one study of patients with intractable PHN.
  6. Gabapentin (Neurontin), a structural analog of gamma-aminobutyric acid (GABA) significantly reduces in daily pain score. Gabapentin is moderately effective for PHN approach to the management of PHN.

IV. Treatment and prevention of herpes zoster

A. Uncomplicated herpes zoster

  1. Antiviral therapy should be initiated within 72 hours in patients older than 50 years of age. Treatment 72 hours after the onset of lesions should be considered if new lesions are still appearing at that time.
  2. The benefit of ACV therapy was less marked in patients under the age of 50 years. Therapy can be considered on an individual basis in younger patients based upon predictors of PHN such as the severity of the acute pain and rash and history of prodromal pain.
  3. Valacyclovir (1000 mg three times per day for seven days) is recommmended because compared to ACV, valacyclovir was associated with more rapid resolution of acute neuritis and a shorter duration of PHN. However, if cost is an issue, then ACV (800 mg every four hours [five times/day] for seven to ten days) may be preferred. If famciclovir is used, the dosage is 500 or 750 mg three times daily.

Treatment Options for Herpes Zoster	
Medication	**Dosage**
Acyclovir (Zovirax)	800 mg orally five times daily for 7 to 10 days 10 mg per kg IV every 8 hours for 7 to 10 days
Famciclovir (Famvir)	500 mg orally three times daily for 7 days
Valacyclovir (Valtrex)	1,000 mg orally three times daily for 7 days

Medication	Dosage
Prednisone (Deltasone)	30 mg orally twice daily on days 1 through 7; then 15 mg twice daily on days 8 through 14; then 7.5 mg twice daily on days 15 through 21 2 (2 to 4) for days 1 through 7 2 (1 to 3) for days 8 through 14 1 (1 to 2) for days 15 to 21

4. **Prednisone** combined with antiviral therapy should be considered only in patients with severe symptoms at initial presentation who do not have a specific contraindication to steroid use. Dosage is 40 mg of prednisone daily with a taper over seven to ten days with the last dose coinciding with the end of antiviral therapy.

5. **Analgesia for herpetic neuralgia.** Nonsteroidal antiinflammatory drugs are usually not effective. Opioid therapy, such as oxycodone/acetaminophen, is preferred.

V. Treatment of postherpetic neuralgia

A. Although postherpetic neuralgia is generally a self-limited condition, it can last indefinitely.

Treatment Options for Postherpetic Neuralgia	
Medication	**Dosage**
Topical agents	
Capsaicin cream (Zostrix)	Apply to affected area three to five times daily.
Lidocaine (Xylocaine) patch	Apply to affected area every 4 to 12 hours as needed.
Tricyclic antidepressants	
Amitriptyline (Elavil)	0 to 25 mg orally at bedtime; increase dosage by 25 mg every 2 to 4 weeks until response is adequate, or to maximum dosage of 150 mg per day.
Nortriptyline (Pamelor)	0 to 25 mg orally at bedtime; increase dosage by 25 mg every 2 to 4 weeks until response is adequate, or to maximum dosage of 125 mg per day.
Imipramine (Tofranil)	25 mg orally at bedtime; increase dosage by 25 mg every 2 to 4 weeks until response is adequate, or to maximum dosage of 150 mg per day.
Desipramine (Norpramin)	25 mg orally at bedtime; increase dosage by 25 mg every 2 to 4 weeks until response is adequate, or to maximum dosage of 150 mg per day.
Anticonvulsants	
Phenytoin (Dilantin)	100 to 300 mg orally at bedtime; increase dosage until response is adequate or blood drug level is 10 to 20 µg per mL (40 to 80 µmol per L).

Medication	Dosage
Carbamazepine (Tegretol)	100 mg orally at bedtime; increase dosage by 100 mg every 3 days until dosage is 200 mg three times daily, response is adequate or blood drug level is 6 to 12 µg per mL (25.4 to 50.8 µmol per L).
Gabapentin (Neurontin)	100 to 300 mg orally at bedtime; increase dosage by 100 to 300 mg every 3 days until dosage is 300 to 900 mg three times daily or response is adequate.

B. Analgesics
  1. Capsaicin is more efficacious than placebo but must be applied to the affected area three to five times daily. Pain will likely increase during the first few days to a week after capsaicin therapy is initiated.
  2. Lidocaine patches reduce pain intensity, with minimal systemic absorption. The effect lasts only four to 12 hours with each application.
  3. Acetaminophen and nonsteroidal anti-inflammatory drugs are useful for potentiating the pain-relieving effects of narcotics.

C. Tricyclic Antidepressants
  1. Tricyclic antidepressants can be effective adjuncts in reducing pain. Tricyclic antidepressants commonly used in the treatment of postherpetic neuralgia include amitriptyline (Elavil), nortriptyline (Pamelor), imipramine (Tofranil) and desipramine (Norpramin).
  2. The tricyclic antidepressants may cause sedation, dry mouth, postural hypotension, blurred vision and urinary retention. Nortriptyline is better tolerated.

D. Gabapentin is effective in treating the pain of postherpetic neuralgia. The dosages required for analgesia are often lower than those used in the treatment of epilepsy.

E. Transcutaneous electric nerve stimulation (TENS), biofeedback and nerve blocks are also sometimes used.

References, see page 372.

Atopic Dermatitis and Eczema

Atopic dermatitis is a chronic inflammation of the skin that occurs in persons of all ages but is more common in children. Atopic dermatitis affects 10 percent of children. The symptoms of atopic dermatitis resolve by adolescence in 50 percent of affected children.

I. Diagnosis
  A. Exposure to aeroallergens, irritating chemicals, foods and emotional stress may worsen the rash.
  B. Acute lesions are papules and vesicles on a background of erythema. Sub-acute lesions may develop scales and lichenification. Chronically involved areas become thick and fibrotic. Lesions can develop secondary infections with crusting and weeping. Xerosis (dry skin) is characteristic.

Diagnostic Features of Atopic Dermatitis

Major features
Pruritus
Chronic or relapsing dermatitis
Personal or family history of atopic disease
Typical distribution and morphology of atopic dermatitis rash:
  Facial and extensor surfaces in infants and young children
  Flexure lichenification in older children and adults

Minor features

Eyes	Nipple eczema
Cataracts (anterior subcapsular)	Positive type I hypersensitivity skin tests
Keratoconus	Propensity for cutaneous infections
Infraorbital folds affected	Elevated serum IgE level
Facial pallor	Food intolerance
Palmar hyperlinearity	Impaired cell-mediated immunity
Xerosis	Erythroderma
Pityriasis alba	Early age of onset
White dermatographism	
Ichthyosis	
Keratosis pilaris	
Nonspecific dermatitis of the hands and feet	

  C. In infants and young children, pruritus commonly is present on the scalp, face (cheeks and chin) and extensor surfaces of the extremities. Older children and adults typically have involvement of the flexor surfaces (antecubital and popliteal fossa), neck, wrists and ankles.

  D. Exposure to pollens, molds, mites and animal dander may be important in some patients.

II. Treatment

  A. Bathing and moisturizers. Bathing should occur once daily with warm water for five to 10 minutes. Soap should not be used unless it is needed for the removal of dirt. A mild cleanser (eg, Dove, Basis, Kiss My Face or Cetaphil) may be used. After bathing, patients should apply a moisturizer liberally (eg, Vaseline, Aquaphor, Eucerin, Moisturel, mineral oil or baby oil). Ointments are superior to creams. Lotions are least effective because of their alcohol content. To avoid injury to the skin from scratching, fingernails should be cut short, and cotton gloves can be worn at night.

  B. Pruritus that is refractory to moisturizers and conservative measures can be treated with sedating agents such as hydroxyzine (Atarax) and diphenhydramine (Benadryl). Tricyclic antidepressants such as doxepin (Sinequan) and amitriptyline (Elavil) also induce sleep and reduce pruritus.

  C. Systemic corticosteroids should be reserved for use in patients with severe treatment-resistant atopic dermatitis.

  D. It is reasonable to use a mild topical steroid initially in infants and for intertriginous areas in patients of any age. If the dermatitis is severe, a more potent steroid is needed.

Commonly Used Topical Corticosteroids	
Preparation	**Size**
Low-Potency Agents	
Hydrocortisone ointment, cream, 1, 2.5% (Hytone)	30 g

Commonly Used Topical Corticosteroids	
Preparation	**Size**
Mild-Potency Agents	
Alclometasone dipropionate cream, ointment, 0.05% (Aclovate)	60 g
Triamcinolone acetonide cream, 0.1% (Aristocort)	60 g
Fluocinolone acetonide cream, 0.01% (Synalar)	60 g
Medium-Potency Agents	
Triamcinolone acetonide ointment (Aristocort A), 0.1%	60 g
Betamethasone dipropionate cream (Diprosone), 0.05%	45 g
Mometasone cream 0.1% (Elocon)	45 g
Fluocinolone acetonide ointment, 0.025% (Synalar)	60 g
Betamethasone valerate cream, 0.1% (Valisone)	45 g
Hydrocortisone valerate cream, ointment, 0.2% (Westcort)	60 g

E. **Immunosuppressants and antineoplastics**
  1. **Pimecrolimus (Elidel)** is a non-steroid cream for the treatment of mild to moderate eczema. Pimecrolimus has anti-inflammatory activity. It does not cause skin atrophy. Topical application is comparable to that of a potent topical steroid. 1% pimecrolimus cream is applied twice daily. It may be used in children ≥2 years old. The FDA has issued warnings about a possible link between the topical calcineurin inhibitors and cancer.
  2. **Tacrolimus (Protopic)** is more potent than pimecrolimus in the treatment of severe or refractory atopic dermatitis, with few adverse effects. Tacrolimus is available in 0.1% and 0.03%. The lower strength may be used in children ≥2 years old. The FDA has issued warnings about a possible link between the topical calcineurin inhibitors and cancer.
  3. **Cyclosporine (Sandimmune)** has been effective in patients with refractory atopic dermatitis. The condition returns after the cessation of therapy, although not always at the original level of severity.

References, see page 372.

Acne Vulgaris

Acne vulgaris affects over 17 million Americans, and 85 percent of the adolescent population experiences acne
I. **Classification of acne**
  A. **Type 1.** Mainly comedones with an occasional small inflamed papule or pustule; no scarring present.
  B. **Type 2.** Comedones and more numerous papules and pustules (mainly facial); mild scarring.
  C. **Type 3.** Numerous comedones, papules, and pustules, spreading to the back, chest, and shoulders, with an occasional cyst or nodule; moderate scarring.
  D. **Type 4.** Numerous large cysts on the face, neck, and upper trunk; severe scarring.

II. Diagnostic evaluation

A. History should exclde polycystic ovary syndrome (PCOS), the most common cause of hyperandrogenism, which is characterized by menstrual irregularity, hirsutism, acne, ovarian cysts, insulin resistance, and acanthosis nigricans. Women with acne and oligomenorrhea should be evaluated for PCOS.

B. The sudden appearance of acne with virilization suggests an adrenal or ovarian tumor; patients with Cushing's disease or syndrome and adult onset congenital adrenal hyperplasia may also have acne vulgaris. Evidence of virilization includes a deepening voice, decreased breast size, clitoromegaly, alopecia, oligomenorrhea, and hirsutism. Imaging studies of the adrenal glands and ovaries, and/or hormonal evaluation may be required.

C. **Medications known to causes of acne** include ACTH, androgens, azathioprine, barbiturates, bromides, corticosteroids, cyclosporine, disulfiram, halogens, iodides, isoniazid, lithium, phenytoin, psoralens, thiourea, and vitamins B2, B6, and B12.

D. **Physical examination** should focus upon the type and location of lesions, scarring, keloids, and postinflammatory pigmentary changes. Hirsutism or virilization should prompt further laboratory and imaging studies.

III. Treatment of comedonal acne

A. Noninflammatory comedones typically develop in the preteen and early teenage years; there are no inflammatory lesions since P. acne colonization has not yet occurred. Treatment of abnormal follicular keratinization is most effective for comedonal acne.

B. **Topical retinoids** (tretinoin, adapalene, tazarotene) are the initial drugs of choice for comedonal acne. These agents halt the progression of comedones to inflammatory lesions by normalizing follicular keratinization.

C. **Tazorotene** does not share the same systemic side effects as oral isotretinoin, but it is still contraindicated in pregnancy.

D. Tretinoin can cause cutaneous irritation; this may be minimized by starting with the lowest strength preparation (0.025 percent cream) and then increasing the potency. The ascending order of potency is as follows: 0.025 percent cream; 0.01 percent gel; 0.05 percent cream; 0.025 percent gel; 0.1 percent cream; and 0.05 percent solution. A microencapsulated form of 0.1 percent tretinoin gel is less irritating. Reduced irritation has been noted with a polyolprepolymer-2 base.

Treatment of Acne			
Medication	**Dose**	**Partial list of preparations**	**Adverse effects**
Topical retinoids			
Tretinoin (Retin-A)	Usually twice daily	0.025 percent cream 0.01 percent gel 0.05 percent cream 0.025 percent gel 0.1 percent cream 0.05 percent solution	Local irritation; photosensitivity (use sunscreen)

Medication	Dose	Partial list of preparations	Adverse effects
Adapalene (Differin)	daily or twice daily	0.1 percent gel	Local irritation (slightly less than tretinoin); photosensitivity (use sunscreen)
Tazarotene (Tazorac)	daily	0.05 percent gel 0.1 percent gel	Local irritation; photosensitivity (use sunscreen); contraindicated in pregnancy, nursing
Benzoyl peroxide	daily or twice daily	2.5, 5, and 10 percent gels, lotions 5 percent solution + 3 percent erythromycin 6 and 10 percent gel + glycolic acid	Local irritation; can bleach hair and clothing
Topical antibiotics			
Metronidazole (Metrogel)	twice daily	1 percent cream 0.75 percent gel	
Clindamycin (Cleocin)	twice daily	10 mg/mL gel 10mg/mL lotion 10 mg/mL topical solution	
Erythromycin (Erycette)	twice daily	1.5 percent solution 2 percent solution 2 percent gel 2 percent ointment 2 percent pledgets	
Azelaic acid (Azelex)	twice daily	20 percent cream	
Oral antibiotics			
Tetracycline	500 mg twice daily (or 250 mg twice daily)		Contraindicated in pregnancy and in children under age 12 due to tooth discoloration
Doxycycline	100 mg twice daily		Phototoxicity; esophageal ulceration
Minocycline	50 to 100 mg twice daily		Vertigo; pseudotumor; tooth discoloration
Erythromycin	250 to 750 mg twice daily		Gastrointestinal complaints

Medication	Dose	Partial list of preparations	Adverse effects
Oral retinoid			
Isotretinoin (Accutane)	0.5 mg/kg, increasing to 1 mg/kg, total dose 120 to 150 mg/kg over 20 weeks		Teratogenicity (absolutely contraindicated in pregnancy, nursing); mucocutaneous effects; hypertriglyceridemia; depression; bone marrow suppression

E. Adapalene produces less cutaneous irritation than tretinoin. However, both drugs increase photosensitivity; they should be applied at bedtime with concurrent use of sunscreen in the morning.

F. Gels have a drying effect; they may be useful in patients with oily skin. Creams and lotions are moisturizing. Solutions are drying but they cover large areas. Most topical medications are applied twice daily, although once daily or alternate day therapy can be used.

G. Salicylic acid and azelaic acid also exhibit comedolytic activity. These preparations are useful for patients who are unable to tolerate the topical retinoids. Salicylic acid is available in a number of nonprescription solutions (0.5 and 2 percent), cleansers, and soaps. Azelaic acid is an antimicrobial agent that reduces cutaneous pigmentation.

H. Comedo extraction can be a useful adjunct to topical therapy in patients with resistant comedones. Excise the roof or enlarge the opening of the comedo with an 18-gauge needle or no. 11 blade. Apply pressure with a comedo extractor.

IV. **Mild to moderate inflammatory acne** responds to benzoyl peroxide, a topical antibiotic, or a combination of the two drugs. Combination therapy is more effective than monotherapy for inflammatory lesions.

A. **Benzoyl peroxide** has both antibacterial and comedolytic properties. It is usually applied twice daily, although when combined with a topical retinoid, benzoyl peroxide is typically applied in the morning and the retinoid at night to limit irritation and photosensitivity.

1. Benzoyl peroxide is available in 2.5, 5, and 10 percent gels and lotions, as a 5 percent solution in combination with 3 percent erythromycin, and as a 6 and 10 percent gel in combination with glycolic acid. Liquids and creams are less irritating than gels, these agents can cause bleaching of the hair and clothing.

B. **Topical antibiotics** are added to eliminate P. acnes and suppress inflammation in papular and inflammatory acne. Topical antibiotics may promote the appearance of resistant strains of P. acne; resistance is diminished by combination use with benzoyl peroxide.

1. Topical antibiotics are available in gels, solutions, and lotions. Erythromycin and clindamycin are most frequently used. All topical antibiotics rarely cause skin irritation. Topical tetracycline can cause yellow staining of the skin and clothing.

V. **Moderate to severe inflammatory acne.** A sequential topical regimen of combination benzoyl peroxide-erythromycin in the morning and topical tretinoin in the evening is often effective. Patients with severe disease should be treated with oral antibiotics or oral isotretinoin in addition to topical therapy. Hormonal therapy may be useful in some women.

A. Oral antibiotics improve inflammatory acne by inhibiting the growth of P. acnes. The tetracyclines also have direct antiinflammatory properties; they inhibit the neutrophil chemotaxis and granuloma formation. Systemic antibiotics may induce vaginal candidiasis, decrease the efficacy of concomitantly administered oral contraceptive pills, and cause gastrointestinal distress.

B. Tetracycline is the preferred oral antibiotic due to its low cost and high efficacy. It is initiated at a dose of 500 mg twice daily, although 250 mg twice daily may also be effective. Absorption is inhibited by food, dairy products, antacids, and iron; it must be taken on an empty stomach. Tetracycline is contraindicated during pregnancy and in children younger than 12 years of age due to its ability to discolor the enamel of developing teeth.

C. Doxycycline and minocycline are more lipid soluble than tetracycline and can therefore be used in lower doses (100 mg twice daily and 50 to 100 mg twice daily, respectively); an extended release formulation of minocycline is also available (45 to 135 mg once daily). Either drug can be taken with meals. Minocycline or doxycycline may be prescribed in those who fail therapy with tetracycline.

1. **Doxycycline** may be photosensitizing, and must be swallowed with ample fluids in order to avoid the development of esophageal ulcerations.

2. **Minocycline** does not cause the phototoxicity seen with both tetracycline and doxycycline, but can cause vertigo, pseudotumor cerebri, tooth discoloration, and a lupus-like syndrome.

D. Erythromycin may be administered as 250 mg to 1500 mg daily in two divided doses. However, it has less antiinflammatory activity than the tetracyclines, and P. acnes often develop resistance, and intolerable gastrointestinal side effects are common.

E. Isotretinoin (Accutane) is a 13-cis retinoic acid that is useful for severe acne. It acts by reducing sebum secretion, an effect that lasts for up to one year after cessation of therapy.

1. The primary indications for therapy with oral isotretinoin include:
   a. Severe nodulocystic acne
   b. Acne that improves less than 50 percent after six months of treatment with oral antibiotics
   c. Relapsing acne
   d. Scarring acne
   e. Acne that causes undue psychological distress

2. Treatment is initiated at a daily dose of 0.5 mg/kg and increased to 1 mg/kg, administered in two divided doses with food, with a total treatment course of 120 to 150 mg/kg over 4 to 7 months (usual duration of treatment 20 weeks).

3. A micronized formulation of isotretinoin offers the advantage of once daily dosing and does not need to be taken with food.

4. The FDA has imposed restrictions on who may prescribe and distribute isotretinoin. Isotretinoin causes both spontaneous abortions and severe life-threatening congenital malformations. Mucocutaneous side effects include cheilitis, dry skin, desquamation, photosensitivity, and pruritus.

5. Arthralgias, myalgias, hyperostosis, pseudotumor cerebri, decreased night vision, corneal opacities, hepatotoxicity, bone marrow suppression, and hypervitaminosis A may occur. Hypertriglyceridemia occurs in up to 45 percent. There is a possible association with depression and suicide.

F. Hormonal and corticosteroid therapy. Therapy with estrogen or an antiandrogen is an alternative to systemic isotretinoin in women with acne that is unresponsive to other methods of treatment.

1. Women with concomitant hirsutism or menstrual irregularity should have a gynecologic and hormonal evaluation.

2. Glucocorticoids are indicated for those with excessive adrenal androgen production, such as in classical congenital adrenal hyperplasia. For those

with nonclassical (late-onset) congenital adrenal hyperplasia, oral contraceptives rather than glucocorticoids are used.

3. Oral contraceptives, particularly those preparations with a low androgenic progestin, are indicated for women with excessive ovarian androgen production (eg, PCOS).

4. Oral contraceptives with a low androgenic progestin may also be useful in some women with normal menses and no evidence of excess androgen production. A triphasic combination pill with norgestimate and ethinylestradiol (Ortho tri-cyclen) has been approved to treat acne vulgaris.

5. Newer oral contraceptives with anti-androgenic properties are being proposed as preferred therapies for women with acne. These include oral contraceptives that contain cyproterone or drospirenone plus an estrogen. Less costly oral contraceptives should be tried before more expensive preparations are prescribed.

6. Antiandrogens act at the peripheral receptor level to decrease sebum production. Spironolactone is most frequently used at a dose of 50 to 150 mg daily. Serum potassium and blood pressure should be monitored.

Androgenic activity of progestins in oral contraceptive pills	
Level of activity	**Brand name**
High	Norgestrel LoOvral Levonorgestrel Nordette Levelen Triphasil Trilevlen
Middle	Norethindrone Genora 1/35 OrthoNovum 1/35 Norinyl 1/35 Ortho 1/11 TriNorinyl Ortho 7/7/7 Modicon Brevicon Ovcon 35 Norethindrone acetate Loestrin 1/20 Loestrin 1.5/30
Low	Ethynodiol Demulen 1/35 Norgestimate Ortho-Cyclen Ortro-Tricyclen Desogestrel Desogen Ortho-Cept Drospirenone Yasmin

References, see page 372.

Dermatophyte (Tinea) Infections

Dermatophytes are the most common type of fungi that cause infection of the skin and nails. Patients often refer to dermatophyte infections of the body or scalp as "ringworm". Three types of superficial fungi/dermatophytes account for the majority of infections: Epidermophyton, Trichophyton, and Microsporum. Dermatophyte infections affect individuals who are healthy, but people with compromised immune systems are particularly susceptible.

I. **Tinea capitis**
   A. Tinea capitis, dermatophyte infection of the scalp, occurs almost always in small children. A clinical diagnosis of tinea capitis in adults is often incorrect, and frequently turns out to be seborrheic dermatitis or syphilis.
   B. Black dot tinea capitis, caused by Trichophyton tonsurans, is the form predominantly seen. Tinea capitis is most often an endothrix infection; nonfluorescent arthroconidia are located within the hair shaft.
   C. Clinical features. The infection begins with an erythematous, scaling, well-demarcated patch on the scalp that spreads centrifugally for a few weeks or months, ceases to spread, and persists indefinitely. The inflammation subsides, and the hairs within the patch break off a millimeter or two above the level of the scalp. The hair stubs take on a frosted appearance. In a few cases the lesions change abruptly to become boggy, elevated, tender nodules (kerion).
   D. **Diagnosis**
      1. **Black dot tinea capitis (BDTC)** is largely a disease of childhood. All ethnic groups may be infected, but African-American children are particularly susceptible. Spread is usually from child to child contact. Fomites (shared hats, combs, brushes, barrettes, rollers, etc) may play an important role. Asymptomatic carriers in the household may also be involved.
      2. **Clinical features.** BDTC usually begins as an asymptomatic, erythematous, scaling patch on the scalp, which slowly enlarges. Lesions may be single or multiple. Hairs within the patches break off flush with the scalp; detritus within the follicular opening formerly occupied by the hair appears as a black dot. In some cases inflammation is prominent, and the lesions can resemble pyoderma or discoid lupus erythematosus. Painful lymphadenopathy can also occur. Left untreated, scarring with permanent alopecia can occur and the disease can last indefinitely. Patches of tinea corporis may appear on glabrous skin, and the nails are sometimes involved. A sudden transition to kerion may occur.
      3. **Diagnosis** of BDTC is made by performing KOH examination of spores on the hair shaft. The infected hairs of BDTC do not fluoresce green under Woods Light. Diagnosis can be confirmed by culture on Sabouraud's medium.
      4. **Treatment.** Griseofulvin remains the drug of choice, although oral therapy with terbinafine or itraconazole are effective alternatives for resistant cases or for patients who are allergic to griseofulvin; oral fluconazole also seems to have similar efficacy to griseofulvin. A meta-analysis suggested that terbinafine is at least as effective as griseofulvin for treating tinea capitis due to Trichophyton infections, while griseofulvin appears to be superior to terbinafine for treating tinea capitis due to Microsporum infections.
         a. **Griseofulvin treatment** schedules are as follows:
            (1) Adults: 250 mg ultramicrosize by mouth twice daily for 6 to 12 weeks. A few cases of the black dot type may require 250 mg three times daily.

        (2) Children: 20 to 25 mg/kg of body weight for 6 to 12 weeks.
     b. Terbinafine (Lamisil) treatment schedules are based on weight:
        (1) 10 to 20 kg: 62.5 mg daily for four weeks
        (2) 20 to 40 kg: 125 mg daily for four weeks
        (3) Above 40 kg: 250 mg daily for four weeks
     c. Itraconazole (Sporanox) can be used in children as continuous therapy at a dose of 3 to 5 mg/kg daily for four to six weeks or as pulse therapy at a dose of 5 mg/kg daily for one week each month for two to three months.
     d. Topical treatment of tinea capitis is futile and a common cause of treatment failure.
     e. Identification of asymptomatic carriers and household fomites is an important part of the management of black dot tinea capitis. Culture on Sabouraud's medium of hairs and scalp dander (collected by brushing the area with a tooth brush) facilitates carrier identification. Carriers should be treated with selenium sulfide shampoo.
     f. Kerion responds best by treating the underlying fungal disorder.

II. Tinea pedis
   A. Tinea pedis (athlete's foot) is the most common dermatophyte infection. It is often accompanied by tinea manuum, onychomycosis (tinea unguium), or tinea cruris (dermatophyte infection of the hands, nails, or groin).
   B. Tinea pedis presents in two readily distinguishable clinical forms, acute and chronic. Both are contagious, contracted by contact with arthrospores shed by infected individuals onto the floor.
   C. Acute tinea pedis
     1. Clinical features. Attacks of acute tinea pedis are self-limited, intermittent, and recurrent. They often follow activities that cause the feet to sweat. Acute tinea pedis begins with the appearance of intensely pruritic, sometimes painful, erythematous vesicular or bullous lesions between the toes and on the soles, frequently extending up the instep. The disease may be unilateral or bilateral. Secondary staphylococcal infections with lymphangitis often complicate the picture.
     2. Secondary eruptions at distant sites may occur simultaneously due to an immunologic reaction to the fungus. This is a sterile vesicular eruption that often occurs on the palms and fingers, referred to as an "id" reaction. This improves as the primary infection is treated.
   D. Diagnosis should be confirmed by KOH examination of scrapings from the lesions. The roof of a vesicle is a good place to look. Culture on Sabouraud's medium is helpful in difficult cases.
   E. Chronic tinea pedis
     1. Clinical features. Chronic tinea pedis is the most common form of tinea pedis encountered in practice. Untreated it usually persists indefinitely. The disease begins with slowly progressive pruritic, erythematous lesions between the toes, especially in the fourth digital interspace. Interdigital fissures are often present. Extension onto the sole follows and later onto the sides or even the top of the foot ("moccasin ringworm"). The border between involved and uninvolved skin is usually quite sharp, and the normal creases and markings of the skin (dermatoglyphs) tend to accumulate scale. In many cases the palms and flexor aspects of the fingers may be involved (tinea manuum). Mycotic nail dystrophy (onychomycosis) is also often present.
     2. Treatment. Tinea pedis can usually be treated with a topical antifungal cream for four weeks; interdigital tinea pedis may only require one week of therapy.

3. Some prescription agents have a broader spectrum of action and may be administered once instead of twice daily, but generally all of the creams are equally effective.

4. Patients with chronic disease or extensive disease may require oral antifungal therapy with griseofulvin (250 to 500 mg of microsize twice daily), terbinafine (250 mg daily), or itraconazole (200 mg daily). Terbinafine is more effective than griseofulvin, while the efficacy of terbinafine and itraconazole are similar. Nail involvement is another indication for oral therapy. Secondary infection should be treated with oral antibiotics.

5. Pediatric dosing options:
   a. Griseofulvin 10 to 15 mg/kg daily or in divided doses
   b. Terbinafine (Lamisil):
      (1) 10 to 20 kg: 62.5 mg daily
      (2) 20 to 40 kg: 125 mg daily
      (3) Above 40 kg: 250 mg daily
   c. Itraconazole 5 mg/kg daily
   d. Fluconazole 6 mg/kg daily
   e. Other adjunctive therapies include use of foot powder to prevent maceration, treatment of shoes with antifungal powders, and avoidance of occlusive footwear.

Topical Antifungal Agents

Drug	Dose	How supplied
Terbinafine (Lamisil)	QD to BID	Cream 1%: 15g, 30g Gel 1%: 5g, 15g, 30g
Clotrimazole (Lotrimin)	BID	Cream 1%: 15g, 30g, 45g, 90g Lotion 1%: 30mL Solution 1%: 10mL, 30mL
Econazole (Spectazole)	QD (BID for candidiasis)	Cream 196: 15g, 30g, 85g
Sulconazole (Exelderm)	QD to BID	Cream 1%: 15g, 30g, 60g Solution 1%: 30mL
Oxiconazole (Oxistat)	QD to BID	Cream 1%: 15g, 30g, 60g Lotion 1%: 30mL
Naftifine (Naftin)	QD (cream), BID (gel)	Cream 1%: 15g, 30g, 60g Gel 1%: 20g, 40g, 60g
Ciclopirox (Loprox)	BID	Cream 1%: 15g, 30g, 90g Lotion 1%: 30mL, 60mL
Ketoconazole (Nizoral)	QD	Cream 2%: 15g, 30g, 60g
Miconazole (Monistat-Derm)	BID	Cream 2%: 15g, 30g, 56.7g, 85g

Drug	Dose	How supplied
Tolnaftate (Tinactin)	BID	Cream 1% : 15g, 30g Gel 1%: 15g Powder 1%: 45g, 90g Topical aerosol: liquid (1%): 59.2mL, 90mL, 120mL powder (1%):56.7g, 100g, 105g, 150g Solution 1%: 10 mL

Oral Antifungal Agents

Terbinafine (Lamisil):
For fingernails — 250 mg daily by mouth for 6 weeks
For toenails — 250 mg daily by mouth for 12 weeks

Itraconazole (Sporanox):
Fixed dosage
For fingernails — 200 mg daily by mouth for 8 weeks
For toenails — 200 mg daily by mouth for 12 weeks
Pulse therapy
For fingernails — 400 mg daily by mouth for one week per month for two months
For toenails — 400 mg daily by mouth for one week per month for three months

III. **Tinea corporis**
   A. Tinea corporis begins as a pruritic circular or oval erythematous scaling lesion that spreads centrifugally. Central clearing follows, while the active advancing border, a few millimeters wide, retains its red color and is slightly raised. The lesion is shaped like a ring.
   B. Extensive presentations suggest an underlying immunologic disorder, such as diabetes mellitus or HIV infection.
   C. Tinea corporis can also occur in outbreaks among athletes who have skin-to-skin contact, such as wrestlers (tinea corporis gladiatorum).
   D. **Treatment.** Tinea corporis usually responds well to the daily application of topical antifungals. For adults with extensive cases or with folliculitis, or in patients who are severely immunocompromised, a systemic agent is preferable.
   E. Appropriate systemic agents include oral terbinafine, fluconazole, and itraconazole; all of these agents appear to have greater efficacy and fewer side effects than oral griseofulvin, however griseofulvin is less expensive. Reasonable regimens in adults include: terbinafine 250 mg daily for one to two weeks; fluconazole 150 mg once weekly for two to four weeks; itraconazole 200 mg daily for one to two weeks; griseofulvin 250 mg three times daily for two weeks.
   F. Patients with tinea corporis gladiatorum should be treated with an oral agent for ten to 15 days along with restricted participation in sports.
IV. **Tinea cruris** (jock itch) is a special form of tinea corporis involving the crural fold. The most common cause is T rubrum. A few cases are caused by E floccosum and occasionally T mentagrophytes.

A. Tinea cruris is far more common in men than women. The disease often begins after physical activity that results in copious sweating, and the source of the infecting fungus is usually the patient's own tinea pedis.

B. Tinea cruris begins with a macular erythematous patch high on the inner aspect of one or both thighs, opposite the scrotum. It spreads centrifugally, with partial central clearing and a slightly elevated, erythematous, sharply demarcated border that may show tiny vesicles.

C. **Diagnosis.** KOH examination of scales scraped from the lesion will show the segmented hyphae and arthrospores. Highest yields are obtained from material taken from the active border of the lesion. Cultures on Sabouraud's medium can also be used to confirm the diagnosis.

D. **Treatment.** Topical antifungal treatment is usually effective. Failure to treat concomitant tinea pedis usually results in prompt recurrence. Lesions resistant to topical medications can be treated with griseofulvin by mouth, 250 mg three times daily for 14 days, or any of the other systemic agents.

References, see page 372.

Common Skin Diseases

I. Alopecia Areata

A. Alopecia areata is characterized by asymptomatic, noninflammatory, non-scarring areas of complete hair loss, most commonly involving the scalp, but the disorder may involve any area of hair-bearing skin.

B. Auto-antibodies to hair follicles are the most likely cause. Emotional stress is sometimes a precipitating factor. The younger the patient and the more widespread the disease, and the poorer the prognosis.

C. Regrowth of hair after the first attack takes place in 6 months in 30% of cases, with 50% regrowing within 1 year, and 80% regrowing within 5 years. Ten to 30% of patients will not regrow hair; 5% progress to total hair loss.

D. Lesions are well defined, single or multiple round or oval areas of total hair loss. Typical "exclamation point" hairs (3-10 mm in size with a tapered, less pigmented proximal shaft) are seen at the margins.

E. **Differential diagnosis** includes tinea capitis, trichotillomania, secondary syphilis, and lupus erythematosus.

F. A VDRL or RPR test for syphilis should be obtained. A CBC, SMAC, sedimentary rate, thyroid function tests, and antinuclear antibody should be completed to screen for pernicious anemia, chronic active hepatitis, thyroid disease, lupus erythematosus, and Addison's disease.

G. **Therapy.** Topical steroids, intralesional steroids, and topical minoxidil may be somewhat effective.

1. Intralesional glucocorticoid injection is the most common therapy for limited involvement. Triamcinolone in a dosage of 10 mg per mL, is the preferred agent.

2. Topical therapy may be beneficial when it is combined with minoxidil, anthralin or injected steroids.

3. Topical minoxidil, 5 percent solution, is 40% effective in stimulating hair growth on the scalp, eyebrows and beard area. Minoxidil solution is applied twice daily and stimulates hair growth within 12 weeks.

4. Anthralin cream is commonly used in children. New hair growth may occur within two to three months after initiation of topical anthralin therapy. In one study, 25 percent of patients had cosmetically acceptable results by six months. Side effects of anthralin include redness, itching and scaling. Removal of the cream after application for 20 to 60 minutes is often recom-

mended. However, overnight application has been shown to be well tolerated by some patients.

5. The investigational technique called topical immunotherapy, or contact sensitization, may be effective.

II. Scabies

A. Scabies is an extremely pruritic eruption usually accentuated in the groin, axillae, navel, breasts and finger webs, with sparing the head.

B. Scabies is spread by skin to skin contact. The diagnosis is established by finding the mite, ova, or feces in scrapings of the skin, usually of the finger webs or genitalia.

C. Treatment of choice for nonpregnant adults and children is lindane (Kwell), applied for 12 hours, then washed off.

D. Elimite, a 5% permethrin cream, applied liberally head to toe and rinsed off in 12 hours, is more effective but more expensive than lindane (Kwell).

E. Treatment should be given to all members of an infected household simultaneously. Clothing and sheets must be washed on the day of treatment.

III. Acne Rosacea

A. This condition commonly presents in fair-skinned individuals and is characterized by papules, erythema, and telangiectasias.

B. Initial treatment consists of doxycycline or tetracycline. Once there has been some clearing, topical metronidazole gel (Metro-gel) can prevent remission. Sunblock should be used because sunlight can exacerbate the condition.

IV. Drug Eruptions

A. Drug eruptions may be type I, type II, type III, or type IV immunologic reactions. Cutaneous drug reactions may start within 7 days of initiation of the drug or within 4-7 days after the offending drug has been stopped.

B. The cutaneous lesions usually become more severe and widespread over the following several days to 1 week and then clear over the next 7-14 days.

C. Lesions most often start first and clear first from the head and upper extremities to the trunk and lower legs. Palms, soles, and mucous membranes may be involved.

D. Most drug reactions appear as a typical maculopapular drug reaction. Tetracycline is associated with a fixed drug eruption. Thiazide diuretics have a tendency for photosensitivity eruptions.

E. Treatment of drug eruptions

1. Oral antihistamines are very useful. Diphenhydramine (Benadryl), 25-50 mg q4-6h. Soothing, tepid water baths in Aveeno or corn starch or cool compresses are useful.

2. **Severe signs and symptoms.** A 2-week course of systemic steroids (prednisone starting at 60 mg/day and then tapering) will usually stop the symptoms.

F. Erythema Multiforme

1. Erythema multiforme presents as dull red macules or papules on the back of hands, palms, wrists, feet, elbows and knees. The periphery is red and the center becomes blue or darker red, hence the characteristic target or iris lesion.

2. The rash is most commonly a drug reaction caused by sulfa medications or phenytoin (Dilantin). It is also seen as a reaction to herpes simplex virus infections, mycoplasma, and Hepatitis B.

3. Erythema multiforme major or Steven's Johnson syndrome is diagnosed when mucous membrane or eye involvement is present.

4. Prednisone 30-60 mg/day is often given with a 2-4 week taper.

5. For HSV-driven erythema multiforme, acyclovir may be helpful. Ophthalmologic consultation is obtained for ocular involvement.

V. Pityriasis Rosea

A. Pityriasis rosea is an acute inflammatory dermatitis characterized by self-limited lesions distributed on the trunk and extremities. A viral cause is hypothesized. It is most common between the ages of 10 and 35.

B. Clinical manifestations

    1. The initial lesion, called the "herald patch," can appear anywhere on the body, and is 2-6 cm in size, and begins a few days to several weeks before the generalized eruption. The hands, face, and feet are usually spared.

    2. The lesions are oval, and the long axes follow the lines of cleavage. Lesions are 2 cm or less, pink, tan, or light brown. The borders of the lesions have a loose rim of scales, peeling peripherally, called the "collarette." Pruritus is usually minimal.

C. Differential diagnosis. Secondary syphilis (a VDRL is indicated for atypical rashes), drug eruptions, viral exanthems, acute papular psoriasis, tinea corporis.

D. Treatment. Topical antipruritic emollients (Caladryl) relieve itching. Ultraviolet therapy may be used. The disease usually resolves in 2-14 weeks and recurrences are unusual.

References, see page 372.

Bacterial Infections of the Skin

Bacterial skin infections most commonly include cellulitis, impetigo, and folliculitis.

I. Cellulitis

A. Cellulitis is a painful, erythematous infection of the dermis and subcutaneous tissues that is characterized by warmth, edema, and advancing borders. Cellulitis commonly occurs near breaks in the skin, such as surgical wounds, trauma, tinea infections, or ulcerations. Patients may have a fever and an elevated white blood cell count. The most common sites of cellulitis are the legs and digits, followed by the face, feet, hands, torso, neck, and buttocks.

B. In otherwise healthy adults, isolation of an etiologic agent is difficult and unrewarding. If the patient has diabetes, an immunocompromising disease, or persistent inflammation, blood cultures or aspiration of the area of maximal inflammation may be useful.

C. Empiric treatment of infection in patients without diabetes:

    1. Penicillinase-resistant penicillin: Dicloxacillin (Pathocil) 40 mg/kg/day in 4 divided doses for 7-12 days; adults: 500 mg qid or

    2. First-generation cephalosporin: Cephalexin (Keflex) 50 mg/kg/day PO in 4 divided doses for 7-10 days; adults: 500 mg PO qid or

    3. Amoxicillin-clavulanate (Augmentin) 500 mg tid or 875 mg bid for 7-10 days.

    4. Azithromycin (Zithromax) 500 mg on day 1, then 250 mg PO qd for 4 days.

    5. Erythromycin ethylsuccinate 40 mg/kg/day in 3 divided doses for 7-10 days; adults: 250-500 mg qid.

    6. Limited disease can be treated orally, but more extensive disease requires parenteral therapy. Marking the margins of erythema with ink is helpful in following the progression or regression of cellulitis.

    7. Outpatient therapy with injected ceftriaxone (Rocephin) provides 24 hours of parenteral coverage and may be an option for some patients.

Descriptions of Bacterial Skin Infections	
Disease	**Description**
Carbuncle	A network of furuncles connected by sinus tracts
Cellulitis	Painful, erythematous infection of deep skin with poorly demarcated borders
Erysipelas	Fiery red, painful infection of superficial skin with sharply demarcated borders
Folliculitis	Papular or pustular inflammation of hair follicles
Furuncle	Painful, firm or fluctuant abscess originating from a hair follicle
Impetigo	Large vesicles and/or honey-crusted sores

D. Antibiotics should be maintained for at least three days after the resolution of acute inflammation. Adjunctive therapy includes cool compresses; appropriate analgesics for pain; tetanus immunization; and immobilization and elevation of the affected extremity.

E. A parenteral second- or third-generation cephalosporin (with or without an aminoglycoside) should be considered in patients who have diabetes, immunocompromised patients, those with unresponsive infections, or in young children. The patient may also require a plain radiograph of the area or surgical debridement to evaluate for gas gangrene, osteomyelitis, or necrotizing fasciitis.

F. Periorbital cellulitis is caused by the same organisms that cause other forms of cellulitis and is treated with warm soaks, oral antibiotics, and close follow-up. Children with periorbital or orbital cellulitis often have underlying sinusitis. If the child is febrile and appears toxic, blood cultures should be performed and lumbar puncture considered.

G. Orbital cellulitis occurs when the infection passes the orbital septum and is manifested by proptosis, orbital pain, restricted eye movement, visual disturbances, and concomitant sinusitis. This ocular emergency requires intravenous antibiotics, otorhinolaryngology, and ophthalmologic consultation.

II. Erysipelas

A. Erysipelas usually presents as an intensely erythematous infection with clearly demarcated raised margins and lymphatic streaking. Common sites are the legs and face.

B. Erysipelas is caused almost exclusively by beta-hemolytic streptococcus and thus can be treated with oral or intravenous penicillin, or this infection may be treated the same as cellulitis. Adjunctive treatment and complications are the same as for cellulitis.

III. Impetigo

A. Impetigo is most commonly seen in children aged two to five years and is classified as bullous or nonbullous. The nonbullous type predominates and presents with an erosion (sore), cluster of erosions, or small vesicles or pustules that have a honey-yellow crust. Impetigo usually appears in areas where there is a break in the skin, such as a wound, herpes simplex infection, or angular cheilitis.

B. The bullous form of impetigo presents as a large thin-walled bulla (2 to 5 cm) containing serous yellow fluid. It often ruptures leaving a denuded area. Both forms of impetigo are primarily caused by *S. aureus* with Streptococcus usually being involved in the nonbullous form.

C. An oral antibiotic with activity against *S. aureus* and group A beta-hemolytic streptococcus is warranted in nonlocalized cases.

1. Azithromycin (Zithromax) for five days and cephalexin (Keflex) for 10 days have been shown to be effective and well-tolerated.
2. Dicloxacillin (Pathocil), 500 mg PO qid for 2 weeks.
3. Oxacillin (Prostaphlin) 1-2 gm IV q4-6h.
4. Cephalexin (Keflex) 250-500 mg PO qid.
5. Amoxicillin-clavulanate (Augmentin) 500 mg tid or 875 mg bid for 7-10 days.
6. Broad-spectrum fluoroquinolones have also been shown to be effective for treating skin and soft tissue infections. These medications have excellent skin penetration and good bioavailability.

IV. Folliculitis

A. The most common form is superficial folliculitis that manifests as a tender or painless pustule that heals without scarring. Multiple or single lesions can appear on any skin bearing hair including the head, neck, trunk, buttocks, and extremities. *S. aureus* is the most likely pathogen. Topical therapy with erythromycin, clindamycin (Cleocin T gel), mupirocin (Bactroban), or benzoyl peroxide can be administered to accelerate the healing process.

B. **Staphylococci** will occasionally invade the deeper portion of the follicle, causing swelling and erythema. These lesions are painful and may scar. This inflammation of the entire follicle or the deeper portion of the hair follicle is called deep folliculitis. Oral antibiotics are usually used and include first-generation cephalosporins, penicillinase-resistant penicillins, macrolides, and fluoroquinolones.

C. Gram-negative folliculitis usually involves the face and affects patients with a history of long-term antibiotic therapy for acne. Pathogens include Klebsiella, Enterobacter, and Proteus species. It can be treated as severe acne with isotretinoin (Accutane).

V. Furuncles and Carbuncles

A. **Furuncles** and carbuncles occur as a follicular infection progresses deeper and extends out from the follicle. Commonly known as an abscess or boil, a furuncle is a tender, erythematous, firm or fluctuant mass of walled-off purulent material, arising from the hair follicle. The pathogen is usually S. aureus. Typically, the furuncle will develop into a fluctuant mass and eventually open to the skin surface.

B. **Carbuncles** are an aggregate of infected hair follicles that form broad, swollen, erythematous, deep, and painful masses that usually open and drain through multiple tracts. Fever and malaise, are commonly associated with these lesions. With both of these lesions, gentle incision and drainage is indicated when lesions "point" (fluctuant). The wound may be packed (usually with iodoform gauze) to encourage further drainage. In severe cases, parenteral antibiotics such as cloxacillin (Tegopen), or a first-generation cephalosporin, such as cefazolin (Ancef), are required.

References, see page 372.

Psoriasis

Approximately 1 percent of the population is affected by psoriasis. The typical clinical findings of erythema and scaling are the result of hyperproliferation and abnormal differentiation of the epidermis, plus inflammatory cell infiltrates and vascular changes.

I. Clinical Manifestations

A. Plaque type psoriasis usually presents in young adults with symmetrically distributed plaques involving the scalp, extensor elbows, knees, and back. The plaques are erythematous with sharply defined, raised margins. A thick silvery scale is usually present. The lesions can range from less than 1 cm to more than 10 cm in diameter. The plaques typically are asymptomatic, although some patients complain of pruritus. Inspection may reveal pitting of the nail plates and involvement of intertriginous areas, such as the umbilicus and intergluteal cleft.

B. **Clinical course.** Most patients with psoriasis tend to have the disease for life. However, there may be marked variability in severity over time, and remissions at some stage are seen in 25 percent of cases. Pruritus may be severe and arthritis can be disabling.

C. **Diagnosis.** The diagnosis of psoriasis is made by physical examination and in some cases skin biopsy. The scalp, umbilicus, intergluteal cleft, and nails should be examined.

II. Treatment

A. **Topical emollients.** Keeping psoriatic skin soft and moist minimizes itching. The most effective are ointments such as petroleum jelly or thick creams.

B. **Topical corticosteroids**

1. Topical corticosteroids remain the mainstay of topical psoriasis treatment despite the development of newer agents.

2. In the scalp, potent steroids in an alcohol solution (eg, fluocinonide 0.05 percent) are frequently indicated. On the face and intertriginous areas, a low-potency cream (eg, hydrocortisone 1 percent) should be used.

3. For thick plaques on extensor surfaces, potent steroid ointments (eg, betamethasone 0.05 percent) with added occlusion by tape or plastic wrap may be required.

4. The typical regimen consists of twice-daily application of topical corticosteroids. Generics include, in order of increasing potency, hydrocortisone (Hytone) 1 percent, triamcinolone (Aristocort) 0.1 percent, fluocinonide (Lidex) 0.05 percent, and betamethasone dipropionate (Diprosone) 0.05 percent.

5. Betamethasone valerate in a foam (Luxiq) has superior efficacy for scalp psoriasis.

Types of Psoriasis, Associated Findings and Treatment Options			
Type of psoriasis	Clinical features	Differential diagnosis	Treatment options
Plaque-type psoriasis	Red, thick, scaly lesions with silvery scale	Atopic dermatitis, irritant dermatitis, cutaneous T-cell lymphoma, pityriasis rubra pilaris, seborrheic dermatitis	Localized: topical therapy with corticosteroids, calcipotriene (Dovonex), coal tars, anthralin (Anthra-Derm) or tazarotene (Tazorac). Generalized: phototherapy, systemic agents, combination therapy

Type of psoriasis	Clinical features	Differential diagnosis	Treatment options
Guttate psoriasis	Teardrop-shaped, pink to salmon, scaly plaques; usually on the trunk, with sparing of palms and soles	Pityriasis rosea, secondary syphilis, drug eruption	Ultraviolet B phototherapy, natural sunlight
Pustular psoriasis, localized	Erythematous papules or plaques studded with pustules; usually on palms or soles (palmoplantar pustular psoriasis)	Pustular drug eruption, dyshidrotic eczema, subcorneal pustular dermatosis	Same as for plaque-type psoriasis
Pustular psoriasis, generalized	Same as localized with a more general involvement; may be associated with systemic symptoms such as fever, malaise and diarrhea	Pustular drug eruption, subcorneal pustular dermatosis	Systemic therapy and/or hospitalization usually required
Erythrodermic psoriasis	Severe, intense, generalized erythema and scaling covering entire body; often associated with systemic symptoms; may or may not have had preexisting psoriasis	Drug eruption, eczematous dermatitis, mycosis fungoides, pityriasis rubra pilaris	Systemic therapy and/or hospitalization usually required

C. Calcipotriol

1. Calcipotriol (Dovonex) has become an established therapy in psoriasis. Calcipotriol affects the growth of keratinocytes via its action at the level of vitamin D receptors. Calcipotriol is at least as effective as potent topical corticosteroids. Skin irritation is the main adverse effect. Topical calcipotriol may be used as an alternative to topical steroid therapy. Twice-daily application is indicated. Other than skin irritation, side effects are usually minimal; the risk of hypercalcemia is low. However, topical calcipotriol is more expensive than potent steroids.

2. **Tazarotene (Tazorac)** is a topical retinoid that appears to be safe and effective for the treatment of mild to moderate plaque psoriasis. Once-daily administration of tazarotene gel, 0.05 or 0.1 percent, compared favorably with topical fluocinonide.

D. Methotrexate

1. Methotrexate is usually administered in an intermittent low-dose regimen, such as once weekly. Administration can be oral, intravenous, intramuscular, or subcutaneous; the usual dose range is between 7.5 mg and 25 mg per week.

2. Folic acid, 1 mg daily, protects against some of the common side effects seen with low-dose MTX such as stomatitis. Monitoring for bone marrow suppression and hepatotoxicity are necessary.

E. **Retinoids.** Systemic retinoids (derivatives of Vitamin A) are indicated in patients with severe psoriasis. The retinoid of choice in psoriasis is acitretin (Soriatane). The usual dose of acitretin is 50 mg daily. Monitoring for hypertriglyceridemia and hepatotoxicity are required with retinoid therapy. Side effects include cheilitis and alopecia. Acitretin is teratogenic and is only indicated in men and in women of nonreproductive potential.

F. **Cyclosporine** is effective in patients with severe psoriasis. Usual doses are in the range of 3 to 5 mg/kg per day orally. Improvement is generally observed within four weeks. Renal toxicity and hypertension are common.

G. **Alefacept (Amevive)**, the first biologic agent for treatment of psoriasis, is fairly effective in moderate to severe disease. Alefacept must be given parenterally (once a week).

References, see page 372.

Allergic Rhinitis

Allergic rhinitis is characterized by paroxysms of sneezing, rhinorrhea, nasal obstruction, and itching of the eyes, nose, and palate. It is also frequently associated with postnasal drip, cough, irritability, and fatigue. Allergic rhinitis is classified as seasonal if symptoms occur at a particular time of the year, or perennial if symptoms occur year round.

I. **Pathophysiology**
   A. Common allergens causing seasonal allergic rhinitis are tree, grass, and weed pollens, and fungi. Dust mites, cockroaches, animal proteins, and fungi are frequently associated with perennial rhinitis.
   B. Perennial allergic rhinitis is associated with nasal symptoms, which occur for more than nine months of the year. Perennial allergic rhinitis usually reflects allergy to indoor allergens like dust mites, cockroaches, or animal dander.
   C. Nine to 40 percent of the population may have some form of allergic rhinitis. The prevalence of allergic rhinitis has a bimodal peak in the early school and early adult years, and declines thereafter.

II. **Clinical manifestations**
   A. The intense nasal itching that occurs in allergic rhinitis is associated with nose rubbing, pushing the tip of the nose up with the hand (the "allergic salute"), and a transverse nasal crease.
   B. Adults and older children frequently have clear mucus. Young children have persistent rhinorrhea and often snort, sniff, cough, and clear their throats. Mouth breathing is common. Allergic rhinitis occurs in association with sinusitis, asthma, eczema and allergic conjunctivitis.

III. **Evaluation**
   A. **Nasal examination.** The nasal mucosa frequently displays a pale bluish hue or pallor along with turbinate edema. In nonallergic or vasomotor rhinitis, the nasal turbinates are erythematous and boggy.
   B. **Identification of allergens.** For patients in whom symptoms are not well controlled with medications and in whom the cause of rhinitis is not evident from the history, skin testing may provide an in vivo assessment of IgE antibodies.
   C. **Skin tests.** Immediate hypersensitivity skin testing is a quick, inexpensive, and safe way to identify the presence of allergen specific IgE.

IV. **Management of allergic rhinitis (rhinosinusitis)**
   A. **Allergen identification and avoidance.** The history frequently identifies involvement of pollens, molds, house dust mites and insects, such as fleas and cockroaches, or animal allergens

B. Allergen avoidance measures:
1. Maintaining the relative humidity at 50 percent or less to limit house dust mite and mold growth and avoiding exposure to irritants, such as cigarette smoke.
2. Air conditioners decrease concentrations of pollen, mold, and dust mite allergens in indoor air.
3. Avoiding exposure to the feces of the house dust mite is facilitated by removing carpets and furry pets, and washing bedding in hot water once weekly.
4. HEPA filters may help reduce animal allergens. Ordinary vacuuming and dusting have little effect.

C. Pharmacologic treatment
1. Nasal decongestant sprays are not recommended in the treatment of allergic rhinitis. Tachyphylaxis develops after three to seven days, rebound nasal congestion results, and continued use causes rhinitis medicamentosa.
2. **Intranasal corticosteroids.** Topical intranasal steroid therapy is presently the most effective single maintenance therapy for allergic rhinitis and causes few side effects. Topical nasal steroids are more effective than cromolyn and second generation antihistamines. Most studies show no effect on growth at recommended doses.
   a. The addition of antihistamine or antihistamine-decongestant combination to nasal corticosteroids offers little additional clinical benefit.
   b. Topical nasal steroids are available in both aqueous and freon-propelled preparations. The aqueous preparations may be particularly useful in patients in whom freon preparations cause mucosal drying, crusting, or epistaxis. Rarely, nasal steroids are associated with nasal septal perforation.
   c. As needed use appears to be almost as effective as daily use in patients with episodic symptoms.
   d. The preparations requiring once-daily dosing are preferred. These include triamcinolone, budesonide, fluticasone, or mometasone. Mometasone is approved for use in children older than two years. For children, mometasone (Nasonex) is the preferred as first-line therapy. Budesonide and fluticasone propionate are approved for use in children older than six years.

Drugs for Allergic Rhinitis		
Drug	**Trade name**	**Dose**
Corticosteroid Nasal Sprays		
Triamcinolone	Nasacort	Two sprays qd
Budesonide	Rhinocort AQ	Two sprays qd
Fluticasone	Flonase	Two sprays qd
Mometasone	Nasonex	Two sprays qd
Beclomethasone	Beconase Vancenase Beconase AQ Vancenase AQ	One spray two to qid One spray bid-qid One to two sprays bid One to two sprays bid
Flunisolide	Nasalide	Two sprays bid

Drug	Trade name	Dose
Oral H$_1$-receptor Blockers		
Citrizine	Zyrtec Zyrtec-D	5 or 10 mg once/d Cetirizine 5 mg, pseudoephedrine 120 mg; 1 tablet bid
Desloratadine	Clarinex	5 mg once/d
Fexofenadine	Allegra	60 mg bid or 180 mg once/d
Loratadine	Claritin Claritin Reditabs Alavert Claritin-D	10 mg once/d Loratadine 5 mg, pseudoephedrine 120 m; 1 tab qAM
Leukotriene Modifier		
Montelukast	Singulair	10 mg once/d

D. Antihistamines

1. Antihistamines are clearly less effective than topical nasal steroids. Antihistamines typically reduce itching, sneezing, and rhinorrhea, but may not completely eliminate the symptoms of nasal congestion.

2. Two second-generation antihistamines are currently available in syrup for young children. Cetirizine (Zyrtec) is approved for children ≥6 months of age. Loratadine (Claritin) is approved for use in children >2 years of age and is available over the counter. Second-generation antihistamines and nasal corticosteroids are not approved for children under two and three years of age, respectively. Rondec (carbinoxamine maleate-pseudoephedrine) drops are approved for children one month and older.

3. In relieving symptoms, second-generation drugs are less efficacious than corticosteroids and equally or more efficacious than cromolyn. The addition of antihistamines to topical nasal steroids may be useful in patients with concomitant allergic conjunctivitis. Oral antihistamine combinations that contain the decongestant, pseudoephedrine, provide better symptom relief than that associated with antihistamine alone.

4. **Adverse effects.**
   a. First-generation antihistamines easily cross the blood brain barrier and cause sedation, making them relatively less desirable. Sedation occurs uncommonly with second-generation antihistamines other than cetirizine and azelastine.
   b. Metabolites of second-generation antihistamines, such as the metabolite of terfenadine, fexofenadine (Allegra), and desloratadine (Clarinex) are classified as "third-generation antihistamines." These compounds avoid potential cardiotoxic effects of the second-generation compounds.
   c. Cetirizine, fexofenadine, desloratadine, and loratadine have not been associated with QT prolongation. However, coadministration with P450-active drugs increases loratadine levels. In addition, licorice ingestion prolongs QT-intervals and may potentially have additive effects.

5. Second-generation antihistamines may be preferable in patients with mild symptoms, or those preferring pills over nose sprays, especially if allergic conjunctivitis is also present. Cetirizine (Zyrtec) is reserved for those who fail loratadine (Claritin) or fexofenadine (Allegra), as cetirizine has sedative properties.

E. **Cromolyn and nedocromil** decrease allergic inflammation by inhibiting mast cell mediator release. Cromolyn, but not nedocromil, is available in the United States. Cromolyn is less effective than topical nasal steroids.

F. **Allergen immunotherapy**

1. Allergen immunotherapy involves the subcutaneous administration of increasing doses of therapeutic vaccines of allergens.

2. **Efficacy.** Allergen immunotherapy to tree, grass and ragweed pollens, Alternaria mold and house dust mite is efficacious in allergic rhinitis. Immunotherapy should be considered in patients in whom pharmacotherapy and avoidance of allergens have failed to resolve symptoms.

References, see page 372.

Renal Disorders

Acute Renal Failure

Acute renal failure is defined as a sudden decrease in renal function sufficient to increase the concentration of nitrogenous wastes in the blood. It is characterized by an increasing BUN and creatinine.

I. **Clinical presentation of acute renal failure**
   A. **Oliguria** is a common indicator of acute renal failure, and it is marked by a decrease in urine output to less than 30 mL/h. Acute renal failure may be oliguric (<500 L/day) or nonoliguric (>30 mL/h). Anuria (<100 mL/day) does not usually occur in renal failure, and its presence suggests obstruction or a vascular cause.
   B. Acute renal failure may also be manifest by encephalopathy, volume overload, pericarditis, bleeding, anemia, hyperkalemia, hyperphosphatemia, hypocalcemia, and metabolic acidemia.

II. **Clinical causes of renal failure**
   A. **Prerenal insult**
      1. Prerenal insult is the most common cause of acute renal failure, accounting for 70% of cases. Prerenal failure is usually caused by reduced renal perfusion secondary to extracellular fluid loss (diarrhea, diuresis, GI hemorrhage) or secondary to extracellular fluid sequestration (pancreatitis, sepsis), inadequate cardiac output, renal vasoconstriction (sepsis, liver disease, drugs), or inadequate fluid intake or replacement.
      2. Most patients with prerenal azotemia have oliguria, a history of large fluid losses (vomiting, diarrhea, burns), and evidence of intravascular volume depletion (thirst, weight loss, orthostatic hypotension, tachycardia, flat neck veins, dry mucous membranes). Patients with congestive heart failure may have total body volume excess (distended neck veins, pulmonary and pedal edema) but still have compromised renal perfusion and prerenal azotemia because of diminished cardiac output.
      3. Causes of prerenal failure are usually reversible if recognized and treated early; otherwise, prolonged renal hypoperfusion can lead to acute tubular necrosis and permanent renal insufficiency.
   B. **Intrarenal insult**
      1. **Acute tubular necrosis (ATN)** is the most common intrinsic renal disease leading to ARF.
         a. **Prolonged renal hypoperfusion** is the most common cause of ATN.
         b. **Nephrotoxic agents** (aminoglycosides, heavy metals, radiocontrast media, ethylene glycol) represent exogenous nephrotoxins. ATN may also occur as a result of endogenous nephrotoxins, such as intratubular pigments (hemoglobinuria), intratubular proteins (myeloma), and intratubular crystals (uric acid).
      2. **Acute interstitial nephritis (AIN)** is an allergic reaction secondary to drugs (NSAIDs, β-lactams).
      3. **Arteriolar injury** occurs secondary to hypertension, vasculitis, microangiopathic disorders.
      4. **Glomerulonephritis** secondary to immunologically mediated inflammation may cause intrarenal damage.

C. **Postrenal insult** results from obstruction of urine flow. Postrenal insult is the least common cause of acute renal failure, accounting for 10%. Postrenal insult may be caused by obstruction secondary to prostate cancer, benign prostatic hypertrophy, or renal calculi. Postrenal insult may be caused by amyloidosis, uric acid crystals, multiple myeloma, methotrexate, or acyclovir.

III. **Clinical evaluation of acute renal failure**

A. **Initial evaluation** of renal failure should determine whether the cause is decreased renal perfusion, obstructed urine flow, or disorders of the renal parenchyma. Volume status (orthostatic pulse, blood pressure, fluid intake and output, daily weights, hemodynamic parameters), nephrotoxic medications, and pattern of urine output should be assessed.

B. **Prerenal azotemia** is likely when there is a history of heart failure or extracellular fluid volume loss or depletion.

C. **Postrenal azotemia** is suggested by a history of decreased size or force of the urine stream, anuria, flank pain, hematuria or pyuria, or cancer of the bladder, prostate or pelvis.

D. **Intrarenal insult** is suggested by a history of prolonged volume depletion (often post-surgical), pigmenturia, hemolysis, rhabdomyolysis, or nephrotoxins. Intrarenal insult is suggested by recent radiocontrast, aminoglycoside use, or vascular catheterization. Interstitial nephritis may be implicated by a history of medication rash, fever, or arthralgias.

E. **Chronic renal failure** is suggested by diabetes mellitus, normochromic normocytic anemia, hypercalcemia, and hyperphosphatemia.

IV. **Physical examination**

A. Cardiac output, volume status, bladder size, and systemic disease manifestations should be assessed.

B. **Prerenal azotemia** is suggested by impaired cardiac output (neck vein distention, pulmonary rales, pedal edema). Volume depletion is suggested by orthostatic blood pressure changes, weight loss, low urine output, or diuretic use.

C. **Flank, suprapubic, or abdominal masses** may indicate an obstructive cause.

D. **Skin rash** suggests drug-induced interstitial nephritis; palpable purpura suggests vasculitis; nonpalpable purpura suggests thrombotic thrombo cytopenic purpura or hemolytic-uremic syndrome.

E. **Bladder catheterization** is useful to rule out suspected bladder outlet obstruction. A residual volume of more than 100 mL suggests bladder outlet obstruction.

F. **Central venous monitoring** is used to measure cardiac output and left ventricular filling pressure if prerenal failure is suspected.

V. **Laboratory evaluation**

A. **Spot urine sodium concentration**

1. Spot urine sodium can help distinguish between prerenal azotemia and acute tubular necrosis.

2. Prerenal failure causes increased reabsorption of salt and water and will manifest as a low spot urine sodium concentration <20 mEq/L and a low fractional sodium excretion <1%, and a urine/plasma creatinine ration of >40. Fractional excretion of sodium (%) = ([urine sodium/plasma sodium] ÷ [urine creatinine/plasma creatinine] x 100).

3. If tubular necrosis is the cause, the spot urine concentration will be >40 mEq/L, and fractional excretion of sodium will be >1%.

B. **Urinalysis**
1. **Normal urine sediment** is a strong indicator of prerenal azotemia or may be an indicator of obstructive uropathy.
2. **Hematuria, pyuria, or crystals** may be associated with postrenal obstructive azotemia.
3. **Abundant cells, casts, or protein** suggests an intrarenal disorder.
4. **Red cells** alone may indicate vascular disorders. RBC casts and abundant protein suggest glomerular disease (glomerulonephritis).
5. **White cell casts and eosinophilic casts** indicate interstitial nephritis.
6. **Renal epithelial cell casts and pigmented granular casts** are associated with acute tubular necrosis.
C. **Ultrasound** is useful for evaluation of suspected postrenal obstruction (nephrolithiasis). The presence of small (<10 cm in length), scarred kidneys is diagnostic of chronic renal insufficiency.

VI. **Management of acute renal failure**
A. Reversible disorders, such as obstruction, should be excluded, and hypovolemia should be corrected with volume replacement. Cardiac output should be maintained. In critically ill patients, a pulmonary artery catheter should be used for evaluation and monitoring.
B. **Extracellular fluid volume expansion.** Infusion of a 1-2 liter crystalloid fluid bolus may confirm suspected volume depletion.
C. If the patient remains oliguric despite euvolemia, IV diuretics may be administered. A large single dose of furosemide (100-200 mg) may be administered intravenously to promote diuresis. If urine flow is not improved, the dose of furosemide may be doubled. Furosemide may be repeated in 2 hours, or a continuous IV infusion of 10-40 mg/hr (max 1000 mg/day) may be used.
D. The dosage or dosing intervals of renally excreted drugs should be modified.
E. **Hyperkalemia** is the most immediately life-threatening complication of renal failure. Serum potassium values greater than 6.5 mEq/L may lead to arrhythmias and cardiac arrest. Potassium should be removed from IV solutions. Hyperkalemia may be treated with sodium polystyrene sulfonate (Kayexalate), 30-60 gm PO/PR every 4-6 hours.
F. **Hyperphosphatemia** can be controlled with aluminum hydroxide antacids (eg, Amphojel or Basaljel), 15-30 ml or one to three capsules PO with meals, should be used.
G. **Fluids.** After normal volume has been restored, fluid intake should be reduced to an amount equal to urinary and other losses plus insensible losses of 300-500 mL/day. In oliguric patients, daily fluid intake may need to be restricted to less than 1 L.
H. **Nutritional therapy.** A renal diet consisting of daily high biologic value protein intake of 0.5 gm/kg/d, sodium 2 g, potassium 40-60 mg/day, and at least 35 kcal/kg of nonprotein calories is recommended. Phosphorus should be restricted to 800 mg/day
I. **Dialysis.** Indications for dialysis include uremic pericarditis, severe hyperkalemia, pulmonary edema, persistent severe metabolic acidosis (pH less than 7.2), and symptomatic uremia.

References, see page 372.

Hematuria

Hematuria may be a sign of urinary tract malignancy or renal parenchymal disease. Up to 18% of normal persons excrete red blood cells into the urine, averaging 2 RBCs per high-power field (HPF).

I. **Clinical evaluation of hematuria**
   A. Dipstick testing detects hemoglobin and myoglobin; therefore, microscopic examination of the urinary sediment is required before a diagnosis of hematuria can be made.
   B. The patient should be asked about frequency, dysuria, pain, colic, fever, fatigue, anorexia, abdominal, flank, or perineal pain. Exercise, jogging, menstruation, or a history of kidney stones should be sought.
   C. The patient should be examined for hypertension, edema, rash, heart murmurs, or abdominal masses (renal tumor, hydronephrosis from obstruction). Costovertebral-angle tenderness may be a sign of renal calculus or pyelonephritis.
   D. Genitourinary examination may reveal a foreign body in the penile urethra or cervical carcinoma invading the urinary tract. Prostatitis, carcinoma, or benign prostatic hyperplasia may be found.

II. **Laboratory evaluation**
   A. At least one of the following criteria should be met before initiating a workup for hematuria.
      1. More than 3 RBCs/HPF on two of three properly collected clean-catch specimens (abstain from exercise for 48 hours before sampling; not during menses).
      2. One episode of gross hematuria.
      3. One episode of high-grade microhematuria (>100 RBCs HPF).
   B. A properly collected, freshly voided specimen should be examined for red blood cell morphology; the character of the sediment and the presence of proteinuria should be determined.
   C. RBC casts are pathognomonic of glomerulonephritis. WBC casts and granular casts are indicative of pyelonephritis.
   D. Urine culture should be completed to rule out urinary tract infection, which may cause hematuria.
   E. Serum blood urea nitrogen and creatinine levels should be evaluated to rule out renal failure. Impaired renal function is seen more commonly with medical causes of hematuria.
   F. Fasting blood glucose levels should be obtained to rule out diabetes; a complete blood count should be obtained to assess severity of blood loss.
   G. Serum coagulation parameters should be measured to screen for coagulopathy. A skin test for tuberculosis should be completed if risk factors are present. A sickle cell prep is recommended for all African-American patients.

III. **Classification of hematuria**
   A. **Medical hematuria** is caused by a glomerular lesion. Plasma proteins are present in the urine out of proportion to the amount of hematuria. Medical hematuria is characterized by glomerular RBCs, which are distorted with crenated membranes and an uneven hemoglobin distribution. Microscopic hematuria and a urine dipstick test of 2+ protein is more likely to have a medical cause.
   B. **Urologic hematuria** is caused by urologic lesions, such as urolithiasis or bladder cancer. It is characterized by minimal proteinuria. Non-glomerular RBCs (disk shaped) and an absence of casts are characteristic.

IV. **Diagnostic evaluation of medical hematuria**
   A. **Renal ultrasound** is used to evaluate kidney size and rule out hydronephrosis or cystic disease.
   B. **24-hour urine.** Creatinine, creatinine clearance and protein should be measured to assess renal failure.
   C. **Immunologic studies** that may suggest a diagnosis include third and fourth complement components, antinuclear antibodies, cryoglobulins, anti-base-

ment membrane antibodies; serum and urine protein electrophoresis (to rule out IgA nephropathy).
  D. **Audiogram** should be obtained if there is a family history of Alport syndrome.
  E. **Skin biopsy** can reveal dermal capillary deposits of IgA in 80% of patients with Berger's disease (IgA nephropathy), which is the most common cause of microhematuria in young adults.

V. **Diagnostic evaluation of urologic hematuria**
  A. **Intravenous pyelography** is the best screening test for upper tract lesions if the serum creatinine is normal. It is usually contraindicated in renal insufficiency. If renal insufficiency is present, renal ultrasound and cystoscopy with retrograde pyelogram should be used to search for stones or malignancy. If the IVP Is normal, cystoscopy with washings for cytology may reveal the cause of bleeding.
  B. **Other tests.** Lesions in the kidney visualized on IVP can be evaluated by renal ultrasound to assess cystic or solid character. CT-guided aspiration of cysts may be considered. Filling defects in the ureter should be evaluated by retrograde pyelogram and ureteral washings.

VI. **Idiopathic hematuria**
  A. Idiopathic hematuria is a diagnosis of exclusion. Five to 10% of patients with significant hematuria will have no diagnosis. Suspected urologic hematuria with a negative initial workup should be followed every 6-12 months with a urinalysis and urine cytology. An IVP should be done every 2-3 years.
  B. Renal function and proteinuria should be monitored. If renal function declines or if proteinuria exceeds 1 gm/day, renal biopsy is indicated.

References, see page 372.

Hyperkalemia

Body potassium is 98% intracellular. Only 2% of total body potassium, about 70 mEq, is in the extracellular fluid, with the normal concentration of 3.5-5 mEq/L.

I. **Pathophysiology of potassium homeostasis**
  A. The normal upper limit of plasma K is 5-5.5 mEq/L, with a mean K level of 4.3.
  B. **External potassium balance.** Normal dietary K intake is 1-1.5 mEq/kg in the form of vegetables and meats. The kidney is the primary organ for preserving external K balance, excreting 90% of the daily K burden.
  C. **Internal potassium balance.** Potassium transfer to and from tissues, is affected by insulin, acid-base status, catecholamines, aldosterone, plasma osmolality, cellular necrosis, and glucagon.

II. **Clinical disorders of external potassium balance**
  A. **Chronic renal failure.** The kidney is able to excrete the dietary intake of potassium until the glomerular filtration rate falls below 10 cc/minute or until urine output falls below 1 L/day. Renal failure is advanced before hyperkalemia occurs.
  B. **Impaired renal tubular function.** Renal diseases may cause hyperkalemia, and the renal tubular acidosis caused by these conditions may worsen hyperkalemia.
  C. **Primary adrenal insufficiency (Addison's disease)** is now a rare cause of hyperkalemia. Diagnosis is indicated by the combination of hyperkalemia and hyponatremia and is confirmed by a low aldosterone and a low plasma cortisol level that does not respond to adrenocorticotropic hormone treatment.
  D. **Drugs** that may cause hyperkalemia include nonsteroidal anti-inflammatory drugs, angiotensin-converting enzyme inhibitors, cyclosporine, and potassium-sparing diuretics. Hyperkalemia is especially common when these drugs are

given to patients at risk for hyperkalemia (diabetics, renal failure, advanced age).

E. **Excessive potassium intake**
1. Long-term potassium supplementation results in hyperkalemia most often when an underlying impairment in renal excretion already exists.
2. Intravenous administration of 0.5 mEq/kg over 1 hour increases serum levels by 0.6 mEq/L. Hyperkalemia often results when infusions of greater than 40 mEq/hour are given.

III. **Clinical disorders of internal potassium balance**
A. **Diabetic patients** are at particular risk for severe hyperkalemia because of renal insufficiency and hyporeninemic hypoaldosteronism.
B. **Systemic acidosis** reduces renal excretion of potassium and moves potassium out of cells, resulting in hyperkalemia.
C. **Endogenous potassium release** from muscle injury, tumor lysis, or chemotherapy may elevate serum potassium.

IV. **Manifestations of hyperkalemia**
A. Hyperkalemia, unless severe, is usually asymptomatic. The effect of hyperkalemia on the heart becomes significant above 6 mEq/L. As levels increase, the initial ECG change is tall peaked T waves. The QT interval is normal or diminished.
B. As K levels rise further, the PR interval becomes prolonged, then the P wave amplitude decreases. The QRS complex eventually widens into a sine wave pattern, with subsequent cardiac standstill.
C. At serum K is >7 mEq/L, muscle weakness may lead to a flaccid paralysis. Sensory abnormalities, impaired speech and respiratory arrest may follow.

V. **Pseudohyperkalemia**
A. Potassium may be falsely elevated by hemolysis during phlebotomy, when K is released from ischemic muscle distal to a tourniquet, and because of erythrocyte fragility disorders.
B. Falsely high laboratory measurement of serum potassium may occur with markedly elevated platelet counts (>10^6 platelet/mm^3) or white blood cell counts (>50,000/mm^3).

VI. **Diagnostic approach to hyperkalemia**
A. The serum K level should be repeat tested to rule out laboratory error. If significant thrombocytosis or leukocytosis is present, a plasma potassium level should be determined.
B. The 24-hour urine output, urinary K excretion, blood urea nitrogen, and serum creatinine should be measured. Renal K retention is diagnosed when urinary K excretion is less than 20 mEq/day.
C. High urinary K, excretion of >20 mEq/day, is indicative of excessive K intake as the cause.

VII. **Renal hyperkalemia**
A. If urinary K excretion is low and urine output is in the oliguric range, and creatinine clearance is lower than 20 cc/minute, renal failure is the probable cause. Prerenal azotemia resulting from volume depletion must be ruled out because the hyperkalemia will respond to volume restoration.
B. When urinary K excretion is low, yet blood urea nitrogen and creatinine levels are not elevated and urine volume is at least 1 L daily and renal sodium excretion is adequate (about 20 mEq/day), then either a defect in the secretion of renin or aldosterone or tubular resistance to aldosterone is likely. Low plasma renin and aldosterone levels, will confirm the diagnosis of hyporeninemic hypoaldosteronism. Addison's disease is suggested by a low serum cortisol, and the diagnosis is confirmed with a ACTH (Cortrosyn) stimulation test.

C. When inadequate K excretion is not caused by hypoaldosteronism, a tubular defect in K clearance is suggested. Urinary tract obstruction, renal transplant, lupus, or a medication should be considered.

VIII. **Extrarenal hyperkalemia**

A. When hyperkalemia occurs along with high urinary K excretion of >20 mEq/day, excessive intake of K is the cause. Potassium excess in IV fluids, diet, or medication should be sought. A concomitant underlying renal defect in K excretion is also likely to be present.

B. Blood sugar should be measured to rule out insulin deficiency; blood pH and serum bicarbonate should be measured to rule out acidosis.

C. Endogenous sources of K, such as tissue necrosis, hypercatabolism, hematoma, gastrointestinal bleeding, or intravascular hemolysis should be excluded.

IX. **Management of hyperkalemia**

A. **Acute treatment of hyperkalemia**

1. **Calcium**

a. If the electrocardiogram shows loss of P waves or widening of QRS complexes, calcium should be given IV; calcium reduces the cell membrane threshold potential.

b. Calcium chloride (10%) 2-3 g should be given over 5 minutes. In patients with circulatory compromise, 1 g of calcium chloride IV should be given over 3 minutes.

c. If the serum K level is greater than 7 mEq/L, calcium should be given. If digitalis intoxication is suspected, calcium must be given cautiously. Coexisting hyponatremia should be treated with hypertonic saline.

2. **Insulin:** If the only ECG abnormalities are peaked T waves and the serum level is under 7 mEq/L, treatment should begin with insulin (regular insulin, 5-10 U by IV push) with 50% dextrose water (D50W) 50 mL IV push. Repeated insulin doses of 10 U and glucose can be given every 15 minutes for maximal effect.

3. **Sodium bicarbonate** promotes cellular uptake of K. It should be given as 1-2 vials (50-mEq/vials) IV push.

4. **Potassium elimination measures**

a. Sodium polystyrene sulfonate (Kayexalate) is a cation exchange resin which binds to potassium in the lower GI tract. Dosage is 30-60 gm premixed with sorbitol 20% PO/PR.

b. Furosemide (Lasix) 100 mg IV should be given to promote kaliuresis.

c. Emergent hemodialysis for hyperkalemia is rarely necessary except when refractory metabolic acidosis is present.

References, see page 372.

Hypokalemia

Hypokalemia is characterized by a serum potassium concentration of less than 3.5 mEq/L. Ninety-eight percent of K is intracellular.

I. **Pathophysiology of hypokalemia**

A. **Cellular redistribution of potassium.** Hypokalemia may result from the intracellular shift of potassium by insulin, beta-2 agonist drugs, stress induced catecholamine release, thyrotoxic periodic paralysis, and alkalosis-induced shift (metabolic or respiratory).

B. **Nonrenal potassium loss**
  1. Gastrointestinal loss can be caused by diarrhea, laxative abuse, villous adenoma, biliary drainage, enteric fistula, clay ingestion, potassium binding resin ingestion, or nasogastric suction.
  2. Sweating, prolonged low-potassium diet, hemodialysis and peritoneal dialysis may also cause nonrenal potassium loss.

C. **Renal potassium loss**
  1. **Hypertensive high renin states.** Malignant hypertension, renal artery stenosis, renin-producing tumors.
  2. **Hypertensive low renin, high aldosterone states.** Primary hyperaldosteronism (adenoma or hyperplasia).
  3. **Hypertensive low renin, low aldosterone states.** Congenital adrenal hyperplasia (11 or 17 hydroxylase deficiency), Cushing's syndrome or disease, exogenous mineralocorticoids (Florinef, licorice, chewing tobacco), Liddle's syndrome.
  4. **Normotensive states**
     a. **Metabolic acidosis.** Renal tubular acidosis (type I or II)
     b. **Metabolic alkalosis (urine chloride <10 mEq/day).** Vomiting
     c. **Metabolic alkalosis (urine chloride >10 mEq/day).** Bartter's syndrome, diuretics, magnesium depletion, normotensive hyperaldosteronism
  5. **Drugs** associated with potassium loss include amphotericin B, ticarcillin, piperacillin, and loop diuretics.

II. **Clinical effects of hypokalemia**
  A. **Cardiac effects.** The most lethal consequence of hypokalemia is cardiac arrhythmia. Electrocardiographic effects include a depressed ST segment, decreased T-wave amplitude, U waves, and a prolonged QT-U interval.
  B. **Musculoskeletal effects.** The initial manifestation of K depletion is muscle weakness, which can lead to paralysis. In severe cases, respiratory muscle paralysis may occur.
  C. **Gastrointestinal effects.** Nausea, vomiting, constipation, and paralytic ileus may develop.

III. **Diagnostic evaluation**
  A. The 24-hour urinary potassium excretion should be measured. If >20 mEq/day, excessive urinary K loss is the cause. If <20 mEq/d, low K intake, or non-urinary K loss is the cause.
  B. In patients with excessive renal K loss and hypertension, plasma renin and aldosterone should be measured to differentiate adrenal from non-adrenal causes of hyperaldosteronism.
  C. If hypertension is absent and serum pH is acidotic, renal tubular acidosis should be considered. If hypertension is absent and serum pH is normal to alkalotic, a high urine chloride (>10 mEq/d) suggests hypokalemia secondary to diuretics or Bartter's syndrome. A low urine chloride (<10 mEq/d) suggests vomiting.

IV. **Emergency treatment of hypokalemia**
  A. **Indications for urgent replacement.** Electrocardiographic abnormalities, myocardial infarction, hypoxia, digitalis intoxication, marked muscle weakness, or respiratory muscle paralysis.
  B. **Intravenous potassium therapy**
    1. Intravenous KCL is usually used unless concomitant hypophosphatemia is present, where potassium phosphate is indicated.
    2. The maximal rate of intravenous K replacement is 30 mEq/hour. The K concentration of IV fluids should be 80 mEq/L or less if given via a peripheral vein. Frequent monitoring of serum K and constant electrocardiographic monitoring is recommended when potassium levels are being replaced.

V. Non-emergent treatment of hypokalemia
A. Attempts should be made to normalize K levels if <3.5 mEq/L.
B. Oral supplementation is significantly safer than IV. Liquid formulations are preferred due to rapid oral absorption, compared to sustained release formulations, which are absorbed over several hours.
1. KCL elixir 20-40 mEq qd-tid PO after meals.
2. Micro-K, 10 mEq tabs, 2-3 tabs tid PO after meals (40-100 mEq/d).

References, see page 372.

Hypermagnesemia

Serum magnesium has a normal range of 0.8-1.2 mmol/L. Magnesium homeostasis is regulated by renal and gastrointestinal mechanisms. Hypermagnesemia is usually iatrogenic and is frequently seen in conjunction with renal insufficiency.

I. Clinical evaluation of hypermagnesemia
A. **Causes of hypermagnesemia**
1. **Renal.** Creatinine clearance <30 mL/minute.
2. **Nonrenal.** Excessive use of magnesium cathartics, especially with renal failure; iatrogenic overtreatment with magnesium sulfate.
B. **Cardiovascular manifestations of hypermagnesemia**
1. **Hypermagnesemia <10 mEq/L.** Delayed interventricular conduction, first-degree heart block, prolongation of the Q-T interval.
2. **Levels greater than 10 mEq/L.** Low-grade heart block progressing to complete heart block and asystole occurs at levels greater than 12.5 mmol/L (>6.25 mmol/L).
C. **Neuromuscular effects**
1. Hyporeflexia occurs at a magnesium level >4 mEq/L (>2 mmol/L); diminution of deep tendon reflexes is an early sign of magnesium toxicity.
2. Respiratory depression due to respiratory muscle paralysis, somnolence and coma occur at levels >13 mEq/L (6.5 mmol/L).
3. Hypermagnesemia should always be considered when these symptoms occur in patients with renal failure, in those receiving therapeutic magnesium, and in laxative abuse.

II. Treatment of hypermagnesemia
A. **Asymptomatic, hemodynamically stable patients.** Moderate hypermagnesemia can be managed by elimination of intake.
B. **Severe hypermagnesemia**
1. Furosemide 20-40 mg IV q3-4h should be given as needed. Saline diuresis should be initiated with 0.9% saline, infused at 120 cc/h to replace urine loss.
2. If ECG abnormalities (peaked T waves, loss of P waves, or widened QRS complexes) or if respiratory depression is present, IV calcium gluconate should be given as 1-3 ampules (10% solution, 1 gm per 10 mL amp), added to saline infusate. Calcium gluconate can be infused to reverse acute cardiovascular toxicity or respiratory failure as 15 mg/kg over a 4-hour period.
3. Parenteral insulin and glucose can be given to shift magnesium into cells. Dialysis is necessary for patients who have severe hypermagnesemia.

References, see page 372.

Hypomagnesemia

Magnesium deficiency occurs in up to 11% of hospitalized patients. The normal range of serum magnesium is 1.5 to 2.0 mEq/L, which is maintained by the kidney, intestine, and bone.

I. Pathophysiology

A. **Decreased magnesium intake.** Protein-calorie malnutrition, prolonged parenteral fluid administration, and catabolic illness are common causes of hypomagnesemia.

B. **Gastrointestinal losses of magnesium** may result from prolonged nasogastric suction, laxative abuse, and pancreatitis.

C. **Renal losses of magnesium**
1. Renal loss of magnesium may occur secondary to renal tubular acidosis, glomerulonephritis, interstitial nephritis, or acute tubular necrosis.
2. Hyperthyroidism, hypercalcemia, and hypophosphatemia may cause magnesium loss.
3. **Agents that enhance renal magnesium excretion** include alcohol, loop and thiazide diuretics, amphotericin B, aminoglycosides, cisplatin, and pentamidine.

D. **Alterations in magnesium distribution**
1. Redistribution of circulating magnesium occurs by extracellular to intracellular shifts, sequestration, hungry bone syndrome, or by acute administration of glucose, insulin, or amino acids.
2. Magnesium depletion can be caused by large quantities of parenteral fluids and pancreatitis-induced sequestration of magnesium.

II. Clinical manifestations of hypomagnesemia

A. **Neuromuscular findings** may include positive Chvostek's and Trousseau's signs, tremors, myoclonic jerks, seizures, and coma.

B. **Cardiovascular.** Ventricular tachycardia, ventricular fibrillation, atrial fibrillation, multifocal atrial tachycardia, ventricular ectopic beats, hypertension, enhancement of digoxin-induced dysrhythmias, and cardiomyopathies.

C. **ECG changes** include ventricular arrhythmias (extrasystoles, tachycardia) and atrial arrhythmias (atrial fibrillation, supraventricular tachycardia, torsades de Pointes). Prolonged PR and QT intervals, ST segment depression, T-wave inversions, wide QRS complexes, and tall T-waves may occur.

III. Clinical evaluation

A. Hypomagnesemia is diagnosed when the serum magnesium is less than 0.7-0.8 mmol/L. Symptoms of magnesium deficiency occur when the serum magnesium concentration is less than 0.5 mmol/L. A 24-hour urine collection for magnesium is the first step in the evaluation of hypomagnesemia. Hypomagnesia caused by renal magnesium loss is associated with magnesium excretion that exceeds 24 mg/day.

B. Low urinary magnesium excretion (<1 mmol/day), with concomitant serum hypomagnesemia, suggests magnesium deficiency due to decreased intake, nonrenal losses, or redistribution of magnesium.

IV. Treatment of hypomagnesemia

A. **Asymptomatic magnesium deficiency**
1. In hospitalized patients, the daily magnesium requirements can be provided through either a balanced diet, as oral magnesium supplements (0.36-0.46 mEq/kg/day), or 16-30 mEq/day in a parenteral nutrition formulation.
2. Magnesium oxide is better absorbed and less likely to cause diarrhea than magnesium sulfate. Magnesium oxide preparations include Mag-Ox 400 (240 mg elemental magnesium per 400 mg tablet), Uro-Mag (84 mg elemental

magnesium per 400 mg tablet), and magnesium chloride (Slo-Mag) 64 mg/tab, 1-2 tabs bid.

B. Symptomatic magnesium deficiency
1. Serum magnesium $\leq$0.5 mmol/L requires IV magnesium repletion with electrocardiographic and respiratory monitoring.
2. Magnesium sulfate 1-6 gm in 500 mL of D5W can be infused IV at 1 gm/hr. An additional 6-9 gm of $MgSO_4$ should be given by continuous infusion over the next 24 hours.

References, see page 372.

Disorders of Water and Sodium Balance

I. Pathophysiology of water and sodium balance
   A. Volitional intake of water is regulated by thirst. Maintenance intake of water is the amount of water sufficient to offset obligatory losses.
   B. Maintenance water needs
   = 100 mL/kg for first 10 kg of body weight
   + 50 mL/kg for next 10 kg
   + 20 mL/kg for weight greater than 20 kg
   C. Clinical signs of hyponatremia. Confusion, agitation, lethargy, seizures, and coma.
   D. Pseudohyponatremia
   1. Elevation of blood glucose may creates an osmotic gradient that pulls water from cells into the extracellular fluid, diluting the extracellular sodium. The contribution of hyperglycemia to hyponatremia can be estimated using the following formula:
   Expected change in serum sodium = (serum glucose - 100) x 0.016
   2. Marked elevation of plasma lipids or protein can also result in erroneous hyponatremia because of laboratory inaccuracy. The percentage of plasma water can be estimated with the following formula:
   % plasma water = 100 - [0.01 x lipids (mg/dL)] - [0.73 x protein (g/dL)]

II. Diagnostic evaluation of hyponatremia
   A. Pseudohyponatremia should be excluded by repeat testing. The cause of the hyponatremia should be determined based on history, physical exam, urine osmolality, serum osmolality, urine sodium and chloride. An assessment of volume status should determine if the patient is volume contracted, normal volume, or volume expanded.
   B. Classification of hyponatremic patients based on urine osmolality
   1. **Low-urine osmolality (50-180 mOsm/L)** indicates primary excessive water intake (psychogenic water drinking).
   2. **High-urine osmolality (urine osmolality >serum osmolality)**
      a. **High-urine sodium (>40 mEq/L) and volume contraction** indicates a renal source of sodium loss and fluid loss (excessive diuretic use, salt-wasting nephropathy, Addison's disease, osmotic diuresis).
      b. **High-urine sodium (>40 mEq/L) and normal volume** is most likely caused by water retention due to a drug effect, hypothyroidism, or the syndrome of inappropriate antidiuretic hormone secretion. In SIADH, the urine sodium level is usually high. SIADH is found in the presence of a malignant tumor or a disorder of the pulmonary or central nervous system.
      c. **Low-urine sodium (<20 mEq/L) and volume contraction,** dry mucous membranes, decreased skin turgor, and orthostatic hypotension indicate an extrarenal source of fluid loss (gastrointestinal disease, burns).

d. **Low-urine sodium (<20 mEq/L) and volume-expansion, and edema** is caused by congestive heart failure, cirrhosis with ascites, or nephrotic syndrome. Effective arterial blood volume is decreased. Decreased renal perfusion causes increased reabsorption of water.

Drugs Associated with SIADH

Acetaminophen	Isoproterenol
Barbiturates	Prostaglandin E$_1$
Carbamazepine	Meperidine
Chlorpropamide	Nicotine
Clofibrate	Tolbutamide
Cyclophosphamide	Vincristine
Indomethacin	

III. Treatment of water excess hyponatremia

A. Determine the volume of water excess

Water excess = total body water x ([140/measured sodium] -1)

B. Treatment of asymptomatic hyponatremia.
Water intake should be restricted to 1,000 mL/day. Food alone in the diet contains this much water, so no liquids should be consumed. If an intravenous solution is needed, an isotonic solution of 0.9% sodium chloride (normal saline) should be used. Dextrose should not be used in the infusion because the dextrose is metabolized into water.

C. Treatment of symptomatic hyponatremia

1. If neurologic symptoms of hyponatremia are present, the serum sodium level should be corrected with hypertonic saline. Excessively rapid correction of sodium may result in a syndrome of central pontine demyelination.
2. The serum sodium should be raised at a rate of 1 mEq/L per hour. If hyponatremia has been chronic, the rate should be limited to 0.5 mEq/L per hour. The goal of initial therapy is a serum sodium of 125-130 mEq/L, then water restriction should be continued until the level normalizes.
3. The amount of hypertonic saline needed is estimated using the following formula:

   Sodium needed (mEq) = 0.6 x wt in kg x (desired sodium - measured sodium)

4. Hypertonic 3% sodium chloride contains 513 mEq/L of sodium. The calculated volume required should be administered over the period required to raise the serum sodium level at a rate of 0.5-1 mEq/L per hour. Concomitant administration of furosemide may be required to lessen the risk of fluid overload.

IV. Hypernatremia

A. Clinical manifestations of hypernatremia:
Clinical manifestations include tremulousness, irritability, ataxia, spasticity, mental confusion, seizures, and coma.

B. Causes of hypernatremia

1. Net sodium gain or net water loss will cause hypernatremia
2. Failure to replace obligate water losses may cause hypernatremia, as in patients unable to obtain water because of an altered mental status or severe debilitating disease.
3. **Diabetes insipidus:** If urine volume is high but urine osmolality is low, diabetes insipidus is the most likely cause.

Drugs Associated with Diabetes Insipidus	
Ethanol	Glyburide
Phenytoin	Amphotericin B
Chlorpromazine	Colchicine
Lithium	Vinblastine

C. Diagnosis of hypernatremia

1. Assessment of urine volume and osmolality are essential in the evaluation of hyperosmolality. The usual renal response to hypernatremia is the excretion of the minimum volume (<500 mL/day) of maximally concentrated urine (urine osmolality >800 mOsm/kg). These findings suggest extrarenal water loss.
2. Diabetes insipidus generally presents with polyuria and hypotonic urine (urine osmolality <250 mOsm/kg).

V. Management of hypernatremia

A. If there is evidence of hemodynamic compromise (eg, orthostatic hypotension, marked oliguria), fluid deficits should be corrected initially with isotonic saline. Once hemodynamic stability is achieved, the remaining free water deficit should be corrected with 5% dextrose water or 0.45% NaCl.

B. The water deficit can be estimated using the following formula:

Water deficit = 0.6 x wt in kg x (1 - [140/measured sodium]).

C. The change in sodium concentration should not exceed 1 mEq/liter/hour. One-half of the calculated water deficit can be administered in the first 24 hours, followed by correction of the remaining deficit over the next 1-2 days. The serum sodium concentration and ECF volume status should be evaluated every 6 hours. Excessively rapid correction of hypernatremia may lead to lethargy and seizures secondary to cerebral edema.

D. Maintenance fluid needs from ongoing renal and insensible losses must also be provided. If the patient is conscious and able to drink, water should be given orally or by nasogastric tube.

E. **Treatment of diabetes insipidus**
1. **Vasopressin (Pitressin)** 5-10 U IV/SQ q6h; fast onset of action with short duration.
2. **Desmopressin (DDAVP)** 2-4 mcg IV/SQ q12h; slow onset of action with long duration of effect.

VI. Mixed disorders

A. **Water excess and saline deficit** occurs when severe vomiting and diarrhea occur in a patient who is given only water. Clinical signs of volume contraction and a low serum sodium are present. Saline deficit is replaced and free water intake restricted until the serum sodium level has normalized.

B. **Water and saline excess** often occurs with heart failure, manifesting as edema and a low serum sodium. An increase in the extracellular fluid volume, as evidenced by edema, is a saline excess. A marked excess of free water expands the extracellular fluid volume, causing apparent hyponatremia. However, the important derangement in edema is an excess of sodium. Sodium and water restriction and use of furosemide are usually indicated in addition to treatment of the underlying disorder.

C. **Water and saline deficit** is frequently caused by vomiting and high fever and is characterized by signs of volume contraction and an elevated serum sodium. Saline and free water should be replaced in addition to maintenance amounts of water.

References, see page 372.

Endocrinologic Disorders

Diabetic Ketoacidosis

Diabetic ketoacidosis is defined by hyperglycemia, metabolic acidosis, and ketosis.

I. **Clinical presentation**
   A. Diabetes is newly diagnosed in 20% of cases of diabetic ketoacidosis. In patients with known diabetes, precipitating factors include infection, noncompliance with insulin, myocardial infarction, and gastrointestinal bleeding.
   B. **Symptoms of DKA** include polyuria, polydipsia, fatigue, nausea, and vomiting, developing over 1 to 2 days. Abdominal pain is prominent in 25%.
   C. **Physical examination**
      1. Patients are typically flushed, tachycardic, tachypneic, and volume depleted with dry mucous membranes. Kussmaul's respiration (rapid, deep breathing and air hunger) occurs when the serum pH is between 7.0 and 7.24.
      2. **A fruity odor** on the breath indicates the presence of acetone, a byproduct of diabetic ketoacidosis.
      3. **Fever**, although seldom present, indicates infection. Eighty percent of patients with diabetic ketoacidosis have altered mental status. Most are awake but confused; 10% are comatose.
   D. **Laboratory findings**
      1. Serum glucose level >300 mg/dL
      2. pH <7.35, pCO_2 <40 mm Hg
      3. Bicarbonate level below normal with an elevated anion gap
      4. Presence of ketones in the serum

II. **Differential diagnosis**
   A. **Differential diagnosis of ketosis-causing conditions**
      1. **Alcoholic ketoacidosis** occurs with heavy drinking and vomiting. It does not cause an elevated glucose.
      2. **Starvation ketosis** occurs after 24 hours without food and is not usually confused with DKA because glucose and serum pH are normal.
   B. **Differential diagnosis of acidosis-causing conditions**
      1. **Metabolic acidoses** are divided into increased anion gap (>14 mEq/L) and normal anion gap; anion gap = sodium - (Cl- + HCO_3-).
      2. **Anion gap acidoses** can be caused by ketoacidoses, lactic acidosis, uremia, salicylate, methanol, ethanol, or ethylene glycol poisoning.
      3. **Non-anion gap acidoses** are associated with a normal glucose level and absent serum ketones. Causes of non-anion gap acidoses include renal or gastrointestinal bicarbonate loss.
   C. **Hyperglycemia caused by hyperosmolar nonketotic coma** occurs in patients with type 2 diabetes with severe hyperglycemia. Patients are usually elderly and have a precipitating illness. Glucose level is markedly elevated (>600 mg/dL), osmolarity is increased, and ketosis is minimal.

III. **Treatment of diabetic ketoacidosis**
   A. **Fluid resuscitation**
      1. Fluid deficits average 5 liters or 50 mL/kg. Resuscitation consists of 1 liter of normal saline over the first hour and a second liter over the second and third hours. Thereafter, 1/2 normal saline should be infused at 100-120 mL/hr.
      2. When the glucose level decreases to 250 mg/dL, 5% dextrose should be added to the replacement fluids to prevent hypoglycemia. If the glucose

level declines rapidly, 10% dextrose should be infused along with regular insulin until the anion gap normalizes.

B. Insulin

1. An initial loading dose consists of 0.1 U/kg IV bolus. Insulin is then infused at 0.1 U/kg per hour. The biologic half-life of IV insulin is less than 20 minutes. The insulin infusion should be adjusted each hour so that the glucose decline does not exceed 100 mg/dL per hour.

2. The insulin infusion rate may be decreased when the bicarbonate level is greater than 20 mEq/L, the anion gap is less than 16 mEq/L, or the glucose is <250 mg/dL.

C. Potassium

1. The most common preventable cause of death in patients with DKA is hypokalemia. The typical deficit is between 300 and 500 mEq.

2. Potassium chloride should be started when fluid therapy is started. In most patients, the initial rate of potassium replacement is 20 mEq/h, but hypokalemia requires more aggressive replacement (40 mEq/h).

3. All patients should receive potassium replacement, except for those with renal failure, no urine output, or an initial serum potassium level greater than 6.0 mEq/L.

D. Sodium. For every 100 mg/dL that glucose is elevated, the sodium level should be assumed to be higher than the measured value by 1.6 mEq/L.

E. Phosphate. Diabetic ketoacidosis depletes phosphate stores. Serum phosphate level should be checked after 4 hours of treatment. If it is below 1.5 mg/dL, potassium phosphate should be added to the IV solution in place of KCl.

F. Bicarbonate therapy is not required unless the arterial pH value is <7.0. For a pH of <7.0, add 50 mEq of sodium bicarbonate to the first liter of IV fluid.

G. Magnesium. The usual magnesium deficit is 2-3 gm. If the patient's magnesium level is less than 1.8 mEq/L or if tetany is present, magnesium sulfate is given as 5g in 500 mL of 0.45% normal saline over 5 hours.

H. Additional therapies

1. **A nasogastric tube** should be inserted in semiconscious patients to protect against aspiration.

2. **Deep vein thrombosis prophylaxis** with subcutaneous heparin should be provided for patients who are elderly, unconscious, or severely hyperosmolar (5,000 U every 12 hours).

IV. **Monitoring of therapy**

A. Serum bicarbonate level and anion gap should be monitored to determine the effectiveness of insulin therapy.

B. Glucose levels should be checked at 1-2 hour intervals during IV insulin administration.

C. Electrolyte levels should be assessed every 2 hours for the first 6-8 hours, and then q8h. Phosphorus and magnesium levels should be checked after 4 hours of treatment.

D. Plasma and urine ketones are helpful in diagnosing diabetic ketoacidosis, but are not necessary during therapy.

V. **Determining the underlying cause**

A. Infection is the underlying cause of diabetic ketoacidosis in 50% of cases. Infection of the urinary tract, respiratory tract, skin, sinuses, ears, or teeth should be sought. Fever is unusual in diabetic ketoacidosis and indicates infection when present. If infection is suspected, antibiotics should be promptly initiated.

B. Omission of insulin doses is often a precipitating factor. Myocardial infarction, ischemic stroke, and abdominal catastrophes may precipitate DKA.

VI. Initiation of subcutaneous insulin
   A. When the serum bicarbonate and anion gap levels are normal, subcutaneous regular insulin can be started.
   B. Intravenous and subcutaneous administration of insulin should overlap to avoid redevelopment of ketoacidosis. The intravenous infusion may be stopped 1 hour after the first subcutaneous injection of insulin.
   C. **Estimation of subcutaneous insulin requirements**
      1. Multiply the final insulin infusion rate times 24 hours. Two-thirds of the total dose is given in the morning as two-thirds NPH and one-third regular insulin. The remaining one-third of the total dose is given before supper as one-half NPH and one-half regular insulin.
      2. Subsequent doses should be adjusted according to the patient's blood glucose response.

References, see page 372.

Type 1 Diabetes Mellitus

Up to 4 percent of Americans have diabetes. The diagnosis of diabetes mellitus is easily established when a patient presents with classic symptoms of hyperglycemia (thirst, polyuria, weight loss, visual blurring), and has a fasting blood glucose concentration of 126 mg/dL or higher, or a random value of 200 mg/dL or higher, and confirmed on another occasion.

I. Definitions from the 2003 ADA report:
   Normal. Fasting plasma glucose (FPG) <100 mg/dL.
   Impaired fasting glucose (IFG). Fasting plasma glucose between 100 and 125 mg/dL.
   Diabetes mellitus. FPG at or above 126 mg/dL, a two-hour value in an OGTT (2-h PG) at or above 200 mg/dL, or a random plasma glucose concentration $\geq$ 200 mg/dL in the presence of symptoms. The diagnosis of diabetes must be confirmed on a subsequent day by measuring any one of the three criteria.

Routine Diabetes Care
History
Review physical activity, diet, self-monitored blood glucose readings, medications
Assess for symptoms of coronary heart disease
Evaluate smoking status, latest eye examination results, foot care
Physical examination
Weight
Blood pressure
Foot examination
Pulse
Sores or callus
Monofilament test for sensation
Insulin injection sites
Refer for dilated retinal examination annually
Laboratory studies
HbA1c every three to six months
Annual fasting lipid panel
Annual urine albumin/creatinine ratio
Annual serum creatinine

Goals of intensive diabetes treatment			
Premeal blood glucose level	Postprandial (ie, mealtime) glucose level	Bedtime glucose level	Hemoglobin A₁c (HbA₁c) level
90 to 130 mg/dL	120 to 180 mg/dL	110 to 150 mg/dL	Less than 6.5%

Pharmacokinetics of insulin preparations			
Insulin type	Onset of action	Time to peak effect	Duration of action
Lispro (Humalog) , aspart (Novolog), glulisine (Apidra)	5 to 15 min	45 to 75 min	2 to 4 h
Regular insulin	About 30 min	2 to 4 h	5 to 8 h
NPH	About 2 h	6 to 10 h	18 to 28 h
Insulin glargine (Lantus)	About 2 h	No peak	20 to >24 h
Insulin detemir (Levemir)	About 2 h	No peak	6 to 24 h

II. Insulin therapy in type 1 diabetes mellitus

A. The Diabetes Control and Complications Trial (DCCT) demonstrated that improved glycemic control with intensive insulin therapy in patients with type 1 diabetes mellitus led to graded reductions in retinopathy, nephropathy, and neuropathy. Intensive therapy is now considered to be standard therapy for management of type 1 diabetes.

B. The term "intensive insulin therapy" describes treatment with three or more injections per day or with continuous subcutaneous insulin infusion with an insulin pump.

C. Choice of insulin regimen. The basic requirements are a stable baseline dose of insulin (basal insulin) (whether an intermediate or long-acting insulin or given via continuous subcutaneous insulin infusion) plus adjustable doses of pre-meal short-acting insulin (regular) or rapid-acting insulin analogs (lispro, aspart, or glulisine).

Multiple daily insulin injection regimens				
Regimen	Breakfast	Lunch	Dinner	Bedtime
1	R + N		R	N
2	R	R	R	N
3	VRA	VRA	VRA	G
4	VRA + G	VRA	VRA	
5	VRA + G	VRA	VRA + G	
R: regular insulin; N: NPH insulin; VRA: any very-rapid-acting analog (lispro, aspart, or glulisine); G: glargine.				

D. Insulin glargine. The time-action profile for insulin glargine has virtually no peak, which makes it a good basal insulin preparation for intensive insulin therapy.

   1. The therapeutic advantage of insulin glargine over NPH is modest, with no real advantage with regard to A1C achieved. Lower fasting blood glucose and fewer hypoglycemic episodes occur when insulin glargine was substituted for once or twice daily NPH insulin, but A1C values have generally not been lower in studies comparing glargine and NPH-based regimens.

   2. Although many patients can achieve stable basal serum insulin concentrations with a single daily injection of insulin glargine given in the morning or evening this is not always the case. About 20 percent of patients with type 1 diabetes need twice-daily glargine.

E. Insulin detemir is the second available long-acting insulin analog. However, its duration of action appears to be substantially shorter than that of insulin glargine, though still longer than NPH. Like NPH, twice-daily injections appear to be necessary in patients with type 1 diabetes. Glycemic control appears to be similar with insulin detemir and NPH; however, insulin detemir may be associated with slightly less nocturnal hypoglycemia and weight gain. These modest advantages of insulin detemir may be offset by its higher cost.

F. Rapid-acting insulins (insulin lispro, aspart, and glulisine) have an onset of action within 5 to 15 minutes, peak action at 30 to 90 minutes, and a duration of action of two to four hours.

G. In patients with type 1 diabetes, rapid-acting insulin has the following advantages when compared to regular insulin:

   1. It decreases the postprandial rise in blood glucose concentration better than regular insulin.

   2. It may modestly reduce the frequency of hypoglycemia in patients with type 1 diabetes.

   3. It is more convenient because it can be injected immediately before meals, whereas regular insulin should be given 30 to 45 minutes before meals. In addition, the action of insulin lispro is not blunted by mixing with NPH insulin just before injection, as is the action of regular insulin.

H. Designing an MDI insulin regimen. Most newly diagnosed patients with type 1 diabetes can be started on a total daily dose of 0.2 to 0.4 units of insulin per kg per day, although most will ultimately require 0.6 to 0.7 units per kg per day. Adolescents, especially during puberty, often need more, but the dose can be adjusted upward every few days based upon blood glucose measurements.

I. In designing an MDI regimen, one-half of the total dose should be given as a basal insulin, either as once per day long-acting insulin (glargine or determir) or as twice per day intermediate-acting insulin (NPH). The long-acting insulin can be given either at bedtime or in the morning; the NPH is usually given as two-thirds of the dose in the morning and one-third at bedtime. The remainder of the total daily dose (TDD) is given as short or rapid-acting insulin, divided before meals. The pre-meal dosing is determined by the usual meal size and content. The sliding-scale that is constructed for premeal use usually takes into account the carbohydrate content and the blood glucose levels before the meal. Regimens that use NPH in the morning may not require a pre-lunch dose of short or rapid-acting insulin.

III. Other management issues

   A. Consistency. The content and timing of meals, the site of insulin injections, and the timing and frequency of exercise should be consistent.

   B. Blood glucose monitoring. Testing at home should to be done four to seven times daily (before breakfast, mid-morning, before lunch, mid-afternoon, before the evening meal, before bedtime, and occasionally at 3 AM). Additionally, it is useful to test blood glucose levels at intervals after certain meals and before, during and after exercise. Chronic glucose control should be monitored with periodic A1C (hemoglobin A1c or HbA1c) levels.

IV. **Screening for microvascular complications in diabetics**

A. **Retinopathy.** Diabetic retinopathy and macular degeneration are the leading causes of blindness in diabetes. Adults with diabetes should receive annual dilated retinal examinations beginning at the time of diagnosis.

B. **Nephropathy.** Diabetes-related nephropathy affects 40% of patients with type 1 disease and 10-20% of those with type 2 disease. Microalbumin may be tested annually by screening with either a specifically sensitive dipstick or a laboratory assay on a spot urine sample, to determine an albumin-to-creatinine ratio. Abnormal results should be repeated at least two or three times over a three to six month period. Screening can be deferred for five years after the onset of disease in patients with type 1 diabetes because microalbuminuria is uncommon before this time.

C. **Peripheral neuropathy** affects many patients with diabetes and causes nocturnal or constant pain, tingling and numbness. The feet should be evaluated regularly for sensation, pulses and sores.

D. **Autonomic neuropathy** is found in many patients with long-standing diabetes, resulting in diarrhea, constipation, gastroparesis, vomiting, orthostatic hypotension, and erectile or ejaculatory dysfunction.

References, see page 372.

Type 2 Diabetes Mellitus

I. **Degree of glycemic control**

A. Measurement of hemoglobin A1C (A1C) provides a better estimate of chronic glycemic control than measurements of fasting blood glucose. The Diabetes Control and Complications Trial (DCCT) demonstrated that achieving near normal blood glucose concentrations markedly reduces the risk of microvascular and neurologic complications in type 1 diabetes.

B. The goal of therapy should be an A1C value of 7.0 percent or less. The goal should be set somewhat higher for older patients. In order to achieve the A1C goal, the glucose goals below are usually necessary:
1. Fasting glucose 70 to 130 mg/dL
2. Postprandial glucose (90 to 120 minutes after a meal) <180 mg/dL

C. Cardiovascular risk factor reduction (smoking cessation, aspirin, blood pressure, reduction in serum lipids, diet, exercise, and, in high-risk patients, an angiotensin converting enzyme inhibitor) should be accomplished for all patients with type 2 diabetes.

II. **Nonpharmacologic treatment**

A. Diet modification can improve obesity, hypertension, and insulin release and responsiveness.

B. Regular exercise leads to improved glycemic control due to increased responsiveness to insulin; it can also delay the progression of impaired glucose tolerance to overt diabetes.

III. **Medications for initial therapy**

A. Sulfonylureas and meglitinides increase insulin release.

B. Biguanides (metformin) and thiazolidinedione increase insulin responsiveness.

C. Alpha-glucosidase inhibitors reduce intestinal absorption of carbohydrate and lipase inhibitors reduce the absorption of fat.

D. **Biguanides.** Metformin (Glucophage) often leads to modest weight reduction and is a reasonable first choice for oral treatment of type 2 diabetes.

1. **Metformin (Glucophage)** is available as 500 and 850 mg tablets, which should be taken with meals; extended release formulations may be convenient once the dose is adjusted. Metformin should not be given to elderly (>80 years) patients unless renal sufficiency is proven with a direct measure of GFR, or to patients who have renal, hepatic or cardiac disease or drink excess alcohol. Patients who are about to receive intravenous iodinated contrast material (with potential for contrast-induced renal failure) or undergo a surgical procedure (with potential compromise of circulation) should have metformin held.

2. Initial dosage is 500 mg once daily with the evening meal and, if tolerated, a second 500 mg dose is added with breakfast. The dose can be increased slowly (one tablet every one to two weeks). The usual maximum effective dose is 850 mg twice per day.

Contraindications to metformin therapy

Renal dysfunction
  Serum creatinine level ≥1.5 mg/dL in men, ≥1.4 mg/dL in women
  Metformin should be temporarily discontinued in patients undergoing radiologic studies involving intravascular administration of iodinated contrast materials. Treatment may be restarted 48 hours after the procedure when normal renal function is documented.
  Treatment should be carefully initiated in patients ≥80 years of age after measurement of creatinine clearance demonstrates that renal function is not reduced.
Congestive heart failure that requires pharmacologic therapy
Hepatic dysfunction
Dehydration
Acute or chronic metabolic acidosis (diabetic ketoacidosis)
Known hypersensitivity to metformin

E. **Sulfonylureas** are moderately effective, lowering blood glucose concentrations by 20 percent and A1C by 1 to 2 percent. Their effectiveness decreases over time.
   1. The choice of sulfonylurea is primarily dependent upon cost, since the efficacy of the available drugs is similar.
F. **Meglitinides.** Repaglinide (Prandin) and nateglinide (Starlix) are short-acting glucose-lowering drugs that act similarly to the sulfonylureas and have similar or slightly less efficacy in decreasing glycemia. Meglitinides may be used in patients who have allergy to sulfonylureas. However, they are considerably more expensive than sulfonylureas, and have no therapeutic advantage.
   1. **Nateglinide (Starlix)** is hepatically metabolized, with renal excretion of active metabolites. With decreased renal function, the accumulation of active metabolites and hypoglycemia has occurred. Repaglinide is principally metabolized by the liver, with less than 10 percent renally excreted.
G. **Thiazolidinediones,** rosiglitazone (Avandia) and pioglitazone (Actos), lower blood glucose concentrations by increasing insulin sensitivity. Hepatotoxicity with rosiglitazone and pioglitazone is very rare.
   1. Pioglitazone and rosiglitazone are approved for monotherapy or in combination with metformin, sulfonylurea or insulin. Combination tablets of metformin and rosiglitazone (Avandamet) are available. Thiazolidinediones are similar to metformin as monotherapy. They are associated with more weight gain than metformin, and are considerably more expensive than any of the other oral hypoglycemic drugs.
   2. Thiazolidinediones are reserved for second-line treatment in combination with other anti-diabetic medications where synergistic effects can lower A1C

substantially. Fluid retention and precipitation or worsening of heart failure are significant concerns.

Pharmacotherapy of Type 2 Diabetes			
Agent	**Starting dose**	**Maximum dose**	**Comments**

Biguanide
  Metformin
  (Glucophage)
	500 mg daily	850 mg three times daily	Do not use if serum creatinine is greater than 1.4 mg/dL in women or 1.5 mg/dL in men or in the presence of heart failure, chronic obstructive pulmonary disease or liver disease; may cause lactic acidosis

Glyburide/ metformin (Glucovance)	25 mg/250 mg; 2.5 mg/500 mg; 5 mg/500 mg	1 tab qAM-bid	

Sulfonylureas
  Glipizide
  (Glucotrol)
  Glyburide
  (DiaBeta,
  Micronase)
  Glimepiride
  (Amaryl)
	5 mg daily
	
	2.5 mg daily
	
	1 mg daily
		20 mg twice daily
		
		10 mg twice daily
		
		8 mg daily
			May cause hypoglycemia, weight gain. Maximum dose should be used only in combination with insulin therapy

Thiazolidinediones
  Pioglitazone
  (Actos)
  Rosiglitazone
  (Avandia)
	15 mg daily
	
	4 mg daily
		45 mg per day
		
		4 mg twice daily
			Should be used only in patients who have contraindications to metformin

**Alpha-glucosidase
inhibitor**
  Acarbose
  (Precose)
  Miglitol (Glyset)
	50 mg tid
	
	50 mg tid
		100 mg three times daily
		100 mg three times daily
			Flatulence; start at low dose to minimize side effects; take at mealtimes

Meglitamide
  Repaglinide
  (Prandin)
  Nateglinide
  (Starlix)
	0.5 mg before meals
	120 mg tid before meals or 60 mg tid before meals
		4 mg tid-qid
		
		120 mg tid
			Take at mealtimes

H. Alpha-glucosidase inhibitors. Because they act by a different mechanism, the alpha-glucosidase inhibitors, acarbose and miglitol, have additive hypoglycemic effects in patients receiving diet, sulfonylurea, metformin, or insulin therapy. This class of drugs is less potent than the sulfonylureas or metformin, lowering A1C by only 0.5 to 1.0 percentage points.
  1. Side effects are flatulence and diarrhea. These agents are not first-line therapy because of low efficacy and poor tolerance.

2. Acarbose is available as 50 and 100 mg tablets which should be taken with the first bite of each meal. Initiate therapy with 50 mg three times daily. Flatulence, diarrhea, and abdominal discomfort resolve if the dose is decreased. Few patients tolerate more than 300 mg daily.

I. **Insulin** should be used early in type 2 diabetes. When treated early with insulin, patients with type 2 diabetes can have remissions of at least several years, during which A1C is normal. A patient who is 20 percent above ideal body weight and has a fasting blood glucose of 180 mg/dL could be started on a total dose of 21 units per day.

IV. Choosing Initial Therapy

A. **Metformin** therapy should be started in most patients at the time of diabetes diagnosis, in the absence of contraindications, along with lifestyle intervention. The dose of metformin should be titrated to its maximally effective dose (usually 850 mg twice per day) over one to two months, as tolerated.

B. Metformin should not be given to elderly (>80 years) patients unless renal sufficiency is proven with a direct measure of GFR, or to patients who have renal, hepatic or cardiac disease or drink excess alcohol. Another oral agent (a sulfonylurea or thiazolidinedione) should be used for initial therapy in these patients.

C. **Patients who are underweight**, are losing weight, or are ketotic should be started on insulin. Insulin should be initial therapy for patients presenting with A1C >10 percent, fasting plasma glucose >250 mg/dL, random glucose consistently >300 mg/dL, or ketonuria.

D. **If inadequate control is achieved** (A1C remains >7 percent), another medication should be added within two to three months of initiation of metformin. The choice of the second medication might be insulin, a sulfonylurea, or a thiazolidinedione. Insulin is recommended for patients whose A1C remains >8.5 percent.

E. Further adjustments of therapy should usually be made every three months, based on the A1C result, aiming for levels as close to the nondiabetic range as possible. Values >7 percent suggest the need for further adjustments in the diabetic regimen.

F. The patient should perform self blood glucose monitoring and keep a record of the fasting blood glucose, obtained after meals and at other times during the day, and when hypoglycemia is suspected.

V. Combination oral therapy for persistent hyperglycemia

A. **Metformin plus sulfonylureas.** Metformin has an additive hypoglycemic effect when given in combination with a sulfonylurea.

1. A combination tablet **(Glucovance)** is now available in the following glyburide/metformin doses: 1.25 mg/250 mg; 2.5 mg/500 mg; 5 mg/500 mg.

B. **Metformin plus a thiazolidinedione.** Patients who fail initial therapy with metformin may benefit from the addition of a thiazolidinedione such as rosiglitazone or pioglitazone.

C. **Insulin** is a reasonable choice for initial therapy in patients who present with symptomatic or poorly controlled diabetes, and is the preferred second-line medication for patients with A1C >8.5 percent or with symptoms of hyperglycemia despite metformin titration. The dose of insulin may be adjusted every three days, until glycemic targets are achieved.

1. Patients with persistent hyperglycemia despite oral hypoglycemic therapy may stop the oral drug and begin insulin, or may add insulin to oral medication.

2. While NPH has been used commonly at bedtime to supplement oral hypoglycemia drug therapy, insulin glargine may be equally effective for reducing A1C values and may cause less nocturnal hypoglycemia. Although

it may be reasonable to administer glargine at bedtime, morning administration may be better.

References: See page 372.

Hypothyroidism

Hypothyroidism is second only to diabetes mellitus as the most common endocrine disorder, and its prevalence may be as high as 18 cases per 1,000 persons in the general population. The disorder becomes increasingly common with advancing age, affecting about 2 to 3 percent of older women.

I. **Etiology**
   A. **Primary hypothyroidism**
      1. The most common cause of hypothyroidism is Hashimoto's (chronic lymphocytic) thyroiditis. Most patients who have Hashimoto's thyroiditis have symmetrical thyroid enlargement, although many older patients with the disease have atrophy of the gland. Anti-thyroid peroxidase (TPO) antibodies are present in almost all patients. Some patients have blocking antibodies to the thyroid-stimulating hormone (TSH) receptor.
      2. Hypothyroidism also occurs after treatment of hyperthyroidism by either surgical removal or radioiodine ablation. Less common causes of hypothyroidism include congenital dyshormonogenesis, external radiotherapy, infiltrative diseases, such as amyloidosis, and peripheral resistance to thyroid hormone action.
   B. **Secondary and central hypothyroidism.** Pituitary and hypothalamic dysfunction can lead to hypothyroidism. Pituitary adenomas, craniopharyngiomas, pinealomas, sarcoidosis, histiocytosis X, metastatic disease, primary central nervous system (CNS) neoplasms (eg, meningioma), and head trauma all may cause hypothyroidism.
   C. **Transient hypothyroidism.** Subacute thyroiditis is frequently associated with a hyperthyroid phase of 4 to 12 weeks' duration; a 2- to 16-week hypothyroid phase follows, before recovery of thyroid function. Subacute granulomatous (de Quervain's) thyroiditis and subacute lymphocytic (painless) thyroiditis are viral and autoimmune disorders, respectively; the latter condition may occur post partum.
II. **Diagnosis**
   A. **Symptoms and signs** of hypothyroidism include fatigue, weight gain, muscle weakness and cramps, fluid retention, constipation, and neuropathy (eg, carpal tunnel syndrome). Severe hypothyroidism may be associated with carotenemia, loss of the lateral aspect of the eyebrows, sleep apnea, hypoventilation, bradycardia, pericardial effusion, anemia, hyponatremia, hyperprolactinemia, hypercholesterolemia, hypothermia, and coma.
   B. In patients with primary hypothyroidism, the thyroid-stimulating hormone (TSH) level is elevated, and free thyroid hormone levels are depressed. In contrast, patients with secondary hypothyroidism have a low or undetectable TSH level.
   C. TSH results have to be interpreted in light of the patient's clinical condition. A low TSH level should not be misinterpreted as hyperthyroidism in the patient with clinical manifestations of hypothyroidism. When symptoms are nonspecific, a follow-up assessment of the free thyroxine (T_4) level can help distinguish between primary and secondary hypothyroidism.

Laboratory Values in Hypothyroidism

TSH level	Free T$_4$ level	Free T$_3$ level	Likely diagnosis
High	Low	Low	Primary hypothyroidism
High (>10 μU per mL)	Normal	Normal	Subclinical hypothyroidism with high risk for future development of overt hypothyroidism
High (6 to 10 μU per mL)	Normal	Normal	Subclinical hypothyroidism with low risk for future development of overt hypothyroidism
High	High	Low	Congenital absence of T$_4$-T$_3$—converting enzyme; amiodarone (Cordarone) effect on T$_4$-T$_3$ conversion
High	High	High	Peripheral thyroid hormone resistance
Low	Low	Low	Pituitary thyroid deficiency or recent withdrawal of thyroxine after excessive replacement therapy

Causes of Hypothyroidism

Primary hypothyroidism (95% of cases)
Idiopathic hypothyroidism
Hashimoto's thyroiditis Irradiation of the thyroid subsequent to Graves' disease
Surgical removal of the thyroid
Late-stage invasive fibrous thyroiditis
Iodine deficiency
Drug therapy (eg, lithium, interferon)
Infiltrative diseases (eg, sarcoidosis, amyloidosis, scleroderma, hemochromatosis)

Secondary hypothyroidism (5% of cases)
Pituitary or hypothalamic neoplasms
Congenital hypopituitarism
Pituitary necrosis (Sheehan's syndrome)

III. Treatment of hypothyroidism
A. Initiating thyroid hormone replacement
1. Most otherwise healthy adult patients with hypothyroidism require thyroid hormone replacement in a dosage of 1.7 mcg per kg per day, with requirements falling to 1 mcg per kg per day in the elderly. Thus, (Synthroid) in a dosage of 0.10 to 0.15 mg per day is needed to achieve euthyroid status. For full replacement, children may require up to 4 mcg per kg per day.
2. In young patients without risk factors for cardiovascular disease, thyroid hormone replacement can start close to the target goal. In most healthy young adults, replacement is initiated using levothyroxine in a dosage of 0.075 mg per day, with the dosage increased slowly as indicated by continued elevation of the TSH level.

3. Levothyroxine (Synthroid) should be initiated in a low dosage in older patients and those at risk for cardiovascular compromise; the usual starting dosage is 0.025 mg per day, increased in increments of 0.025 to 0.050 mg every four to six weeks until the TSH level returns to normal.

Commonly Prescribed Thyroid Hormone Preparations			
Generic Name	**Brand Name(s)**	**Approximate Equivalent Dose**	**Preparations**
Levothyroxine	Synthroid Levothroid Levoxyl Eltroxin	100 mcg	Tablets: 25, 50, 75, 88, 100, 112, 125, 137, 150, 175, 200, 300 mcg

IV. Monitoring thyroid function
A. In patients with an intact hypothalamic-pituitary axis, the adequacy of thyroid hormone replacement can be followed with serial TSH assessments. The TSH level should be evaluated no earlier than four weeks after an adjustment in the levothyroxine dosage. The full effects of thyroid hormone replacement on the TSH level may not become apparent until after eight weeks of therapy.
B. In patients with pituitary insufficiency, measurements of free T_4 and T_3 levels can be performed to determine whether patients remain euthyroid. TSH or free T_4 levels are monitored annually in most patients with hypothyroidism.

V. Subclinical Hypothyroidism
A. The TSH level can be mildly elevated when the free T_4 and T_3 levels are normal, a situation that occurs most often in women and becomes increasingly common with advancing age. This condition has been termed "subclinical hypothyroidism."
B. In patients at higher risk for osteoporosis or fractures, the deleterious effects of excessive thyroid hormone can be avoided by withholding replacement until the free T_4 and T_3 levels drop below normal.

References, see page 372.

Obesity

Evaluation of the obese patient should include determination of the body mass index (BMI), the distribution of fat based upon the waist circumference, and investigations for comorbid conditions such as diabetes mellitus, dyslipidemia, hypertension, and heart disease. Anti-obesity drugs can be useful adjuncts to diet and exercise for obese subjects with a BMI greater than 30 kg/m^2.

I. Goals of therapy and criteria for success
A. Weight loss should exceed 2 kg during the first month of drug therapy (1 pound per week), fall more than 5 percent below baseline by three to six months, and remain at this level to be considered effective. A weight loss of 5 to 10 percent can significantly reduce the risk factors for diabetes and cardiovascular disease.
B. Weight loss of 10 to 15 percent is considered a very good response and weight loss exceeding 15 percent is considered an excellent response. This degree of weight loss may lower blood pressure and serum lipid concentrations, increase insulin sensitivity, and reduce hyperglycemia.

II. Practice guidelines

A. Counsel all obese patients (BMI $\geq$30 kg/m^2) on diet, lifestyle, and goals for weight loss.

B. Pharmacologic therapy may be offered to those who have failed to achieve weight loss goals through diet and exercise alone. Bariatric surgery should be considered for patients with BMI $\geq$40 kg/m^2 who have failed diet and exercise (with or without drug therapy) and who have obesity-related co-morbidities (hypertension, impaired glucose tolerance, diabetes mellitus, dyslipidemia, sleep apnea).

C. Noradrenergic sympathomimetic drugs:

1. Stimulate the release of norepinephrine or inhibit its reuptake into nerve terminals
2. Block norepinephrine and serotonin reuptake (sibutramine)
3. May increase blood pressure
4. Sympathomimetic drugs reduce food intake by causing early satiety.

D. Sibutramine (Meridia) is a specific inhibitor of norepinephrine, serotonin and to a lesser degree dopamine reuptake into nerve terminals. It inhibits food intake. Sibutramine result is weight loss of about 9.5 percent.

1. Sympathomimetic drugs can increase blood pressure. Sibutramine may increase systolic and diastolic blood pressure increased on average by 1 to 3 mmHg, and pulse increases by four to five beats per minute. Thus, sibutramine should be given cautiously to subjects receiving other drugs that may increase blood pressure.
2. Sibutramine produces a significant overall weight loss and significant increase in both systolic and diastolic blood pressure.
3. **Sibutramine should be avoided in:**
   a. Patients with a history of coronary heart disease, congestive heart failure, cardiac arrhythmia, or stroke.
   b. Patients receiving a monoamine oxidase inhibitor or selective serotonin reuptake inhibitor (risk of serotonin syndrome).
   c. Patients taking erythromycin and ketoconazole (sibutramine is metabolized by the cytochrome P450 enzyme system [isozyme CYP3A4])
4. Sibutramine is available in 5, 10, and 15 mg tablets. The recommended starting dose is 10 mg daily, with titration up or down based upon the response. Doses above 15 mg daily are not recommended.
5. Phentermine leads to more weight loss than placebo. Weight loss slowed during the drug-free periods in the intermittently-treated patients, but accelerated when treatment was resumed.

III. Drugs that alter fat digestion

A. Orlistat (Xenical) inhibits pancreatic lipases. As a result, ingested fat is not completely hydrolyzed to fatty acids and glycerol, and fecal fat excretion is increased.

B. Pharmacology. Orlistat does not alter the pharmacokinetics of digoxin, phenytoin, warfarin, glyburide, oral contraceptives, alcohol, furosemide, captopril, nifedipine, or atenolol. However, absorption of fat-soluble vitamins may be decreased by orlistat.

Anorectic Medication for Obesity Treatment				
Medication	**Sched ule**	**Trade Name(s)**	**Dosage (mg)**	**Common Use**
Phentermine	IV		8, 15, 30	Initial dose: 8-15 mg/d Higher dose: 15 mg bid or 30 mg q AM
		Adipex-P	37.5	Initial dose: ½ tablet/d Higher dose: ½ tablet bid or 37.5-mg tablet q AM
		Fastin	30	1 capsule q AM
Phentermine resin	IV	Ionamin	15, 30	Initial dose: 15 mg/d Higher dose: 15 mg bid or 30 mg q AM
Diethylpropion	IV	Tenuate Tenuate Dospan (sustained-r elease form)	25 75	25 mg tid 75 mg qd
Sibutramine	IV	Meridia	5, 10, 15	Initial dose: 5-10 mg/d Higher dose: 15-25 mg/d
Orlistat	IV	Xenical	120	Initial dose: 1 capsule with a fatty meal qd; bid; or tid

    C. Efficacy. The mean weight loss due to orlistat is 2.89 kg. Weight loss at one year varies from 8.5 to 10.2 percent.

    D. Side effects. Orlistat is generally well-tolerated. Major side effects are intestinal borborygmi and cramps, flatus, fecal incontinence, oily spotting, and flatus with discharge occur in15 to 30 percent. These gastrointestinal complaints are usually mild and subside after the first several weeks of treatment.

    E. Absorption of vitamins A and E and beta-carotene may be slightly reduced. Vitamin supplements should be given to patients treated with this drug.

    F. Orlistat is available in 120 mg capsules. The recommended dose is 120 mg three times daily.

IV. Diabetes drugs

    A. Metformin is a biguanide that is approved for the treatment of diabetes mellitus. Patients receiving metformin lose 1 to 2 kg.

    B. Although metformin does not produce enough weight loss (5 percent) to qualify as a "weight-loss drug," it is very useful for overweight individuals at high risk for diabetes.

V. Recommendations

    A. Diet and lifestyle

        1. All patients who are overweight (BMI $\geq$27 kg/m^2) or obese (BMI $\geq$30 kg/m^2), should receive counseling on diet, lifestyle, and goals for weight loss.

        2. Patients with a BMI of 25 to 29.9 kg/m^2 who have an increased waist circumference (>40 inches in men or >35 inches in women) or those with a BMI 27 to 30 kg/m^2 with comorbidities deserve the same consideration for obesity intervention as those with BMI >30 kg/m^2.

B. Pharmacotherapy
1. For patients who have failed to achieve weight loss goals through diet and exercise alone, pharmacologic therapy should be initiated.
2. For obese patients with elevated blood pressure, cardiovascular disease, or dyslipidemia, orlistat is first line pharmacologic therapy.
3. For otherwise healthy obese patients, sibutramine should be given because of the efficacy and easy tolerability of this agent.
4. For patients with type 2 diabetes, in addition to lifestyle modifications, metformin should be prescribed both for glycemic control and for weight reduction. If the patient has coexisting hypertension, sibutramine should not be used. Orlistat is recommended if further weight reduction is needed.

C. Bariatric surgery
1. For patients with BMI $\geq$40 kg/m^2 who have failed diet and exercise (with or without drug therapy) or for patients with BMI >35 kg/m^2 and obesity-related co-morbidities (hypertension, impaired glucose tolerance, diabetes mellitus, dyslipidemia, sleep apnea), bariatric surgery is recommended.

References, see page 372.

Rheumatic and Hematologic Disorders

Osteoarthritis

Approximately 40 million Americans of are affected by osteoarthritis, and 70 to 90 percent of Americans older than 75 years have at least one involved joint. The prevalence of osteoarthritis ranges from 30 to 90 percent.

Clinical Features of Osteoarthritis	
Symptoms Joint pain Morning stiffness lasting less than 30 minutes Joint instability or buckling Loss of function	**Pattern of joint involvement** **Axial:** cervical and lumbar spine **Peripheral:** distal interphalangeal joint proximal interphalangeal joint first carpometacarpal joints, knees, hips
Signs Bony enlargement at affected joints Limitation of range of motion Crepitus on motion Pain with motion Malalignment and/or joint deformity	

I. **Clinical evaluation**
   A. **Pathogenesis.** Osteoarthritis is caused by a combination of mechanical, cellular, and biochemical processes leading to changes in the composition and mechanical properties of the articular cartilage and degenerative changes and an abnormal repair response.
   B. The typical patient with osteoarthritis is middle-aged or elderly and complains of pain in the knee, hip, hand or spine. The usual presenting symptom is pain involving one or only a few joints. Joint involvement is usually symmetric. The patient usually has pain, stiffness, and some limitation of function. Pain typically worsens with use of the affected joint and is alleviated with rest. Morning stiffness lasting less than 30 minutes is common. (morning stiffness in rheumatoid arthritis lasts longer than 45 minutes.)
   C. Patients with osteoarthritis of the hip may complain of pain in the buttock, groin, thigh or knee. Hip stiffness is common, particularly after inactivity. Involvement of the apophyseal or facet joints of the lower cervical spine may cause neck symptoms, and involvement of the lumbar spine may cause pain in the lower back. Patients may have radicular symptoms, including pain, weakness and numbness.
   D. The physical examination should include an assessment of the affected joints, surrounding soft tissue and bursal areas. Joint enlargement may become evident. Crepitus, or a grating sensation in the joint, is a late manifestation.
   E. Laboratory work may include erythrocyte sedimentation rate and rheumatoid factor.
   F. Radiographic findings consistent with osteoarthritis include presence of joint space narrowing, osteophyte formation, pseudocyst in subchondral bone, and increased density of subchondral bone. The absence of radiographic changes does not exclude the diagnosis of osteoarthritis. Radiographs are recommended for patients with trauma, joint pain at night, progressive joint pain,

significant family history of inflammatory arthritis, and children younger than 18 years.

Distinction Between Rheumatoid Arthritis and Osteoarthritis		
Feature	**Rheumatoid arthritis**	**Osteoarthritis**
Primary joints affected	Metacarpophalangeal Proximal interphalangeal	Distal interphalangeal Carpometacarpal
Heberden's nodes	Absent	Frequently present
Joint characteristics	Soft, warm, and tender	Hard and bony
Stiffness	Worse after resting (eg, morning stiffness)	Worse after effort
Laboratory findings	Positive rheumatoid factor Elevated ESR and C reactive protein	Rheumatoid factor negative Normal ESR and C reactive protein

II. Treatment of osteoarthritis

A. Analgesics. Acetaminophen at doses of up to 4 g/day is the drug of choice for pain relief. Hepatotoxicity is primarily seen only in patients who consume excessive amounts of alcohol. Combination analgesics (eg, acetaminophen with aspirin) increase the risk for renal failure.

1. Opioid analgesics, such as codeine, oxycodone, or propoxyphene may be beneficial for short-term use.
2. Tramadol (Ultram) alone or in combination with acetaminophen are useful when added to an NSAID or COX-2 inhibitor. The combination of tramadol and acetaminophen (37.5 mg/325 mg) is roughly equivalent to 30 mg codeine and 325 mg of acetaminophen.

B. Nonsteroidal anti-inflammatory drugs (NSAIDs) are indicated in patients with OA who fail to respond to acetaminophen. NSAIDs are more efficacious than acetaminophen. Gastrointestinal symptoms were more frequent with use of nonselective NSAIDs than with acetaminophen. Nonacetylated salicylates (salsalate, choline magnesium trisalicylate), sulindac, and perhaps nabumetone appear to have less renal toxicity. The nonacetylated salicylates and nabumetone (Relafen) have less antiplatelet activity. Low-dose ibuprofen (less than 1600 mg/day) may have less serious gastrointestinal toxicity.

C. COX-2 inhibitors have a 200 to 300 fold selectivity for inhibition of COX-2 over COX-1. Celecoxib (Celebrex) is available.

1. Selective COX-2 inhibitors are an option for patients with a history of peptic ulcer, gastrointestinal bleeding, or gastrointestinal intolerance to NSAIDs (including salicylates). These agents are contraindicated in cardiovascular disease or with multiple risk factors for atherosclerotic coronary heart disease. An alternative approach is the use of a nonselective NSAID and misoprostol or a proton pump inhibitor. Selective COX-2 and nonselective NSAIDs should be avoided in renal disease, congestive heart failure,

cirrhosis, and volume depletion. Celecoxib (Celebrex) dosage is 100 mg twice daily and 200 mg once daily.

D. Adverse effects. NSAID use is often limited by toxicity. Among the side effects that can occur are:

1. Rash and hypersensitivity reactions.
2. Abdominal pain and gastrointestinal bleeding.
3. Impairment of renal, hepatic, and bone marrow function, and platelet aggregation.
4. Central nervous system dysfunction in the elderly.
5. NSAIDs are contraindicated in patients with active peptic ulcer disease. Non-specific COX inhibitors should be avoided in patients with a history of peptic ulcer disease. Specific COX-2 inhibitors are preferred in these individuals.
6. Non-specific COX-2 inhibitors must be used with caution in patients on warfarin. NSAID-induced platelet dysfunction can increase the risk of bleeding. Specific COX-2 inhibitors can be used in this setting.
7. Patients with intrinsic renal disease, congestive heart failure, and those receiving diuretic therapy are at risk for developing reversible renal failure while using an NSAID, resulting in an elevation in the plasma creatinine. Nonacetylated salicylates and sulindac (Clinoril) in low doses appear to relatively spare renal prostaglandin synthesis and can be used in these settings.
8. NSAIDs may interfere with the control of hypertension, usually resulting in a modest rise in blood pressure of 5 mm Hg.
9. Some patients with diminished cardiac function may develop overt congestive heart failure when given NSAIDs.
10. NSAIDs can be safely used in combination with low-dose aspirin (81 to 325 mg/day) that is prescribed for cardiovascular protection. NSAIDs should be avoided in patients with aspirin sensitivity.

Dosage of nonsteroidal anti-inflammatory drugs (NSAIDs)				
Agent	**Brand name(s)**	**Dosing**	**Daily use**	**Specific benefits**
Salicylates				
Aspirin		BID-QID	500-4000 mg	Titrate dose by serum levels
Choline magnesium trisalicylate	Trilisate	BID-QID	975-3600 mg	Decreased GI toxicity, titrate dose by serum levels
Salsalate	Disalcid, Salflex, Monogesic	BID-QID	975-3600 mg	Decreased GI toxicity, titrate dose by serum levels

Agent	Brand name(s)	Dosing	Daily use	Specific benefits
Short half-life NSAID				
Fenoprofen calcium	Nalfon	TID-QID	900-2400 mg	Generally fewer side effects
Ibuprofen	Motrin, Advil, Midol, Nuprin	TID-QID	600-3600 mg	
Indometha-cin	Indocin	TID-QID	75-200 mg	Excellent efficacy if tol-erated
Ketoprofen	Orudis	TID-QID	75-300 mg	Dialyzable
Meclofena-mate sodium	Meclomen	TID-QID	150-400 mg	
Tolmetin	Tolectin	TID-QID	600-2000 mg	
Intermediate half-life NSAID				
Diclofenac	Cataflam, Voltaren	BID-QID	100-200 mg	
Etodolac	Lodine	BID-QID	400-1200 mg	
Flurbiprofen	Ansaid	BID-QID	100-300 mg	
Naproxen	Naproxyn, Napron X	BID-TID	500-1500 mg	
Naproxen-sodium	Anaprox, Aleve	BID-TID	550-1650 mg	
Sulindac	Clinoril	BID	150-1000 mg	Decreased renal prosta-glandin effect
Diflunisal	Dolobid	BID	500-1000 mg	Most uricosuric NSAID
Long half-life NSAID				
Nabumetone	Relafen	QD-BID	1000-2000 mg	Decreased GI side ef-fects
Oxaprozin	Daypro	QD-BID	600-1800 mg	
Piroxicam	Feldene	QD	10-20 mg	

Cyclooxygenase-2 inhibitor		
Celecoxib (Celebrex)	100 mg twice daily or 200 mg daily for osteoarthritis 100 to 200 mg twice daily for rheumatoid arthritis	100 mg 200 mg

E. Choice of NSAID
  1. None of the available NSAIDs is more effective than any other. It is preferable to use a NSAID on a periodic basis in patients with noninflammatory OA since the presence and intensity of symptoms usually vary with time; a short-acting agent is ideal in this setting. Continuous therapy with a long-acting agent is indicated if this regimen does not provide adequate symptom control.
  2. A short-acting NSAID is generally used initially. An over-the-counter agent (ibuprofen or naproxen) is a reasonable choice. If there is inadequate control with the initial dose, then the dose should be gradually increased toward the maximum for that drug. If one NSAID is not effective after two to four weeks on a maximal dosage, then another NSAID or nonacetylated salicylate should be tried. If there is a history of gastroduodenal disease, a specific COX-2 inhibitor is preferred
  3. **Misoprostol (Cytotec)** can also be used as prophylaxis for the development of upper gastrointestinal bleeding in patients who receive non-specific COX-2 inhibitors. Misoprostol dose is 100 µg twice daily.
F. Intraarticular corticosteroid injections may be appropriate in patients with OA who have one or several joints that are painful despite the use of a NSAIDs and in patients with monoarticular or pauciarticular inflammatory osteoarthritis in whom NSAIDs are contraindicated. Intraarticular corticosteroids are effective for short-term pain relief.
  1. Common corticosteroid suspensions used for intraarticular injection include triamcinolone acetonide, hexacetonide, and Depo-Medrol:
     a. 10 mg for small joints (interphalangeal, metacarpophalangeal and metatarsophalangeal joints).
     b. 20 mg for medium-sized joints (wrists, elbows, ankles).
     c. 40 mg for larger joints (shoulders, knees, hips).
     d. Corticosteroid injections in a weight-bearing joint should be limited to three to four per year.
G. Intraarticular hyaluronic acid derivatives are more efficacious than intraarticular placebo. However, the magnitude of the benefit is modest.
H. Joint irrigation may be warranted in patients with inflammatory symptoms who are refractory to NSAIDs or intraarticular corticosteroid injections.
I. Colchicine may be a reasonable treatment option in patients with inflammatory OA who have symptoms that are unresponsive to nonpharmacologic interventions and NSAIDs.
J. Arthroscopic debridement. Patients who will benefit from arthroscopic lavage and debridement have predominantly mechanical symptoms.
K. Surgical intervention should be considered in patients with severe symptomatic OA who have failed to respond to medical management (including arthroscopic procedures), and who have marked limitations in activities of daily living. Total joint arthroplasty replacement provides marked pain relief and functional improvement in patients with severe hip or knee OA.
L. The risk of NSAID-induced renal and hepatic toxicity is increased in older patients and in patients with preexisting renal or hepatic insufficiency. Choline

magnesium trisalicylate (Trilisate) and salsalate (Disalcid) cause less renal toxicity. Liver function tests and serum hemoglobin, creatinine and potassium measurements should be performed initially and after six months of treatment.
References, see page 372.

Low Back Pain

Approximately 90 percent of adults experience back pain at some time in life, and 50 percent of persons in the working population have back pain every year.

I. Evaluation of low back pain

A. A comprehensive history and physical examination can identify the small percentage of patients with serious conditions such as infection, malignancy, rheumatologic diseases and neurologic disorders.

B. The history and review of systems include patient age, constitutional symptoms and the presence of night pain, bone pain or morning stiffness. The patient should be asked about the occurrence of visceral pain, claudication, numbness, weakness, radiating pain, and bowel and bladder dysfunction.

History and Physical Examination in the Patient with Acute Low Back Pain

History
Onset of pain (eg, time of day, activity)
Location of pain (eg, specific site, radiation of pain)
Type and character of pain (sharp, dull)
Aggravating and relieving factors
Medical history, including previous injuries
Psychosocial stressors at home or work
"Red flags": age greater than 50 years, fever, weight loss
Incontinence, constipation
Physical examination
Informal observation (eg, patient's posture, expressions, pain behavior)
Physical examination, with attention to specific areas as indicated by the history
Neurologic evaluation
Back examination
    Palpation
    Range of motion or painful arc
    Stance
    Gait
    Mobility (test by having the patient sit, lie down and stand up)
    Straight leg raise test

C. Specific characteristics and severity of the pain, a history of trauma, previous therapy and its efficacy, and the functional impact of the pain on the patient's work and activities of daily living should be assessed.

D. The most common levels for a herniated disc are L4-5 and L5-S1. The onset of symptoms is characterized by a sharp, burning, stabbing pain radiating down the posterior or lateral aspect of the leg, to below the knee. Pain is generally superficial and localized, and is often associated with numbness or tingling. In more advanced cases, motor deficit, diminished reflexes or weakness may occur.

E. If a disc herniation is responsible for the back pain, the patient can usually recall the time of onset and contributing factors, whereas if the pain is of a gradual onset, other degenerative diseases are more probable than disc herniation.

F. Rheumatoid arthritis often begins in the appendicular skeleton before progressing to the spine. Inflammatory arthritides, such as ankylosing spondylitis, cause generalized pain and stiffness that are worse in the morning and relieved somewhat throughout the day.

G. **Cauda equina syndrome.** Only the relatively uncommon central disc herniation provokes low back pain and saddle pain in the S1 and S2 distributions. A central herniated disc may also compress nerve roots of the cauda equina, resulting in difficult urination, incontinence or impotence. If bowel or bladder dysfunction is present, immediate referral to a specialist is required for emergency surgery to prevent permanent loss of function.

II. **Physical and neurologic examination of the lumbar spine**

A. **External manifestations of pain**, including an abnormal stance, should be noted. The patient's posture and gait should be examined for sciatic list, which is indicative of disc herniation. The spinous processes and interspinous ligaments should be palpated for tenderness.

B. **Range of motion** should be evaluated. Pain during lumbar flexion suggests discogenic pain, while pain on lumbar extension suggests facet disease. Ligamentous or muscular strain can cause pain when the patient bends contralaterally.

C. **Motor, sensory and reflex function** should be assessed to determine the affected nerve root level. Muscle strength is graded from zero (no evidence of contractility) to 5 (motion against resistance).

D. **Specific movements and positions that reproduce the symptoms** should be sought. The upper lumbar region (L1, L2 and L3) controls the iliopsoas muscles, which can be evaluated by testing resistance to hip flexion. While seated, the patient should attempt to raise each thigh. Pain and weakness are indicative of upper lumbar nerve root involvement. The L2, L3 and L4 nerve roots control the quadriceps muscle, which can be evaluated by manually trying to flex the actively extended knee. The L4 nerve root also controls the tibialis anterior muscle, which can be tested by heel walking.

Indications for Radiographs in the Patient with Acute Low Back Pain

History of significant trauma
Neurologic deficits
Systemic symptoms
Temperature greater than 38°C (100.4°F)
Unexplained weight loss
Medical history
  Cancer
  Corticosteroid use
  Drug or alcohol abuse
Ankylosing spondylitis suspected

Waddell Signs: Nonorganic Signs Indicating the Presence of a Functional Component of Back Pain

Superficial, nonanatomic tenderness
Pain with simulated testing (eg, axial loading or pelvic rotation)
Inconsistent responses with distraction (eg, straight leg raises while the patient is sitting)
Nonorganic regional disturbances (eg, nondermatomal sensory loss)
Overreaction

Differential Diagnosis of Acute Low Back Pain

Disease or condition	Patient age (years)	Location of pain	Quality of pain	Aggravating or relieving factors	Signs
Back strain	20 to 40	Low back, buttock, posterior thigh	Ache, spasm	Increased with activity or bending	Local tenderness, limited spinal motion
Acute disc herniation	30 to 50	Low back to lower leg	Sharp, shooting or burning pain, paresthesia in leg	Decreased with standing; increased with bending or sitting	Positive straight leg raise test, weakness, asymmetric reflexes
Osteoarthritis or spinal stenosis	>50	Low back to lower leg; often bilateral	Ache, shooting pain, "pins and needles" sensation	Increased with walking, especially up an incline; decreased with sitting	Mild decrease in extension of spine; may have weakness or asymmetric reflexes
Spondylolisthesis	Any age	Back, posterior thigh	Ache	Increased with activity or bending	Exaggeration of the lumbar curve, palpable "step off" (defect between spinous processes), tight hamstrings
Ankylosing spondylitis	15 to 40	Sacroiliac joints, lumbar spine	Ache	Morning stiffness	Decreased back motion, tenderness over sacroiliac joints
Infection	Any age	Lumbar spine, sacrum	Sharp pain, ache	Varies	Fever, percussive tenderness; may have neurologic abnormalities or decreased motion
Malignancy	>50	Affected bone(s)	Dull ache, throbbing pain; slowly progressive	Increased with recumbency or cough	May have localized tenderness, neurologic signs or fever

| Location of Pain and Motor Deficits in Association with Nerve Root Involvement |||
Disc level	Location of pain	Motor deficit
T12-L1	Pain in inguinal region and medial thigh	None
L1-2	Pain in anterior and medial aspect of upper thigh	Slight weakness in quadriceps; slightly diminished suprapatellar reflex
L2-3	Pain in anterolateral thigh	Weakened quadriceps; diminished patellar or suprapatellar reflex
L3-4	Pain in posterolateral thigh and anterior tibial area	Weakened quadriceps; diminished patellar reflex
L4-5	Pain in dorsum of foot	Extensor weakness of big toe and foot
L5-S1	Pain in lateral aspect of foot	Diminished or absent Achilles reflex

E. **The L5 nerve root** controls the extensor hallucis longus, which can be tested with the patient seated and moving both great toes in a dorsiflexed position against resistance. The L5 nerve root also innervates the hip abductors, which are evaluated by the Trendelenburg test. This test requires the patient to stand on one leg; the physician stands behind the patient and puts his or her hands on the patient's hips. A positive test is characterized by any drop in the pelvis and suggests L5 nerve root pathology.

F. **Cauda equina syndrome** can be identified by unexpected laxity of the anal sphincter, perianal or perineal sensory loss, or major motor loss in the lower extremities.

G. **Nerve root tension signs** are evaluated with the straight-leg raising test in the supine position. The physician raises the patient's legs to 90 degrees. If nerve root compression is present, this test causes severe pain in the back of the affected leg and can reveal a disorder of the L5 or S1 nerve root.

H. **The most common sites for a herniated lumbar disc** are L4-5 and L5-S1, resulting in back pain and pain radiating down the posterior and lateral leg, to below the knee.

I. **A crossed straight-leg raising test** may suggest nerve root compression. In this test, straight-leg raising of the contralateral limb reproduces more specific but less intense pain on the affected side. In addition, the femoral stretch test can be used to evaluate the reproducibility of pain. The patient lies in either the prone or the lateral decubitus position, and the thigh is extended at the hip, and the knee is flexed. Reproduction of pain suggests upper nerve root (L2, L3 and L4) disorders.

J. **Laboratory tests**
   1. Evaluation may include a complete blood count, determination of erythrocyte sedimentation rate.
   2. **Radiographic evaluation.** Plain-film radiography is rarely useful in the initial evaluation of patients with acute-onset low back pain. Plain-film radiographs are normal or equivocal in more than 75 percent of patients

with low back pain. Views of the spine uncover useful information in fewer than 3 percent of patients. Anteroposterior and lateral radiographs should be considered in patients who have a history of trauma, neurologic deficits, or systemic symptoms.

3. **Magnetic resonance imaging and computed tomographic scanning**
   a. Magnetic resonance imaging (MRI) and computed tomographic (CT) scanning often demonstrate abnormalities in "normal" asymptomatic people. Thus, positive findings in patients with back pain are frequently of questionable clinical significance.
   b. MRI is better at imaging soft tissue (eg, herniated discs, tumors). CT scanning provides better imaging of bone (eg, osteoarthritis). MRI has the ability to demonstrate disc damage. MRI or CT studies should be considered in patients with worsening neurologic deficits or a suspected systemic cause of back pain such as infection or neoplasm.

4. **Bone scintigraphy** or bone scanning, can be useful when radiographs of the spine are normal, but the clinical findings are suspicious for osteomyelitis, bony neoplasm or occult fracture.

5. **Physiologic assessment**. Electrodiagnostic assessments such as needle electromyography and nerve conduction studies are useful in differentiating peripheral neuropathy from radiculopathy or myopathy.

III. Management of acute low back pain

A. Pharmacologic therapy

1. The mainstay of pharmacologic therapy for acute low back pain is acetaminophen or a nonsteroidal anti-inflammatory drug (NSAID). If no medical contraindications are present, a two- to four-week course of medication at anti-inflammatory levels is suggested.
2. Naproxen (Naprosyn) 500 mg, followed by 250 mg PO tid-qid prn [250, 375,500 mg].
3. Naproxen sodium (Aleve) 200 mg PO tid prn.
4. Naproxen sodium (Anaprox) 550 mg, followed by 275 mg PO tid-qid prn.
5. Ibuprofen (Motrin, Advil) 800 mg, then 400 mg PO q4-6h prn.
6. Diclofenac (Voltaren) 50 mg bid-tid or 75 mg bid.
7. Gastrointestinal prophylaxis, using a histamine H_2 antagonist or misoprostol (Cytotec), should be prescribed for patients who are at risk for peptic ulcer disease.
8. Celecoxib (Celebrex) are NSAIDs with selective cyclo-oxygenase-2 inhibition. These agents have fewer gastrointestinal side effects.
9. Celecoxib (Celebrex) is given as 200 mg qd or 100 mg bid.
10. For relief of acute pain, short-term use of a narcotic may be considered.

B. Rest.
Two to three days of bed rest in a supine position may be recommended for patients with acute radiculopathy.

C. Physical therapy modalities

1. Superficial heat, ultrasound (deep heat), cold packs and massage are useful for relieving symptoms in the acute phase after the onset of low back pain.
2. No convincing evidence has demonstrated the long-term effectiveness of lumbar traction and transcutaneous electrical stimulation.

D. Aerobic exercise
has been reported to improve or prevent back pain. Exercise programs that facilitate weight loss, trunk strengthening and the stretching of musculotendinous structures appear to be most helpful. Exercises should promote the strengthening of muscles that support the spine.

E. Trigger point injections
can provide extended relief for localized pain sources. An injection of 1 to 2 mL of 1 percent lidocaine (Xylocaine) without epinephrine is usually administered. Epidural steroid injection therapy has been reported to be effective in patients with lumbar disc herniation.

F. **Indications for herniated disc surgery.** Most patients with a herniated disc may be effectively treated conservatively. Indications for referral include the following: (1) cauda equina syndrome, (2) progressive neurologic deficit, (3) profound neurologic deficit and (4) severe and disabling pain refractory to four to six weeks of conservative treatment.

References, see page 372.

Gout

Gout comprises a heterogeneous group of disorders characterized by deposition of uric acid crystals in the joints and tendons. Gout has a prevalence of 5.0 to 6.6 cases per 1,000 men and 1.0 to 3.0 cases per 1,000 women.

I. **Clinical features**
   A. **Asymptomatic hyperuricemia** is defined as an abnormally high serum urate level, without gouty arthritis or nephrolithiasis. Hyperuricemia is defined as a serum urate concentration greater than 7 mg/dL. Hyperuricemia predisposes patients to both gout and nephrolithiasis, but therapy is generally not warranted in the asymptomatic patient.
   B. **Acute gout** is characterized by the sudden onset of pain, erythema, limited range of motion and swelling of the involved joint. The peak incidence of acute gout occurs between 30 and 50 years of age. First attacks are monoarticular in 90 percent. In more than one-half of patients, the first metatarsophalangeal joint is the initial joint involved, a condition known as podagra. Joint involvement includes the metatarsophalangeal joint, the instep/forefoot, the ankle, the knee, the wrist and the fingers.
   C. **Intercritical gout** consists of the asymptomatic phase of the disease following recovery from acute gouty arthritis.
   D. **Recurrent gouty arthritis.** Approximately 60 percent of patients have a second attack within the first year, and 78 percent have a second attack within two years.
   E. **Chronic tophaceous gout.** Tophi are deposits of sodium urate that are large enough to be seen on radiographs and may occur at virtually any site. Common sites include the joints of the hands or feet, the helix of the ear, the olecranon bursa, and the Achilles tendon.

II. **Diagnosis**
   A. Definitive diagnosis of gout requires aspiration and examination of synovial fluid for monosodium urate crystals. Monosodium urate crystals are identified by polarized light microscopy.
   B. If a polarizing microscope is not available, the characteristic needle shape of the monosodium urate crystals, especially when found within white blood cells, can be identified with conventional light microscopy. The appearance resembles a toothpick piercing an olive.

III. **Treatment of gout**
   A. **Asymptomatic hyperuricemia.** Urate-lowering drugs should not be used to treat patients with asymptomatic hyperuricemia. If hyperuricemia is identified, associated factors such as obesity, hypercholesterolemia, alcohol consumption and hypertension should be addressed.
   B. **Acute gout**
      1. **NSAIDs** are the preferred therapy for the treatment of acute gout. Indomethacin (Indocin), ibuprofen (Motrin), naproxen (Naprosyn), sulindac (Clinoril), piroxicam (Feldene) and ketoprofen (Orudis) are effective. More than 90 percent of patients have a resolution of the attack within five to eight days.

Drugs Used in the Management of Acute Gout		
Drug	**Dosage**	**Side effects/comments**
NSAIDS		
Indomethacin (Indocin) Naproxen (Naprosyn) Ibuprofen (Motrin) Sulindac (Clinoril) Ketoprofen (Orudis)	25 to 50 mg four times daily 500 mg two times daily 800 mg four times daily 200 mg two times daily 75 mg four times daily	Contraindicated with peptic ulcer disease or systemic anticoagulation; side effects include gastropathy, nephropathy, liver dysfunction, and reversible platelet dysfunction; may cause fluid overload in patients with heart failure
Corticosteroids		
Oral	Prednisone, 0.5 mg per kg on day 1, taper by 5.0 mg each day thereafter	Fluid retention; impaired wound healing
Intramuscular	Triamcinolone acetonide (Kenalog), 60 mg intramuscularly, repeat in 24 hours if necessary	May require repeat injections; risk of soft tissue atrophy
Intra-articular	Large joints: 10 to 40 mg Small joints: 5 to 20 mg	Preferable route for monoarticular involvement
ACTH	40 to 80 IU intramuscularly; repeat every 8 hours as necessary	Repeat injections are commonly needed; requires intact pituitary-adrenal axis; stimulation of mineralocorticoid release may cause volume overload
Colchicine	0.5 to 0.6 mg PO every hour until relief or side effects occur, or until a maximum dosage of 6 mg is reached	Dose-dependent gastrointestinal side effects; improper intravenous dosing has caused bone marrow suppression, renal failure and death

2. **Corticosteroids**
   a. **Intra-articular, intravenous, intramuscular or oral corticosteroids** are effective in acute gout. In cases where one or two joints are involved, intra-articular injection of corticosteroid can be used.
   b. **Intramuscular triamcinolone acetonide** (60 mg) is as effective as indomethacin in relieving acute gouty arthritis. Triamcinolone acetonide is especially useful in patients with contraindications to NSAIDs.
   c. **Oral prednisone** is an option when repeat dosing is anticipated. Prednisone, 0.5 mg per kg on day 1 and tapered by 5 mg each day is very effective.
3. **Colchicine** is effective in treating acute gout; however, 80 percent of patients experience gastrointestinal side effects, including nausea, vomiting and diarrhea. Intravenous colchicine is available but is highly toxic and not recommended.

C. Treatment of intercritical gout

1. Prophylactic colchicine (from 0.6 mg to 1.2 mg) should be administered at the same time urate-lowering drug therapy is initiate. Colchicine should be used for prophylaxis only with concurrent use of urate-lowering agents. Colchicine is used for prophylaxis until the serum urate concentration is at the desired level and the patient has been free from acute gouty attacks for three to six months.

2. **Urate-lowering agents**

   a. After the acute gouty attack is treated and prophylactic therapy is initiated, sources of hyperuricemia should be eliminated to lower the serum urate level without the use of medication.

   b. Medications that may aggravate the patient's condition (eg, diuretics) should be discontinued; purine-rich foods and alcohol consumption should be curtailed, and the patient should gradually lose weight, if obese.

Purine Content of Foods and Beverages

High

    Avoid: Liver, kidney, anchovies, sardines, herring, mussels, bacon, codfish, scallops, trout, haddock, veal, venison, turkey, alcoholic beverages

Moderate

    May eat occasionally: Asparagus, beef, bouillon, chicken, crab, duck, ham, kidney beans, lentils, lima beans, mushrooms, lobster, oysters, pork, shrimp, spinach

---

3. **24-hour urine uric acid excretion measurement** is essential to identify the most appropriate urate-lowering medication and to check for significant preexisting renal insufficiency.

   a. Uricosuric agents should be used in most patients with gout because most are "underexcretors" of uric acid. Inhibitors of uric acid synthesis are more toxic and should be reserved for use in "overproducers" of urate (urine excretion >800 mg in 24 hours).

   b. Urate-lowering therapy should not be initiated until the acute attack has resolved, since they may exacerbate the attack.

Urate-Lowering Drugs for the Treatment of Gout and Hyperuricemia

Drug	Dosage	Indications	Side effects/comments
Probenecid (Benemid)	Begin with 250 mg twice daily, gradually titrating upward until the serum urate level is <6 mg per dL; maximum: 3 g per day	Recurrent gout may be combined with allopurinol in resistant hyperuricemia	Uricosuric agent; creatinine clearance must be >60 mL per minute; therapeutic effect reversed by aspirin therapy; avoid concurrent daily aspirin use; contraindicated in urolithiasis; may precipitate gouty attack at start of therapy; rash or gastrointestinal side effects may occur

Drug	Dosage	Indications	Side effects/comments
Allopurinol (Zyloprim)	Begin with 50 to 100 mg daily, gradually titrating upward until the serum urate level is <6 mg per dL; typical dosage: 200 to 300 mg daily	Chronic gouty arthritis; secondary hyper-uricemia related to the use of cytolytics in the treatment of hematologic ma-lignancies; gout complicated by renal disease or renal calculi	Inhibits uric acid synthesis; side effects include rash, gastrointesti-nal symptoms, headache, urticaria and interstitial nephritis; rare, po-tentially fatal hypersensitivity syn-drome

4. **Probenecid (Benemid)** is the most frequently used uricosuric medication. Candidates for probenecid therapy must have hyperuricemia attributed to undersecretion of urate (ie, <800 mg in 24 hours), a creatinine clearance of >60 mL/minute and no history of nephrolithiasis. Probenecid should be initiated at a dosage of 250 mg twice daily and increased as needed, up to 3 g per day, to achieve a serum urate level of less than 6 mg per dL. Side effects include precipitation of an acute gouty attack, renal calculi, rash, and gastrointestinal problems.

5. **Allopurinol (Zyloprim)** is an inhibitor of uric acid synthesis. Allopurinol is initiated at a dosage of 100 mg per day and increased in increments of 50 to 100 mg per day every two weeks until the urate level is <6 mg per dL. Side effects include rash, gastrointestinal problems, headache, urticaria and interstitial nephritis. A hypersensitivity syndrome associated with fever, bone marrow suppression, hepatic toxicity, renal failure and a systemic hypersensitivity vasculitis is rare.

References, see page 372.

Rheumatoid Arthritis

Rheumatoid arthritis (RA) is a chronic, polyarticular, symmetric, inflammatory disease that affects about 2.5 million people in the United States. The disease has a predilection for small proximal joints, although virtually every peripheral joint in the body can be involved. RA strikes women, usually of childbearing age, three times more often than it does men. This process causes the immune system to attack the synovium of various joints, leading to synovitis.

I. Clinical manifestations
A. RA is a chronic, symmetric polyarthritis. The polyarthritis is often deforming. About 80% of patients describe a slowly progressive onset over weeks or months.

B. Inflammatory features
1. The joints in RA are swollen, tender, slightly warm, and stiff. Synovial fluid is cloudy and has an increased number of inflammatory white blood cells.
2. Patients with RA usually have profound and prolonged morning stiffness. Fatigue, anemia of chronic disease, fever, vasculitis, pericarditis, and myocarditis, are common.

C. Joint involvement. RA may begin in one or two joints, but it almost invariably progresses to affect 20 or more. In some cases, joint involvement is nearly symmetric. Initially, the disease typically involves the metacarpophalangeal, proximal interphalangeal, wrist, and metatarsophalangeal joints, either alone or in combination with others.

D. Proliferative/erosive features. The inflamed synovial tissue evolves into a thickened, boggy mass known as a pannus. Pannus can eat through joint cartilage and into adjacent bone.

E. Joint deformity. Deformities of RA are more likely to be the result of damage to ligaments, tendons, and joint capsule.

II. Diagnosis

A. RA is a clinical diagnosis. The presence of arthritis excludes the many forms of soft tissue rheumatism (eg, tendinitis, bursitis). The degree of inflammation excludes osteoarthritis and traumatic arthritis. Polyarticular involvement of the appropriate joints makes the spondyloarthropathies unlikely. The pannus is often palpable as a rubbery mass of tissue around a joint.

B. **Rheumatoid factor testing** helps to confirm the diagnosis of RA. Rheumatoid factor serves as a marker for RA, but it is not reliable because 1-2% of the normal population have rheumatoid factor. Chronic infections, other inflammatory conditions and malignancies may trigger formation of rheumatoid factor. Conversely, 15% of patients with RA are seronegative for rheumatoid factor.

C. **Radiography.** Typical erosions around joint margins help confirm the diagnosis of RA.

III. Treatment of mild disease rheumatoid arthritis

A. **NSAIDs.** Appropriate initial therapy of patients with mild disease consists of an NSAID at full therapeutic dose.

   1. Initial therapy consists of an NSAID rather than a salicylate, because fewer tablets are required each day. Full anti-inflammatory doses should be administered, such as the equivalent of 3200 mg of ibuprofen,1000 mg of naproxen (Naprosyn), or 200 mg of celecoxib (Celebrex) per day in divided doses, or a single-daily dose of longer-acting agents, such as piroxicam (Feldene,10 mg bid or 20 mg qd) may be used.

   2. Selective COX-2 inhibitors, which have equivalent efficacy to NSAIDs but markedly lower gastroduodenal toxicity, are recommended for patients with a history of peptic ulcer, gastrointestinal bleeding, or gastrointestinal intolerance to NSAIDs (including salicylates); celecoxib (Celebrex) 100-200 bid.

B. **Disease modifying anti-rheumatic drugs (DMARDs).** The addition of hydroxychloroquine (200 mg BID) or sulfasalazine (1000 mg BID or TID) is frequently employed for mild disease. Sulfasalazine is utilized among those with active synovitis.

C. **Adjunctive therapies.** Additional initial therapies may include:

   1. Acetaminophen for pain relief

   2. Patient education concerning joint protection

   3. Physical therapy to enhance muscle tone and help maintain full range of motion

   4. Intraarticular injection of steroids. When the disease is oligoarticular, joint injection with a depo-corticosteroid preparation, such as triamcinolone hexacetonide, may lead to prolonged local disease control

IV. Treatment of moderate disease rheumatoid arthritis

A. Patients presenting with moderate disease should receive DMARD therapy in addition to an NSAID.

B. **NSAIDs.** Full anti-inflammatory doses should be administered, such as the equivalent of 3200 mg of ibuprofen,1000 mg of naproxen (Naprosyn), or 200 mg of celecoxib (Celebrex) per day in divided doses, or a single-daily dose of longer-acting agents, such as piroxicam (Feldene) may be used.

C. DMARDs

1. Hydroxychloroquine (200 mg BID) is initiated if the disease is more mild, or sulfasalazine 1000 BID-TID if the disease is intermediate.

2. Methotrexate (MTX) is commonly selected as early therapy for active disease. Methotrexate is used, except in women who may become pregnant and patients with liver disease. The dose is 7.5 mg per week. Folic acid (1 to 2 mg/day) or folinic acid (2.5 to 5 mg per week, 8 to 12 hours after methotrexate) should be administered concurrently to reduce potential MTX toxicity.

3. For those with contraindications to the use of methotrexate, the following agents can be considered:

   a. Leflunomide (Arava) alone
   b. Etanercept (Enbrel) alone
   c. Adalimumab (Humira) alone
   d. Infliximab (Remicade) alone
   e. Combination of hydroxychloroquine and sulfasalazine
   f. Anakinra (Kineret) alone

D. Begin with either leflunomide or TNF-alpha-blockade in this setting. Leflunomide can cause fetal harm and is contraindicated in women who are or may become pregnant. Etanercept, adalimumab, and infliximab are contraindicated in women who are pregnant or nursing, patients with active infection, and those at high risk of reactivation of tuberculosis unless given prophylactic antituberculous therapy.

E. Anticytokine therapy. Etanercept, infliximab, adalimumab, or anakinra alone are alternatives for the patient in whom methotrexate is contraindicated. Addition of one of these agents to ongoing methotrexate therapy is an option for patients with moderate disease.

Antirheumatic drugs used in treatment of rheumatoid arthritis			
Drug	**Delivery**	**Dose**	**Side effects**
Methotrexate (Rheumatrex Dose Pack)	PO or SC	5-20 mg/wk	Marrow suppression, mucositis, hepatotoxicity, pulmonary disease, susceptibility to infection
Cyclosporine (Neoral)	PO	2-4 mg/kg daily	Marrow suppression, renal toxicity, hyperuricemia, susceptibility to infection
Azathioprine (Imuran)	PO	50-250 mg/day	Marrow suppression, GI intolerance, hepatotoxicity, tumors, susceptibility to infection
Chlorambucil (Leukeran)	PO	2-8 mg/day	Marrow suppression (particularly thrombocytopenia), tumors, susceptibility to infection
Cyclophosphamide (Cytoxan, Neosar)	PO	25-150 mg/day	Marrow suppression, hemorrhagic cystitis, transitional cell carcinoma and other tumors, susceptibility to infection

Drug	Delivery	Dose	Side effects
Leflunomide (Arava)	PO	100 mg/day for 3 days, then 20 mg/day	Diarrhea, dyspepsia, rash, alopecia, hepatotoxicity, marrow suppression
Infliximab (Remicade)	IV	10 mg/kg infusions sporadically	Susceptibility to infection, autoimmune phenomenon, diarrhea, rash, infusion reactions
Etanercept (Enbrel)	SC	25 mg twice/wk	Injection site reactions, upper respiratory tract infections; theoretically, sepsis or tumors
Adalimumab (Humira)	SC	40 mg, every other week	Injection site reactions, upper respiratory tract infections; theoretically, sepsis or tumors

    F. Adjunctive therapies
        1. If the disease remains active (as demonstrated by inflamed joints) and/or the NSAID has produced toxicity, consider the following:
        2. Change NSAID
    G. Add prednisone or prednisolone
        1. Administer intraarticular steroids
        2. Prednisone can be added at a dose of up to 7.5 mg/day.
V. Severe disease
    A. NSAIDs. Therapy initially involves a NSAID in full antiinflammatory doses.
    B. DMARDs
        1. Unless contraindicated, methotrexate (MTX) is the DMARD of first choice for those with severe disease. The dose is 7.5 mg per week.
        2. Folic acid that can competitively inhibit the binding of dihydrofolic acid. Folic acid (1 to 2 mg/day) or folinic acid (2.5 to 5 mg per week, 8 to 12 hours after methotrexate) should be administered concurrently to reduce potential toxicity.
    C. Anticytokine therapy
        1. Etanercept (Enbrel). Etanercept is extremely effective in controlling symptoms and slowing the rate of radiographic progression in early severe RA (10 or 25 mg twice a week). Etanercept is contraindicated in women who are pregnant or nursing, and in patients with active infection.
        2. Infliximab (Remicade.) Unlike etanercept, which may be used alone, infliximab, a chimeric anti-TNF monoclonal antibody, is generally given in combination with methotrexate. It is therefore usually reserved for use in patients with moderate or severe disease who tolerate, but have had an inadequate response to, methotrexate.
        3. Adalimumab (Humira). The fully human anti-TNF monoclonal antibody, adalimumab, administered subcutaneously every two weeks is efficacious and can be used alone or combined with methotrexate treatment for RA.
        4. Anakinra (Kineret). Anakinra, a human interleukin-1 receptor antagonist, also may be of value in patients with active RA. It can be given alone or in combination with methotrexate. However, anakinra should not be given with anti-TNF therapy due to an increased risk of serious infections.
    D. Prednisone. If the patient is febrile, toxic or experiencing a rapid decline in function, prednisone (5 to 20 mg/day) is frequently added to the regimen of an NSAID and an DMARD. However, once the patient responds sufficiently, the

dose of prednisone should be tapered as rapidly as possible to less than 10 mg/day (usually by 8 to 12 weeks).
References, see page 372.

Deep Vein Thrombosis

The incidence of first-time venous thromboembolism (VTE) is 1.92 per 1000 person-years. Rates are higher in men than women, and increase with age. Most cases are of secondary VTE are associated with more than one underlying condition, such as cancer (48 percent), hospitalization (52 percent), surgery (42 percent), and major trauma (6 percent).

I. Initial approach to venous thromboembolism
  A. Risk factors for venous thromboembolism:
    1. History of immobilization or prolonged hospitalization/bed rest
    2. Recent surgery
    3. Obesity
    4. Prior episode(s) of venous thromboembolism
    5. Lower extremity trauma
    6. Malignancy
    7. Use of oral contraceptives or hormone replacement therapy
    8. Pregnancy or postpartum status
    9. Stroke

Causes of Venous Thrombosis

Inherited thrombophilia. May be present in 24% of cases

Factor V Leiden mutation
Prothrombin gene mutation
Protein S deficiency
Protein C deficiency
Antithrombin (AT) deficiency
Rare disorders
  Dysfibrinogenemia
  Increased factor VIII coagulant activity

Acquired disorders	

Malignancy
  Tissue factor
  Cancer procoagulant
Presence of a central venous catheter
Surgery, especially orthopedic
Trauma
Pregnancy
Oral contraceptives
Hormone replacement therapy
Tamoxifen
Immobilization
Congestive heart failure
Hyperhomocyst(e)inemia
	Antiphospholipid antibody syndrome
	Myeloproliferative disorders
	  Polycythemia vera
	  Essential thrombocythemia
	Paroxysmal nocturnal hemoglobinuria
	Inflammatory bowel disease
	Nephrotic syndrome
	Hyperviscosity
	  Waldenstrom's macroglobulinemia
	  Multiple myeloma
	  Polycythemia vera
	Marked leukocytosis in acute leuke-
	mia
	Sickle cell anemia

B. History. Classic symptoms of DVT include swelling, pain, and discoloration of the extremity.

1. Assess the age of onset, location of prior thromboses, and results of diagnostic studies documenting thrombotic episodes in the patient, as well as in any family members. A history of venous thrombosis in one or more first-degree relatives strongly suggests the presence of a hereditary defect.

2. Potential precipitating conditions: Surgical procedures, trauma, pregnancy, heart failure, and immobility. Women should be questioned about use of oral contraceptives or hormone replacement therapy as well as their obstetric history. The presence of recurrent fetal loss suggests the possible presence of an inherited thrombophilia or antiphospholipid antibodies.

3. Events proximate to the time of thrombosis, previous outcome of situations that predispose to thrombosis, such as pregnancy, caesarian section, and surgery. If the patient has undergone these events without thrombosis, then it suggests the presence of an acquired hypercoagulable state, such antiphospholipid syndrome or malignancy, rather than a hereditary defect.

4. Collagen-vascular disease, myeloproliferative disease, atherosclerotic disease, or nephrotic syndrome and the use of drugs which can induce antiphospholipid antibodies such as hydralazine, procainamide, and phenothiazines.

5. Past history of cancer, and the results of regular screening examinations for cancer (eg, mammography, colonoscopy, pelvic examinations). Other findings that may suggest an underlying malignancy are loss of appetite, weight loss, fatigue, pain, hematochezia, hemoptysis, and hematuria.

C. Physical examination may reveal a palpable cord (reflecting a thrombosed vein), ipsilateral edema, warmth, and/or superficial venous dilation.

1. Signs of superficial or deep vein thrombosis: Skin necrosis, livedo reticularis, pain and tenderness in the thigh along the course of the major veins ("painful deep vein syndrome"). Tenderness on deep palpation of the calf muscles is suggestive, but not diagnostic. Homan's sign, pain with dorsiflexion of the ankle, is unreliable.

2. Other signs and symptoms have variable sensitivity and specificity for DVT:
   a. Edema — 97, 33 percent
   b. Pain — 86, 19 percent
   c. Warmth — 72 percent

3. The physical examination also may reveal signs of hepatic vein thrombosis (Budd-Chiari syndrome), such as ascites and hepatomegaly, or edema due to the nephrotic syndrome.

4. **Screening for malignancy.** Venous thromboembolism may be the first manifestation of an underlying malignancy; therefore, rectal examination and stool testing for occult blood should be performed and women should undergo a pelvic examination to rule out the presence of a previously unsuspected pelvic mass or malignancy.

II. Differential diagnosis

A. Common causes of leg pain and swelling

1. Muscle strain, tear, or twisting injury to the leg — 40 percent
2. Leg swelling in a paralyzed limb — 9 percent
3. Lymphangitis or lymph obstruction — 7 percent
4. Venous insufficiency — 7 percent
5. Popliteal (Baker's) cyst — 5 percent
6. Cellulitis — 3 percent
7. Knee abnormality — 2 percent
8. Unknown — 26 percent

B. Cellulitis.
Bacterial cellulitis is a frequent complication in the leg with chronic swelling due to venous insufficiency or lymphedema.

C. Superficial thrombophlebitis
is most likely in the presence of palpable, tender superficial veins.

D. Venous valvular insufficiency.
Chronic venous insufficiency is the most common cause of chronic unilateral leg edema and is usually associated with a past history of DVT.

E. Lymphedema
is an important cause of chronic edema of the extremities.

F. Popliteal (Baker's) cyst.
The majority of popliteal cysts in adults are caused by either distention of a bursa by fluid. A popliteal cyst that causes calf symptoms is usually leaking or has ruptured.

G. Internal derangement of the knee.
Pain, inflammation, and swelling can accompany knee joint inflammation.

H. Drug-induced edema.
Leg swelling is a side effect of calcium channel blockers. The edema is usually bilateral; signs of inflammation are not present.

I. Calf muscle pull or tear
is frequently induced by strenuous physical activity. There may be signs of bleeding within muscle compartments of the affected leg.

III. Laboratory testing.
A complete blood count, coagulation studies (eg, prothrombin time, activated partial thromboplastin time), renal function tests, and urinalysis. A prostate-specific antigen measurement in men over the age of 50.

IV. Diagnostic testing

A. Contrast venography
is not recommended as an initial screening due to patient discomfort and difficulty in obtaining an adequate study. Venography is reserved for situations in which ultrasound or impedance plethysmography is not feasible, when noninvasive studies are equivocal, or when noninvasive studies are discordant with a strong clinical impression.

B. Noninvasive tests.

1. **Impedance plethysmography** requires the patient to lie still while a thigh cuff is inflated. The change in blood volume at the calf is measured from the impedance of the calf as determined by electrodes wrapped around it. After rapid deflation of the cuff, the proportional change of impedance over the subsequent three seconds is used to measure venous outflow obstruction. Many facilities do not have the equipment to perform impedance plethysmography, while the availability of ultrasonography is more wide-

spread. Impedance plethysmography is the preferred test for the evaluation of suspected recurrent DVT.

2. **Compression ultrasonography.** The chronicity of the thrombus may be inferred from the echogenicity of the clot.

   a. **Procedure.** The diagnosis of venous thrombosis using compression ultrasonography is made by the findings such as:

      (1) Abnormal compressibility of the vein

      (2) Abnormal Doppler color flow

      (3) The presence of an echogenic band

      (4) Abnormal change in diameter during the Valsalva maneuver

   b. **Accuracy.** Compression ultrasonography has a sensitivity and specificity of 100 and 99 percent, respectively.

3. **D-dimer**, is a degradation product of cross-linked fibrin. D-dimers are detectable at levels greater than 500 ng/mL of fibrinogen equivalent units in nearly all patients with venous thromboembolism.

   a. However, the finding of elevated D-dimer concentrations alone is insufficient to establish the diagnosis of venous thromboembolism, because elevated D-dimer levels are not specific for VTE and are commonly present in hospitalized patients, particularly the elderly, those with malignancy, recent surgery, and other conditions.

   b. **Addition of Wells score.** A D-dimer level less than 200 to 500 ng/mL by ELISA or a negative SimpliRED assay in conjunction with a low clinical probability of DVT appears to be useful and cost-effective in excluding DVT without the need for an ultrasound examination.

Disorders associated with increased fibrin D-dimer

Arterial thromboembolic disease
Myocardial infarction
Stroke
Acute limb ischemia
Atrial fibrillation
Intracardiac thrombus
Venous thromboembolic disease
Deep vein thrombosis
Pulmonary embolism
Disseminated intravascular coagulation
Preeclampsia and eclampsia
Abnormal fibrinolysis; use of thrombolytic agents
Cardiovascular disease, congestive failure
Severe infection/sepsis/inflammation
Surgery/trauma (eg, tissue ischemia, necrosis)
Systemic inflammatory response syndrome
Vasoocclusive episode of sickle cell disease
Severe liver disease (decreased clearance)
Malignancy
Renal disease
Nephrotic syndrome (eg, renal vein thrombosis)
Acute renal failure
Chronic renal failure and underlying cardiovascular disease
Normal pregnancy

Pretest probability of deep vein thrombosis (Modified Wells score)	
Clinical feature	**Score**
Active cancer (treatment ongoing or within the previous 6 months or palliative)	1
Paralysis, paresis, or recent plaster immobilization of the lower extremities	1
Recently bedridden for more than 3 days or major surgery, within 4 weeks	1
Localized tenderness along the distribution of the deep venous system	1
Entire leg swollen	1
Calf swelling by more than 3 cm when compared to the asymptomatic leg (measured below tibial tuberosity)	1
Pitting edema (greater in the symptomatic leg)	1
Collateral superficial veins (nonvaricose)	1
Previously documented deep vein thrombosis (DVT)	1
Alternative diagnosis as likely or more likely than that of deep venous thrombosis	-2
DVT likely	2 or greater
DVT unlikely	1 or less

C. **Approach to diagnosis of deep vein thrombosis.**

1. Initial evaluation should assess the probability of DVT using the Wells score and D-dimer. If the probability of DVT is likely, obtain a compression ultrasound.

2. In selected patients with a low pretest probability of DVT according to the Wells score and a negative D-dimer, the likelihood of DVT is low, and further testing (eg, ultrasonography) is not be needed.

3. If the probability of DVT is likely according to the Wells score, ultrasound evaluation is recommended. Repeat ultrasound or venography may be required for those with suspected calf vein DVT and a negative initial ultrasound investigation.

4. Compression ultrasonography is the noninvasive approach of choice for the diagnosis of patients with suspected DVT. Impedance plethysmography with serial studies is an acceptable alternative. Impedance plethysmography is preferred for possible recurrent DVT since it normalizes more quickly after a previous episode than compression ultrasonography.

5. A positive noninvasive study in patients with a first episode of DVT usually establishes the diagnosis, with positive predictive values for compression ultrasonography and impedance plethysmography of 94 percent and 83 percent, respectively. If the initial study is negative and the clinical suspicion of DVT is high, a repeat study should be obtained on day 5 to 7. Venography is currently used only when noninvasive testing is not clinically feasible or the results are equivocal.

V. Treatment of deep vein thrombosis
A. Treatment of DVT prevents the following complications:
1. Prevent further clot extension
2. Prevention of acute pulmonary embolism
3. Reducing the risk of recurrent thrombosis
4. Treatment of massive iliofemoral thrombosis with acute lower limb ischemia and/or venous gangrene (ie, phlegmasia cerulea dolens)
5. Limiting the development of late complications, such as the postphlebitic syndrome, chronic venous insufficiency, and chronic thromboembolic pulmonary hypertension.
6. Anticoagulant therapy is indicated for patients with symptomatic proximal DVT, since pulmonary embolism will occur in 50 percent of untreated individuals, most often within days or weeks of the event.

B. Anticoagulation.
Patients with DVT or pulmonary embolism should be treated immediately with LMW heparin, unfractionated intravenous heparin, or adjusted-dose subcutaneous heparin.
1. Enoxaparin (Lovenox) 1.0 mg/kg SQ q12h
2. When unfractionated heparin is used, the dose should be sufficient to prolong the activated partial thromboplastin time (aPTT) to 1.5 to 2.5 times the mean of the control value, or the upper limit of the normal aPTT range.
3. **Treatment with LMW heparin or heparin** should be continued for at least five days and oral anticoagulation should be overlapped with LMW heparin or unfractionated heparin for at least four to five days. Warfarin can be initiated simultaneously with the heparin, at an initial oral dose not exceeding 5 to 10 mg per day. Heparin can be discontinued on day five or six if the INR has been therapeutic for two consecutive days.
4. For patients receiving unfractionated heparin (UFH), platelet counts be obtained regularly to monitor for thrombocytopenia. The heparin product should be stopped if the platelet count falls, or a platelet count <100,000/microL.

Management of Deep Venous Thrombosis

Superficial Venous Thrombosis
- Use compression ultrasound to screen for involvement of deep system
- Elevation, nonsteroidal anti-inflammatory drugs

Deep Venous Thrombosis
- Begin warfarin on the first hospital day
- Low-molecular-weight heparin--more effective and safer than standard heparin. Enoxaparin 1.0 mg/kg SQ q12h

Phlegmasia Dolens
- Enoxaparin (Lovenox) 1.0 mg/kg SQ q12h
- Heparin 80 U/kg load, 18 U/kg/hr drip
- Thrombolysis for severe disease in young adults
- Vena cava filter if thrombosis in presence of adequate anticoagulation

Exclusions for Home Treatment for DVT

Medical Exclusions
  Concurrent Pulmonary Embolism (PE)
  Serious co-morbid condition
  Cancer, infection, stroke
  Prior DVT or PE
  Contraindications to anticoagulation
  Familial bleeding disorder
  Known deficiency of Antithrombin III, Protein C, Protein S Pregnancy
Social Exclusions
  No phone
  Lives far from hospital
  Unable to understand instructions or comply with follow-up
  Family or patient resistance to home therapy

Low Molecular Weight Heparin Protocol

Subcutaneous enoxaparin (Lovenox) 1 mg/kg q12hours for a minimum of five days and achieving INR of 2-3 (from warfarin therapy)
Warfarin to be started on first day of therapy
INR should be monitored during outpatient treatment
Warn patients to return immediately for shortness of breath, hemorrhage, or clinical decomposition

Weight-based nomogram for intravenous heparin infusion

Initial dose	80 U/kg bolus, then 18 U/kg per hour
aPTT* <35 sec (<1.2 x control)	80 U/kg bolus, then increase infusion rate by 4 U/kg per hour
aPTT	40 U/kg per hour, then increase infusion by 2 U/kg per hour
aPTT	No change
aPTT	Decrease infusion rate by 2q U/kg per hour
aPTT	Hold infusion 1 hour, then decrease infusion rate by 3 U/kg per hour
*aPTT = activated partial thromboplastin time	

C. **Thrombolytic agents** are initiated in patients with hemodynamically unstable PE or massive iliofemoral thrombosis (ie, phlegmasia cerulea dolens), and who are also at low risk to bleed.
  1. **Recombinant tissue type plasminogen activator (tPA, Activase).** tPA binds to fibrin, which increases its affinity for plasminogen and enhances plasminogen activation. tPA is recommended because it has an infusion time that is short (two hours), and it is not associated with allergic reactions or hypotension. Administer 100 mg intravenously over two hours.
D. **Inferior vena caval filter** placement is recommended when there is a contraindication to, or a complication of, anticoagulant therapy in an individual with, or

at high risk for, proximal vein thrombosis or PE. It is also recommended in patients with recurrent thromboembolism despite adequate anticoagulation.
  E. Oral anticoagulation with warfarin should prolong the INR to a target of 2.5 (range: 2.0 to 3.0).
   1. Patients with a first thromboembolic event in the context of a reversible risk factor should be treated for at least three months. Patients with a first idiopathic thromboembolic event should be treated for at least six to twelve months. Most patients with advanced malignancy should be treated indefinitely or until the cancer resolves.
   2. Indefinite anticoagulation is recommended in high risk patients. This includes patients with two or more spontaneous thromboses, one spontaneous life-threatening thrombosis, one spontaneous thrombosis at an unusual site (eg, mesenteric or cerebral vein), or one spontaneous thrombosis in the presence of laboratory markers of the antiphospholipid syndrome, two or more genetic defects predisposing to a thromboembolic event, or hereditary antithrombin deficiency.
   3. Once anticoagulation has been started and the patient's symptoms (ie, pain, swelling) are under control, the patient is encouraged to ambulate. During initial ambulation, and for the first two years following an episode of VTE, use of an elastic compression stocking is recommended to prevent the postphlebitic syndrome.

References, see page 372.

Acute Pulmonary Embolism

More than 500,000 cases of pulmonary emboli occur annually, resulting in 200,000 deaths each year. Pulmonary embolism is associated with a mortality rate of 30 percent if untreated. Diagnosis followed by therapy with anticoagulants significantly decreases the mortality rate to 2 to 8 percent.

I. Definitions
  A. Massive pulmonary embolism (PE) has been defined as a PE associated with a systolic blood pressure <90 mmHg or a drop in systolic blood pressure of 40 mmHg from baseline for a period >15 minutes, which is not otherwise explained by hypovolemia, sepsis, or a new arrhythmia. It often results in acute right ventricular failure and death.
  B. All PE not meeting the definition of massive PE are considered submassive PE.
  C. Pulmonary embolism (PE) is associated with a mortality rate of 30 percent without treatment, primarily the result of recurrent embolism. Accurate diagnosis and effective therapy with anticoagulants decreases the mortality rate to 2 to 8 percent.

II. Pathophysiology
  A. 65 to 90 percent of pulmonary emboli (PE) arise from thrombi in the deep venous system of the lower extremities; however, they may also originate in the pelvic, renal, or upper extremity veins and in the right heart.
  B. Iliofemoral thrombi are the source of most clinically recognized PE. 50 to 80 percent of iliac, femoral, and popliteal vein thrombi (proximal vein thrombi) originate below the popliteal vein (calf vein thrombi) and propagate proximally.
  C. After traveling to the lung, large thrombi may lodge at the bifurcation of the main pulmonary artery or the lobar branches and cause hemodynamic compromise. Ten percent of emboli cause pulmonary infarction.

III. Risk factors

A. Patients with pulmonary emboli (PE) usually have identifiable risk factors for the development of venous thrombosis.

B. Risk factors for pulmonary embolism:
   1. Immobilization
   2. Surgery within the last three months
   3. Stroke
   4. History of venous thromboembolism
   5. Malignancy
   6. Preexisting respiratory disease
   7. Chronic heart disease

C. Additional risk factors for pulmonary embolism in women:
   1. Obesity (BMI 29 kg/m^2)
   2. Heavy cigarette smoking (>25 cigarettes per day)
   3. Hypertension

D. Patients with PE without identifiable risk factors (ie, idiopathic or primary venous thromboembolism) may have unsuspected abnormalities that favor the development of thromboembolic disease:
   1. Factor V Leiden mutation (40 percent of cases)
   2. Increased factor VIII (11 percent of population)
   3. Some patients have more than one type of inherited thrombophilia, or have a combination of inherited plus acquired thrombophila, which places them at even greater risk.
   4. Malignancy is eventually detected in 17 percent of patients who have recurrent idiopathic venous thromboembolism. When PE complicates cancer, it is more likely to be the presenting sign of pancreatic or prostate cancer and to occur later in the course of breast, lung, uterine, or brain cancer.

IV. Clinical evaluation

A. Common symptoms of pulmonary embolism are dyspnea (73 percent), pleuritic pain (66 percent), cough (37 percent) and hemoptysis (13 percent). Hemoptysis is blood tinged, blood streaked, or pure blood.

B. Common signs of pulmonary embolism are tachypnea (70 percent), rales (51 percent), tachycardia (30 percent), a fourth heart sound (24 percent), and an accentuated pulmonic component of the second heart sound (23 percent). Circulatory collapse is uncommon (8 percent).

C. Fever, usually with a temperature <102.0°F (38.9°C), occurs in 14 percent of patients.

D. In patients with massive PE, acute right ventricular failure may be manifested by increased jugular venous pressure, a right-sided S3, and a parasternal lift.

E. Most patients with PE have no leg symptoms at the time of diagnosis. Less than 30 percent of patients with PE have symptoms or signs of lower extremity venous thrombosis.

F. Patients with symptomatic deep venous thrombosis (DVT) may have asymptomatic PE. In patients with DVT, pulmonary embolism is present in 56 percent.

Frequency of Symptoms and Signs in Pulmonary Embolism			
Symptoms	**Frequency (%)**	**Signs**	**Frequency (%)**
Dyspnea	84	Tachypnea (>16/min)	92
Pleuritic chest pain	74	Rales	58
Apprehension	59	Accentuated S2	53
Cough	53	Tachycardia	44
Hemoptysis	30	Fever (>37.8°C)	43
Sweating	27	Diaphoresis	36
Non-pleuritic chest pain	14	S3 or S4 gallop	34
		Thrombophlebitis	32

Modified Wells criteria: clinical assessment for pulmonary embolism	
Clinical symptoms of DVT (leg swelling, pain with palpation)	3.0
Other diagnosis less likely than pulmonary embolism	3.0
Heart rate >100	1.5
Immobilization (≥3 days) or surgery in the previous four weeks	1.5
Previous DVT/PE	1.5
Hemoptysis	1.0
Malignancy	1.0
Probability	Score
Simplified clinical probability assessment	
PE likely	>4.0
PE unlikely	≤4.0

V. Diagnostic tests

A. **Laboratory** findings are nonspecific and include leukocytosis, an increase in the erythrocyte sedimentation rate (ESR), and an elevated serum LDH or AST with a normal serum bilirubin.

B. **Arterial blood gas (ABG)** usually reveal hypoxemia, hypocapnia, and respiratory alkalosis.

   1. Typical arterial blood gas findings are not always seen. Massive PE with hypotension and respiratory collapse can cause hypercapnia and a combined respiratory and metabolic acidosis. In addition, hypoxemia can be minimal or absent. A PaO2 between 85 and 105 mmHg exists in approximately 18 percent of patients with PE and up to six percent may have a normal alveolar-arterial gradient for oxygen.

C. **Brain natriuretic peptide (BNP)** levels are typically greater in patients with PE compared to patients without PE; however, many patients with PE do not have elevated BNP levels (ie, it is insensitive) and there are many alternative causes of an elevated BNP level (ie, it is nonspecific), limiting its usefulness as a diagnostic test.

    1. BNP has a sensitivity and specificity of only 60 and 62 percent for acute PE.

D. Troponin. Serum troponin I and troponin T are elevated in 30 to 50 percent of patients with a moderate to large pulmonary embolism because of acute right heart overload.

E. Electrocardiography. 70 percent of patients have ECG abnormalities, most commonly nonspecific ST-segment and T-wave changes.

F. Chest radiography. Radiographic abnormalities are common in patients with PE; however, they are also common in patients without PE.

    1. Atelectasis is noted in 69 and 58 percent of patients with and without PE, respectively.

    2. Pleural effusion is detected in 47 and 39 percent of patients with and without PE, respectively.

G. Ventilation/Perfusion Scan

    1. Patients with high clinical probability and a high-probability V/Q scan have a 95 percent likelihood of having PE.

    2. Patients with low clinical probability and a low-probability V/Q scan have only a 4 percent likelihood of having PE.

    3. A normal V/Q scan virtually excludes PE.

H. D-dimer is a degradation product of cross-linked fibrin. A new rapid ELISA is quick and accurate. A level >500 ng/mL is considered abnormal.

    1. Use of D-dimer assays for the diagnosis of PE has a good sensitivity and negative predictive value, but poor specificity:

    2. Sensitivity. D-dimer levels are abnormal in 95 percent of patients with PE.

    3. Negative predictive value. Patients with normal D-dimer levels have a 95 percent likelihood of not having PE.

    4. Specificity. D-dimer levels are normal in only 25 percent of patients without PE.

Disorders associated with increased fibrin D-dimer

Arterial thromboembolic disease
Myocardial infarction
Stroke
Acute limb ischemia
Atrial fibrillation
Intracardiac thrombus
Venous thromboembolic disease
Deep vein thrombosis
Pulmonary embolism
Disseminated intravascular coagulation
Preeclampsia and eclampsia
Abnormal fibrinolysis; use of thrombolytic agents
Cardiovascular disease, congestive failure
Severe infection, sepsis, inflammation
Surgery, trauma (eg, tissue ischemia, necrosis)
Systemic inflammatory response syndrome
Vasoocclusive episode of sickle cell disease
Severe liver disease (decreased clearance)
Malignancy
Renal disease
Nephrotic syndrome (eg, renal vein thrombosis)
Acute renal failure

Chronic renal failure and underlying cardiovascular disease
Normal pregnancy

A. **Pulmonary angiography** is the definitive diagnostic technique or "gold standard" in the diagnosis of acute PE. It is performed by injecting contrast into a pulmonary artery. Mortality of the procedure is two percent. Morbidity occurs in five percent, usually related to catheter insertion, contrast reactions, cardiac arrhythmia, or respiratory insufficiency.

B. **Spiral CT.** Spiral (helical) CT scanning with intravenous contrast (ie, CT pulmonary angiography or CT-PA) is being used increasingly. One of the benefits of CT-PA is the ability to detect alternative pulmonary abnormalities.

   1. 87 percent of patients with PE are detected by CT-PA. The frequency of negative CT-PA among patients without PE has been more consistent (90 percent).

   2. In the largest study to date (824 patients), the accuracy of CT-PA with and without clinical probability assessment (using the Well's criteria) prior to the CT-PA was determined by comparison against a composite reference standard. Key findings included:

      a. 83 percent of patients with PE had a positive CT-PA. Conversely, 96 percent of patients without PE had a negative CT-PA. Addition of venous-phase imaging improved the sensitivity (90 percent) with similar specificity (95 percent).

      b. There is a low risk of PE following a negative CT-PA. However, CT-PA results that are discordant with clinical suspicion should be viewed with skepticism and additional testing performed.

II. **Diagnostic approach to pulmonary embolism.** When PE is suspected because of sudden onset of dyspnea, or sudden onset of pleuritic chest pain without another apparent cause, CT-pulmonary angiogram is the most accessible diagnostic modality.

A. When PE is suspected, the modified Wells criteria should be applied to determine if PE is unlikely (score <4) or likely (score >4). The modified Wells Criteria include the following:

   1. Clinical symptoms of DVT (3 points)
   2. Other diagnosis less likely than PE (3 points)
   3. Heart rate >100 (1.5 points)
   4. Immobilization or surgery in previous four weeks (1.5 points)
   5. Previous DVT/PE (1.5 points)
   6. Hemoptysis (1 point)
   7. Malignancy (1 point)

B. Patients classified as PE unlikely should undergo quantitative D-dimer testing. If the D-dimer level is <500 ng/mL, the diagnosis of PE can be excluded.

C. Patients classified as PE likely should undergo CT-PA.

D. Patients classified as PE unlikely who have a D-dimer level >500 ng/mL should undergo CT-PA. A positive CT-PA confirms the diagnosis of PE. Alternatively, a negative CT-PA excludes the diagnosis of PE. In those rare instances in which the CT-PA is inconclusive, pulmonary angiography should be performed.

III. **Treatment of acute pulmonary embolism**

A. **Resuscitation**

   1. **Respiratory support.** Supplemental oxygen should be administered if hypoxemia exists. Severe hypoxemia and/or respiratory failure requires intubation and mechanical ventilation.

2. **Hemodynamic support.** PE that causes persistent hypotension (systolic <90 mmHg) is referred to as massive PE. Hemodynamic support should be started immediately.
   a. Intravenous fluid administration may be beneficial, but should be administered cautiously because intravenous fluids can precipitate right ventricular (RV) failure. Intravenous fluids should be administered cautiously. Clinicians should usually avoid administering more than 500 to 1000 mL during the initial resuscitation period.
   b. If the patient's hypotension does not resolve with intravenous fluids, vasopressor therapy should be initiated immediately:
      (1) Norepinephrine is least likely to cause tachycardia. Dopamine is least expensive and often most readily available.
3. **Anticoagulation.** Initiation of PE-directed therapy should be considered during the resuscitative period.
   a. For a patient in whom there is a high clinical suspicion of PE, empiric anticoagulant therapy should be initiated. The high incidence of mortality due to recurrent PE in untreated patients (30 percent) outweighs the risk of major bleeding (less than three percent).

Weight-based nomogram for intravenous heparin infusion	
Initial dose	80 U/kg bolus, then 18 U/kg per hour
aPTT* <35 sec (<1.2 x control)	80 U/kg bolus, then increase infusion rate by 4 U/kg per hour
aPTT	40 U/kg per hour, then increase infusion by 2 U/kg per hour
aPTT	No change
aPTT	Decrease infusion rate by 2q U/kg per hour
aPTT	Hold infusion 1 hour, then decrease infusion rate by 3 U/kg per hour
*aPTT = activated partial thromboplastin time	

B. General approach
1. Patients in whom anticoagulation was initiated during the resuscitative period should remain anticoagulated during the diagnostic evaluation. Long-term anticoagulation is indicated if PE is confirmed. Anticoagulation should be discontinued of PE is excluded.
2. Thrombolysis should be considered once PE is confirmed. If thrombolysis is chosen, anticoagulation should be temporarily discontinued during the thrombolytic infusion, then resumed.
3. If anticoagulation is contraindicated, fails, or causes severe bleeding, inferior vena caval filter placement should be considered.
4. Patients whose presentation is severe enough to warrant thrombolysis (eg, persistent hypotension) should be considered for embolectomy if thrombolysis is contraindicated or unsuccessful.

C. **Anticoagulation** reduces mortality due to pulmonary embolism; thus, it is the primary therapy. The goal of anticoagulation is to decrease mortality by preventing recurrent PE.

1. Anticoagulation should be initiated using subcutaneous low molecular weight heparin (SC LMWH) or intravenous unfractionated heparin (IV UFH). Hemodynamically stable patients with PE should receive, SC LMWH should be used. Patients with persistent hypotension caused by PE (ie, massive PE) or severe renal failure IV UFH should be used.
2. Enoxaparin (Lovenox) 1.0 mg/kg SC bid
3. Tinzaparin (Innohep) 175 Xa U/kg sc once daily
4. Dalteparin (Fragmin) 200 Xa U/kg sc once daily

D. **Thrombolytic therapy** accelerates the lysis of acute pulmonary emboli (PE) but may be associated with major hemorrhage, (intracranial hemorrhage, retroperitoneal hemorrhage, or bleeding leading directly to death, hospitalization, or transfusion).

1. Persistent hypotension due to PE (ie, massive PE) is an indication for thrombolytic therapy. Thrombolysis should be considered for severe hypoxemia, large perfusion defects, right ventricular dysfunction, free floating right ventricular thrombus, and patent foramen ovale.
2. Recombinant tissue type plasminogen activator (tPA, Activase). tPA binds to fibrin, which increases its affinity for plasminogen and enhances plasminogen activation. tPA is recommended because it has an infusion time that is short (two hours), and it is not associated with allergic reactions or hypotension. Administer 100 mg intravenously over two hours.

E. **Inferior vena caval (IVC) filters** obstruct the inferior vena cava, allowing blood to pass through while preventing large emboli from traveling from the pelvis or lower extremities to the lung.

1. **Indications for an inferior vena cava (IVC) filter after pulmonary embolism**:
   a. Absolute contraindication to anticoagulation (eg, active bleeding).
   b. Recurrent PE during adequate anticoagulant therapy.
   c. Complication of anticoagulation (eg, severe bleeding).
   d. Patients with PE who have poor cardiopulmonary reserve (ie, recurrent PE likely to be fatal) and patients who have undergone embolectomy (surgical or catheter).
2. **Outcome.** IVC filters decrease recurrent PE. However, a reduction in mortality has not been conclusively demonstrated.

F. **Embolectomy** can be performed using catheters or surgically. It should be considered when a patient's presentation is severe enough (eg, persistent hypotension due to PE) to warrant thrombolysis and thrombolysis either fails or is contraindicated.

References, see page 372.

Anemia

The prevalence of anemia is about 29 to 30 cases per 1,000 females of all ages and six cases per 1,000 males under the age of 45 Deficiencies of iron, vitamin B12 and folic acid are the most common causes.

I. **Clinical manifestations.** Severe anemia may be tolerated well if it develops gradually. Patients with an Hb of less than 7 g/dL will have symptoms of tissue hypoxia (fatigue, headache, dyspnea, light-headedness, angina). Pallor, syncope and tachycardia may signal hypovolemia and impending shock.

II. History and physical examination

A. The evaluation should determine if the anemia is of acute or chronic onset, and clues to any underlying systemic process should be sought. A history of drug exposure, blood loss, or a family history of anemia should be sought.

B. Lymphadenopathy, hepatic or splenic enlargement, jaundice, bone tenderness, neurologic symptoms or blood in the feces should be sought.

III. Laboratory evaluation

A. **Hemoglobin and hematocrit** serve as an estimate of the RBC mass.

B. **Reticulocyte count** reflects the rate of marrow production of RBCs. Absolute reticulocyte count = (% reticulocytes/100) × RBC count. An increase of reticulocytes to greater than 100,000/mm^3 suggests a hyperproliferative bone marrow.

C. **Mean corpuscular volume (MCV)** is used in classifying anemia as microcytic, normocytic or macrocytic.

Normal Hematologic Values			
Age of patient	Hemoglobin	Hematocrit (%)	Mean corpuscular volume (pm^3)
One to three days	14.5-22.5 g per dL	45-67	95-121
Six months to two years	10.5-13.5 g per dL	33-39	70-86
12 to 18 years (male)	13.0-16.0 g per dL	37-49	78-98
12 to 18 years (female)	12.0-16.0 g per dL	36-46	78-102
>18 years (male)	13.5-17.5 g per dL	41-53	78-98
>18 years (female)	12.0-16.0 g per dL	36-46	78-98

IV. Iron deficiency anemia

A. Iron deficiency is the most common cause of anemia. In children, the deficiency is typically caused by diet. In adults, the cause should be considered to be a result of chronic blood loss until a definitive diagnosis is established.

B. **Laboratory results**

1. The MCV is normal in early iron deficiency. As the hematocrit falls below 30%, hypochromic microcytic cells appear, followed by a decrease in the MCV.

2. **A serum ferritin level** of less than 10 ng/mL in women or 20 ng/mL in men is indicative of low iron stores. A serum ferritin level of more than 200 ng/mL indicates adequate iron stores.

C. **Treatment of iron deficiency anemia**

1. Ferrous salts of iron are absorbed much more readily and are preferred. Commonly available oral preparations include ferrous sulfate, ferrous gluconate and ferrous fumarate (Hemocyte). All three forms are well absorbed. Ferrous sulfate is the least expensive and most commonly used oral iron supplement.

Oral Iron Preparations			
Preparation	Elemental iron (%)	Typical dosage	Elemental iron per dose
Ferrous sulfate	20	325 mg three times daily	65 mg
Ferrous sulfate, exsiccated (Feosol)	30	200 mg three times daily	65 mg
Ferrous gluconate	12	325 mg three times daily	36 mg
Ferrous fumarate (Hemocyte)	33	325 mg twice daily	106 mg

2. For iron replacement therapy, a dosage equivalent to 150 to 200 mg of elemental iron per day is recommended.

3. Ferrous sulfate, 325 mg of three times a day, will provide the necessary elemental iron for replacement therapy. Hematocrit levels should show improvement within one to two months.

4. Depending on the cause and severity of the anemia, replacement of low iron stores usually requires four to six months of iron supplementation. A daily dosage of 325 mg of ferrous sulfate is necessary for maintenance therapy.

5. **Side effects** from oral iron replacement therapy are common and include nausea, constipation, diarrhea and abdominal pain. Iron supplements should be taken with food; however, this may decrease iron absorption by 40 to 66 percent. Changing to a different iron salt or to a controlled-release preparation may also reduce side effects.

6. For optimum delivery, oral iron supplements must dissolve rapidly in the stomach so that the iron can be absorbed in the duodenum and upper jejunum. Enteric-coated preparations are ineffective since they do not dissolve in the stomach.

7. Causes of resistance to iron therapy include continuing blood loss, ineffective intake and ineffective absorption. Continuing blood loss may be overt (eg, menstruation, hemorrhoids) or occult (e.g., gastrointestinal malignancies, intestinal parasites, nonsteroidal anti-inflammatory drugs).

V. Vitamin B12 deficiency anemia

A. Since body stores of vitamin B12 are adequate for up to five years, deficiency is generally the result of failure to absorb it. Pernicious anemia, Crohn's disease and other intestinal disorders are the most frequent causes of vitamin B12 deficiency.

B. Symptoms are attributable primarily to anemia, although glossitis, jaundice, and splenomegaly may be present. Vitamin B12 deficiency may cause decreased vibratory and positional sense, ataxia, paresthesias, confusion, and dementia. Neurologic complications may occur in the absence of anemia and may not resolve completely despite adequate treatment. Folic acid deficiency does not cause neurologic disease.

C. Laboratory results

1. A macrocytic anemia usually is present, and leukopenia and thrombocytopenia may occur. Lactate dehydrogenase (LDH) and indirect bilirubin typically are elevated.

    2. Vitamin B12 levels are low. RBC folate levels should be measured to exclude folate deficiency.

  D. Treatment of vitamin B12 deficiency anemia. Intramuscular, oral or intranasal preparations are available for B12 replacement. In patients with severe vitamin B12 deficiency, daily IM injections of 1,000 mcg of cyanocobalamin are recommended for five days, followed by weekly injections for four weeks. Hematologic improvement should begin within five to seven days, and the deficiency should resolve after three to four weeks.

Vitamin B12 and Folic Acid Preparations	
Preparation	**Dosage**
Cyanocobalamin tablets	1,000 µg daily
Cyanocobalamin injection	1,000 µg weekly
Cyanocobalamin nasal gel (Nascobal)	500 µg weekly
Folic acid (Folvite)	1 mg daily

VI. Folate deficiency anemia

  A. Folate deficiency is characterized by megaloblastic anemia and low serum folate levels. Most patients with folate deficiency have inadequate intake. Lactate dehydrogenase (LDH) and indirect bilirubin typically are elevated, reflecting ineffective erythropoiesis and premature destruction of RBCs.

  B. RBC folate and serum vitamin B_{12} levels should be measured. RBC folate is a more accurate indicator of body folate stores than is serum folate, particularly if measured after folate therapy has been initiated.

  C. Treatment of folate deficiency anemia

    1. A once-daily dosage of 1 mg of folic acid given PO will replenish body stores in about three weeks.

    2. Folate supplementation is also recommended for women of child-bearing age to reduce the incidence of fetal neural tube defects. Folic acid should be initiated at 0.4 mg daily before conception. Prenatal vitamins contain this amount. Women who have previously given birth to a child with a neural tube defect should take 4 to 5 mg of folic acid daily.

References, see page 372.

Gynecologic Disorders

Osteoporosis

Over 1.3 million osteoporotic fractures occur each year in the United States. The risk of all fractures increases with age; among persons who survive until age 90, 33% of women will have a hip fracture. The lifetime risk of hip fracture for white women at age 50 is 16%. Osteoporosis is characterized by low bone mass, micro-architectural disruption, and increased skeletal fragility.

Risk Factors for Osteoporotic Fractures	
Personal history of fracture as an adult	White race
History of fracture in a first-degree relative	Advanced age
Current cigarette smoking	Lifelong low calcium intake
Low body weight (less than 58 kg [127 lb])	Alcoholism
Female sex	Inadequate physical activity
Estrogen deficiency (menopause before age 45 years or bilateral ovariectomy, prolonged premenopausal amenorrhea [>one year])	Recurrent falls
	Dementia
	Impaired eyesight despite adequate correction
	Poor health/frailty

I. **Screening for osteoporosis and osteopenia**
   A. **Normal bone density** is defined as a bone mineral density (BMD) value within one standard deviation of the mean value in young adults of the same sex and race.
   B. **Osteopenia** is defined as a BMD between 1 and 2.5 standard deviations below the mean.
   C. **Osteoporosis** is defined as a value more than 2.5 standard deviations below the mean; this level is the fracture threshold. These values are referred to as T-scores (number of standard deviations above or below the mean value).
   D. **Dual x-ray absorptiometry**. In dual x-ray absorptiometry (DXA), two photons are emitted from an x-ray tube. DXA is the most commonly used method for measuring bone density because it gives very precise measurements with minimal radiation. DXA measurements of the spine and hip are recommended.
II. **Recommendations for screening for osteoporosis of the National Osteoporosis Foundation**
   A. All women should be counseled about the risk factors for osteoporosis, especially smoking cessation and limiting alcohol. All women should be encouraged to participate in regular weight-bearing and exercise.
   B. Measurement of BMD is recommended for all women 65 years and older regardless of risk factors. BMD should also be measured in all women under the age of 65 years who have one or more risk factors for osteoporosis (in addition to menopause). The hip is the recommended site of measurement.
   C. All adults should be advised to consume at least 1,200 mg of calcium per day and 400 to 800 IU of vitamin D per day. A daily multivitamin (which provides 400 IU) is recommended. In patients with documented vitamin D deficiency, osteoporosis, or previous fracture, two multivitamins may be reasonable, particularly if dietary intake is inadequate and access to sunlight is poor.

    D. Treatment is recommended for women without risk factors who have a BMD that is 2 SD below the mean for young women, and in women with risk factors who have a BMD that is 1.5 SD below the mean.

III. Nonpharmacologic therapy of osteoporosis in women

    A. Diet. An optimal diet for treatment (or prevention) of osteoporosis includes an adequate intake of calories (to avoid malnutrition), calcium, and vitamin D.

    B. Calcium. Postmenopausal women should be advised to take 1000 to 1500 mg/day of elemental calcium, in divided doses, with meals.

    C. Vitamin D total of 800 IU daily should be taken.

    D. Exercise. Women should exercise for at least 30 minutes three times per week. Any weight-bearing exercise regimen, including walking, is acceptable.

    E. Cessation of smoking is recommended for all women because smoking cigarettes accelerates bone loss.

IV. Drug therapy of osteoporosis in women

    A. Selected postmenopausal women with osteoporosis or at high risk for the disease should be considered for drug therapy. Particular attention should be paid to treating women with a recent fragility fracture, including hip fracture, because they are at high risk for a second fracture.

    B. Candidates for drug therapy are women who already have postmenopausal osteoporosis (less than -2.5) and women with osteopenia (T score -1 to -2.5) soon after menopause.

    C. Bisphosphonates

        1. Alendronate (Fosamax) (10 mg/day or 70 mg once weekly) or **risedronate (Actonel)** (5 mg/day or 35 mg once weekly) are good choices for the treatment of osteoporosis. Bisphosphonate therapy increases bone mass and reduces the incidence of vertebral and nonvertebral fractures.

        2. Alendronate (5 mg/day or 35 mg once weekly) and risedronate (5 mg/day or 35 mg once weekly) have been approved for prevention of osteoporosis.

        3. Alendronate or risedronate should be taken with a full glass of water 30 minutes before the first meal or beverage of the day. Patients should not lie down for at least 30 minutes after taking the dose to avoid the unusual complication of pill-induced esophagitis.

        4. Alendronate is well tolerated and effective for at least seven years.

        5. The bisphosphonates (alendronate or risedronate) and raloxifene are first-line treatments for *prevention* of osteoporosis. The bisphosphonates are first-line therapy for *treatment* of osteoporosis. Bisphosphonates are preferred for prevention and treatment of osteoporosis because they increase bone mineral density more than raloxifene.

    D. Selective estrogen receptor modulators

        1. Raloxifene (Evista) (5 mg daily or a once-a-week preparation) is a selective estrogen receptor modulator (SERM) for prevention and treatment of osteoporosis. It increases bone mineral density and reduces serum total and low-density-lipoprotein (LDL) cholesterol. It also appears to reduce the incidence of vertebral fractures and is one of the first-line drugs for prevention of osteoporosis.

        2. Raloxifene is somewhat less effective than the bisphosphonates for the prevention and treatment of osteoporosis. Venous thromboembolism is a risk.

Treatment Guidelines for Osteoporosis
Calcium supplements with or without vitamin D supplements or calcium-rich diet Weight-bearing exercise Avoidance of alcohol tobacco products Alendronate (Fosamax) Risedronate (Actonel) Raloxifene (Evista)

Agents for Treating Osteoporosis		
Medication	**Dosage**	**Route**
Calcium	1,000 to 1,500 mg per day	Oral
Vitamin D	400 IU per day (800 IU per day in winter in northern latitudes)	Oral
Alendronate (Fosamax)	**Prevention:** 5 mg per day or 35 mg once-a-week **Treatment:** 10 mg per day or 70 mg once-a-week	Oral
Risedronate (Actonel)	5 mg daily or 35 mg once weekly	Oral
Raloxifene (Evista)	60 mg per day	Oral

E. **Monitoring the response to therapy**
   1. Bone mineral density and a marker of bone turnover should be measured at baseline, followed by a repeat measurement of the marker in three months.
   2. If the marker falls appropriately, the drug is having the desired effect, and therapy should be continued for two years, at which time bone mineral density can be measured again. The anticipated three-month decline in markers is 50% with alendronate.

F. **Estrogen/progestin therapy**
   1. Estrogen-progestin therapy is no longer a first-line approach for the treatment of osteoporosis in postmenopausal women because of increases in the risk of breast cancer, stroke, venous thromboembolism, and coronary disease.
   2. Indications for estrogen-progestin in postmenopausal women include persistent menopausal symptoms and patients with an indication for antiresorptive therapy who cannot tolerate the other drugs.

References, see page 372.

Screening for Cervical Cancer

Cervical cancer screening should be started three years after the onset of sexual activity, but no later than age 21. The basis of this recommendation is that high grade cervical intraepithelial lesions (HSIL) are almost entirely related to acquisition of human papillomavirus (HPV) infection through genital skin to skin contact and these lesions usually do not occur until three to five years after exposure to HPV. HSIL is a precursor to cervical cancer.

I. Screening interval

A. Cervical cancer screening should be started three years after the onset of sexual activity, but no later than age 21.

B. The American Cancer Society recommends that initial cervical screening should be performed annually if conventional cervical cytology smears (Pap) are used and every two years with liquid-based cytology tests until age 30. The screening interval can then be increased to every two to three years in women with three or more consecutive normal cytology results who are $\geq$30 years old.

C. The American College of Obstetricians and Gynecologists recommends annual screening for women younger than 30 years of age regardless of testing method (conventional or liquid-based cytology). Women aged 30 and over who have had three negative smears, no history of CIN II/III, and are not immunocompromised or DES exposed in utero may extend the interval between tests to two to three years. Women aged 30 and over may also consider the option of a combined cervical cytology and HPV test. Women who test negative by both tests should not be screened more frequently than every three years.

D. Exceptions. Women at increased risk of CIN, such as those with in utero DES exposure, immunocompromise, or a history of CIN II/III or cancer, should continue to be screened at least annually. More frequent surveillance should also be considered in women whose smears do not contain endocervical cells or are partially obscured.

E. Discontinuing screening

   1. The United States Preventive Services Task Force stated screening may stop at age 65 if the woman has had recent normal smears and is not at high risk for cervical cancer.

   2. The American Cancer Society guideline stated that women age 70 or older may elect to stop cervical cancer screening if they have had three consecutive satisfactory, normal/negative test results and no abnormal test results within the prior 10 years.

   3. Cervical cancer screening is not recommended in women who have had total hysterectomies for benign indications (presence of CIN II or III excludes benign categorization). Screening of women with CIN II/III who undergo hysterectomy may be discontinued after three consecutive negative results have been obtained. However, screening should be performed if the woman acquires risk factors for intraepithelial neoplasia, such as new sexual partners or immunosuppression.

Bethesda 2001 Pap Smear Report

Interpretation Result
Negative for intraepithelial lesion or malignancy
Infection (Trichomonas vaginalis, Candida spp., shift in flora suggestive of bacterial vaginosis, Actinomyces spp., cellular changes consistent with Herpes simplex virus)
Other Non-neoplastic Findings:
    Reactive cellular changes associated with inflammation (includes typical repair) radiation, intrauterine contraceptive device (IUD)
    Glandular cells status post-hysterectomy
    Atrophy
Other
    Endometrial cells (in a woman $\geq$40 years of age)
Epithelial Cell Abnormalities
    Squamous Cell
        Atypical squamous cells
            -of undetermined significance (ASC-US)
            -cannot exclude HSIL (ASC-H)
        Low-grade squamous intraepithelial lesion (LSIL) encompassing: HPV/mild dysplasia/CIN 1
        High-grade squamous intraepithelial lesion (HSIL) encompassing: moderate and severe dysplasia, CIS/CIN 2 and CIN 3 with features suspicious for invasion (if invasion is suspected)
        Squamous cell carcinoma
    Glandular Cell
        Atypical
            -Endocervical cells (not otherwise specified or specify in comments)
            -Glandular cell (not otherwise specified or specify in comments)
            -Endometrial cells (not otherwise specified or specify in comments)
            -Glandular cells (not otherwise specified or specify in comments)
        Atypical
            -Endocervical cells, favor neoplastic
            -Glandular cells, favor neoplastic
        Endocervical adenocarcinoma in situ
        Adenocarcinoma (endocervical, endometrial, extrauterine, not otherwise specified (not otherwise specified)
Other Malignant Neoplasms (specify)

Management of the Abnormal Papanicolaou Smear	
Result	**Action**
Specimen adequacy	
Satisfactory for evaluation	Routine follow-up
Unsatisfactory for evaluation	Repeat smear
No endocervical cells	Follow-up in one year for low-risk women with a previously normal smear; repeat in 4-6 months for high-risk women

Result	Action
Atypical cells	
Atypical squamous cells of undetermined significance (ASC-US)	HPV testing with referral to colposcopy if positive for high-risk HPV type; if negative for high-risk HPV type, then repeat cytology in 12 months
Special circumstances	Postmenopausal women with atrophic epitheliium may be treated with topical estrogen followed by repeat cervical cytology one week after completing treatment
ASC-H	Immediate referral to colposcopy
Atypical glandular cells (AGS)	Immediate referral to colposcopy with sampling of the endocervical canal. Women over age 35 and any woman with unexplained vaginal bleeding should also have an endometrial biopsy
Intraepithelial neoplasia	
High grade	Immediate referral for colposcopy
Low grade	Immediate referral for colposcopy, except adolescents and postmenopausal women
Endometrial cells	Endometrial biopsy in selected cases
Other malignant cells	Referral to a gynecologic oncologist

References, see page 372.

Atypical Squamous Cells on Cervical Cytology

Atypical squamous cells are commonly caused by self-limited disease, which resolves spontaneously. The risk of invasive cancer in patients with atypical squamous cells is low, 0.1 to 0.2%. However, 5 to 17% of patients with atypical squamous cells and 24 to 94% of those with ASC-high grade will have precancerous lesions at biopsy, therefore, further evaluation is necessary to determine if high-grade dysplasia is present.

I. **Evaluation of atypical squamous cells of undetermined significance (ASC-US).**
   A. Reflex HPV testing with triage of women with high risk HPV types to colposcopy is the recommended approach. Reflex testing refers to concurrent collection of cytology and HPV samples with actual testing for HPV only if indicated by abnormal cytology results.
      1. If liquid-based cytology is used, reflex HPV testing can be performed on the same specimen. If a conventional Papanicolaou (Pap) smear is obtained, a second specimen is collected for HPV DNA testing. If high risk subtypes are found, colposcopy is performed.

Risk of cervical cancer with human papilloma virus
High-risk (oncogenic or cancer-associated) types Common types: 16, 18, 31, 33, 35, 39, 45, 51, 52, 56, 58, 59, 68, 69, 82
Low-risk (non-oncogenic) types Common types: 6, 11, 40, 42, 43, 44, 54, 61, 72, 81

Management of women with combined test screening	
Results of cytology/HPV	**Recommended follow-up**
Negative / Negative	Routine screening in 3 years
Negative / Positive	Repeat combined test in 6 to 12 months
ASCUS / Negative	Repeat cytology in 12 months
ASCUS / Positive	Colposcopy
Greater than ASCUS / Positive or negative	Colposcopy

- B. **Special circumstances and populations**
    1. **Pregnant women** with ASC are managed in the same way as nonpregnant women, except endocervical sampling is not performed.
    2. **Infection or reactive changes.** When an infectious organism is identified or suggested, the patient should be contacted to determine if she is symptomatic. Antibiotic therapy is indicated for symptomatic infections, as well as some asymptomatic infections. After treatment of the infection, women with high risk HPV types are referred to colposcopy.
    3. **Atrophic epithelium** (a normal finding in postmenopausal women) is often characterized by nuclear enlargement, which meets one of the pathologic criteria for ASC. Administration of estrogen (eg, 0.3 mg conjugated estrogen applied as vaginal cream nightly for four weeks [1/8th of the applicator]) causes atypical atrophic, but not dysplastic, epithelium to mature into normal squamous epithelium. Hormonal therapy given for vaginal atrophy should be followed by repeat cervical cytology one week after completing treatment. If negative, cytology should be repeated again in six months. If both tests are negative, the woman can return to routine screening intervals, but if either test is positive for ASC-US or greater colposcopy should be completed.
    4. **Immunosuppressed women**, including all women who are HIV positive, with ASC-US should be referred for immediate colposcopy instead of HPV testing or serial cytology.
    5. **Adolescents.** Initial colposcopy or reflex HPV testing may be deferred in adolescents because the risk of invasive cancer is near zero and the prevalence of transient HPV infection is very high . Instead, serial cytology should be completed at six and 12 months or HPV DNA testing at 12 months with referral to colposcopy for positive results (ASC or greater, high risk HPV DNA types).
- C. **Management after colposcopy/biopsy.** Colposcopy/biopsy of women with ASC-US will either yield a histologic abnormality (eg, CIN II or III), which should be treated as appropriate, or show no abnormal findings. If no abnormal findings are found and HPV testing was not performed or showed a low-risk type, then follow-up cytological testing in 12 months is recommended.

     D. Women who test positive for high risk HPV types, but have CIN I or less on colposcopy/biopsy require a repeat cervical cytology at 6 and 12 months, or perform an HPV test at 12 months, with colposcopy for ASC or higher or a positive HPV test.

II. **Evaluation of atypical squamous cells–cannot exclude high-grade squamous intraepithelial lesion (ASC-H)**

     A. Most women with ASC-H on cytological examination should be referred for colposcopy and ECC (ECC is not performed in pregnancy), without HPV testing. Twenty-four to 94% of these women will have CIN II or higher. Biopsy proven CIN II or III is treated, as appropriate.

     B. If no lesion or a CIN I lesion is identified, the cytology sample, colposcopy, and any biopsy specimens should be reviewed, if possible, to address any possible cytological-histological discordancy, with further management dependent upon the results. If review of cytology confirms ASC-H, follow-up cytology in six and 12 months or HPV DNA testing in 12 months is acceptable. Colposcopy should be repeated for ASC-US or greater on cytology or a positive test for high risk HPV DNA.

     C. In women age 30 or older with ASC-H, an acceptable alternative is to perform HPV testing for initial triaging. If high risk HPV types are present, the patient is referred for colposcopy.

References: See page 372.

Atypical and Malignant Glandular Cells on Cervical Cytology

Cervical Pap smear cytology showing atypical glandular (AGC) or endometrial carcinoma cells indicates the presence of glandular cells that could originate from the endocervical or endometrial region. The Bethesda 2001 system classifies AGC into two subcategories:

     AGC (specify endocervical, endometrial, or glandular cells not otherwise specified [NOS])

     AGC, favor neoplastic (specify endocervical or NOS)

Additional categories for glandular cell abnormalities are:

     Endocervical adenocarcinoma in situ (AIS)

     Adenocarcinoma

I. **Atypical glandular cells**

     A. A smear with AGC is associated with a premalignant or malignant lesion of the endocervix or endometrium in 10 to 40% of cases.

     B. Women over age 50 with AGC are at higher risk of having uterine cancer than younger women (8 and 1%, respectively). Conversely, premenopausal women with AGC are more likely to have CIN II/III or AIS than postmenopausal women.

     C. **Evaluation.** Presence of AGC or AIS on cervical cytology is a significant marker for neoplasia of the endometrium, as well as the squamous and glandular epithelium of the cervix. All women with atypical glandular cells or AIS should be referred for colposcopy with directed cervical biopsies and sampling of the endocervical canal. An endometrial biopsy should be performed on all women over age 35 and on younger women with unexplained or anovulatory bleeding, morbid obesity, oligomenorrhea, or an increased risk of endometrial cancer.

     D. Women with only atypical endometrial cells on cytology can be initially evaluated with endometrial biopsy only, rather than colposcopy. If endometrial sampling is normal, then colposcopy and endocervical curettage should be performed.

   E. Positive findings, such as any grade of CIN on biopsy, should be managed as appropriate.
   F. **Negative colposcopy/endocervical curettage.** The management of women with AGC and a negative initial colposcopy/endocervical sampling depends upon AGC subclassification.
      1. **AGC NOS.** Women with AGC NOS who have a normal initial colposcopic evaluation and endocervical biopsy can be followed with cervical cytology at four to six month intervals until four consecutive tests are negative for intraepithelial lesions or malignancy. They are then followed with routine surveillance. However, if any abnormality (ASC or greater) is noted on follow-up cytology smears, another colposcopy is required. Women with persistent AGC NOS (two or more cytology results) are at especially high risk of significant glandular disease and need conization if repeat colposcopy and endometrial biopsy are nondiagnostic.
      2. In women with AGC NOS and normal colposcopic evaluation and biopsies, HPV studies may be used for further monitoring and, if negative, repeat cytology and endocervical sampling can be done in one year rather than in four visits over two years.
      3. AGC favor neoplasia or AIS. A cold-knife conization is the best procedure for subsequent evaluation of AGC lesions at high risk of associated adenocarcinoma, such as AGC favor neoplasia or AIS or persistent AGC NOS.
      4. If conization and endometrial biopsies are also negative, the patient should be evaluated for primary or metastatic disease involving the fallopian tube, ovary, and other pelvic and abdominal organs with pelvic ultrasound examination, colonoscopy, and computed tomography of the abdomen.
II. **Endocervical adenocarcinoma**
   A. Endocervical adenocarcinoma in situ (AIS) and adenocarcinoma requires evaluation and will show invasive cancer in a proportion of women with AIS on cytology. An intermediate category: atypical endocervical cells, favor neoplastic suggests some features of AIS but without criteria for a definitive diagnosis.
   B. Colposcopy with directed biopsy is required. A diagnostic excisional procedure is often needed because colposcopy/biopsy can miss small lesions of AIS or adenocarcinoma and lesions high in the canal.
References: See page 372.

Pelvic Inflammatory Disease

Pelvic inflammatory disease (PID) is an acute infection of the upper genital tract structures in women, involving the uterus, oviducts, and ovaries. PID usually is a community-acquired infection initiated by a sexually transmitted agent. The estimated number of cases of PID in women 15 to 44 years of age in the United States was 168,837 in 2003.

I. **Clinical features**
   A. **Lower abdominal pain** is the cardinal presenting symptom in women with PID. The recent onset of pain that worsens during coitus or with jarring movement may be the only presenting symptom of PID; the onset of pain during or shortly after menses is particularly suggestive. The abdominal pain is usually bilateral and rarely of more than two weeks' duration.

B. **Abnormal uterine bleeding** occurs in one-third or more of patients with PID. New vaginal discharge, urethritis, proctitis, fever, and chills can be associated signs. The presence of PID is less likely if symptoms referable to the bowel or urinary tract predominate.

C. **Risk factors for sexually transmitted diseases:**
   1. Age less than 25 years
   2. Young age at first sex
   3. Nonbarrier contraception
   4. New, multiple, or symptomatic sexual partners
   5. Oral contraception
   6. Cervical ectopy

D. **Factors that facilitate pelvic inflammatory disease:**
   1. Previous episode of PID
   2. Sex during menses
   3. Vaginal douching
   4. Bacterial vaginosis
   5. Intrauterine device

E. **Physical examination.** Only one-half of patients with PID have fever. Abdominal examination reveals diffuse tenderness greatest in the lower quadrants, which may or may not be symmetrical. Rebound tenderness and decreased bowel sounds are common. Marked tenderness in the right upper quadrant does not exclude PID, since 10% of these patients have perihepatitis (Fitz-Hugh Curtis syndrome).

F. **Pelvic examination.** Purulent endocervical discharge and/or acute cervical motion and adnexal tenderness with bimanual examination is strongly suggestive of PID. Significant lateralization of adnexal tenderness is uncommon in PID.

G. **Subclinical pelvic inflammatory disease.** Lower genital tract infection with gonorrhea, chlamydia, or bacterial vaginosis is a risk factor for subclinical PID, defined by the presence of neutrophils and plasma cells in endometrial tissue.

II. Diagnostic considerations

A. Laparoscopy is recommended for the following:
   1. A sick patient with high suspicion of a competing diagnosis (appendicitis)
   2. An acutely ill patient who has failed outpatient treatment for PID
   3. Any patient not clearly improving after 72 hours of inpatient treatment for PID. Consent for laparotomy at the same procedure should be obtained in advance for these patients.

B. **Diagnostic criteria.** The index of suspicion for the clinical diagnosis of PID should be high, especially in adolescent women, even if they deny sexual activity. Empiric treatment is recommended for women with abdominal pain who have at least one of the following:
   1. Cervical motion tenderness or uterine/adnexal tenderness
   2. Oral temperature >101 F (>38.3 C)
   3. Peripheral leukocytosis/left shift
   4. Abnormal cervical or vaginal mucopurulent discharge
   5. Presence of white blood cells (WBCs) on saline microscopy of vaginal secretions
   6. Elevated erythrocyte sedimentation rate
   7. Elevated C-reactive protein

III. **Differential diagnosis.** In addition to PID, the differential diagnosis of lower abdominal pain in a young woman includes the following conditions:

A. Gastrointestinal: Appendicitis, cholecystitis, constipation, gastroenteritis, inflammatory bowel disease

B. Renal: Cystitis, pyelonephritis, nephrolithiasis, urethritis

C. Obstetric/Gynecologic: Dysmenorrhea, ectopic pregnancy, intrauterine pregnancy complication, ovarian cyst, ovarian torsion, ovarian tumor.

Differential Diagnosis of Pelvic Inflammatory Disease	
Appendicitis	Irritable bowel syndrome
Ectopic pregnancy	Somatization
Hemorrhagic ovarian cyst	Gastroenteritis
Ovarian torsion	Cholecystitis
Endometriosis	Nephrolithiasis
Urinary tract Infection	

IV. Diagnostic testing

A. Laboratory testing for patients suspected of PID always begins with a pregnancy test to rule out ectopic pregnancy and complications of an intrauterine pregnancy. A urinalysis (preferably on a catheterized specimen) and a stool for occult blood should be obtained since abnormalities in either lessen the probability of PID. Although PID is usually an acute process, fewer than one-half of PID patients exhibit leukocytosis. A hematocrit of less than 0.30 makes PID less likely.

B. Gram stain and microscopic examination of vaginal discharge. If a cervical Gram stain is positive for Gram negative intracellular diplococci, the probability of PID greatly increases; if negative, it is of little use.

C. Increased white blood cells (WBC) in vaginal fluid is the most sensitive single laboratory test for PID (78% for $\geq$3 WBC per high power field. However, the specificity is only 39%.

D. Recommended laboratory tests:
1. Pregnancy test
2. Microscopic exam of vaginal discharge in saline
3. Complete blood counts
4. Nucleic acid amplification tests for chlamydia and gonococcus
5. Urinalysis
6. Fecal occult blood test
7. C-reactive protein (optional)
8. Ultrasounds are reserved for acutely ill patients with PID in whom a pelvic abscess is a consideration.

V. Treatment and sequelae of pelvic inflammatory disease

A. Outpatient therapy. The CDC recommends either oral ofloxacin (Floxin, 400 mg twice daily) or levofloxacin (Levaquin, 500 mg once daily) with or without metronidazole (Flagyl) 500 mg twice daily) for 14 days. Metronidazole is added when anaerobic coverage is of concern. Beyond 48 hours of symptoms, the most frequent isolates are anaerobes.

B. An alternative is an initial single dose of ceftriaxone (Rocephin, 250 mg IM), cefoxitin (Mefoxin, 2 g IM plus probenecid 1 g orally), or another parenteral third-generation cephalosporin, followed by doxycycline (100 mg orally twice daily) with or without metronidazole for 14 days. The combination of amoxicillin-clavulanate and doxycycline is also an alternative that has achieved short-term clinical response. For patients younger than 18 years of age, one of the alternative regimens should be used since neither ofloxacin nor levofloxacin is approved for systemic use in this age group.

C. For women younger than 18 years treatment consists of an initial single dose of ceftriaxone (Rocephin, 250 mg IM) or cefoxitin (Mefoxin, 2 g IM plus probenecid 1 g orally), or another parenteral third-generation cephalosporin, followed by doxycycline (100 mg orally twice daily) with or without metronidazole for 14 days. For those who are unlikely to complete at least seven days of doxycycline, some providers suggest administration of azithromycin 1 g PO should be given at the time of parenteral adminstration of cephalosporin to ensure eradication of chlamydia.

D. **For women ≥18 years azithromycin (Zithromax)** 1 g PO should be given for Chlamydia coverage, and either cefixime (Suprax) 400 mg PO or ceftriaxone (Rocephin) 125 mg IM (for gonococcus coverage) given for one dose by directly observed therapy, followed by amoxicillin-clavulanate 875 mg PO twice daily for 7 to 10 days. For penicillin-allergic patients, a fluoroquinolone or spectinomycin may be used for initial single-dose gonococcus coverage, followed by doxycycline and metronidazole for 14 days.

E. Reevaluation two to three days after the initiation of therapy to assure accuracy of diagnosis and response to therapy is an extremely important aspect of outpatient treatment of PID.

F. **Inpatient therapy.** The CDC suggest either of the following regimens:
   1. Cefotetan (Cefotan, 2 g IV every12h) or cefoxitin (Mefoxin, 2 g IV every 6h) plus doxycycline (100 mg IV or PO every 12h), or
   2. Clindamycin (900 mg IV every 8h) plus gentamicin loading dose (2 mg/kg of body weight) followed by a maintenance dose (1.5 mg/kg) every 8 hours. Single daily dosing of gentamicin may be substituted.
   3. **Alternative regimens:**
      a. Ofloxacin (Floxin, 400 mg IV every12h) or levofloxacin (Levoquin, 500 mg IV daily) with or without metronidazole (Flagyl, 500 mg IV every 8h), or
      b. Ampicillin-sulbactam (Unasyn, 3 g IV every 6h) plus doxycycline (100 mg IV or PO every12h).
      c. Ofloxacin has been studied as monotherapy for the treatment of PID; however, due to concerns regarding its lack of activity against anaerobic flora, some clinicians prefer to also add metronidazole. Ampicillin-sulbactam plus oral doxycycline is effective coverage against Chlamydia trachomatis, Neisseria gonorrhoeae, and anaerobes.
   4. Parenteral administration of antibiotics should be continued for 24 hours after a clear clinical response, followed by doxycycline (100 mg PO BID) or clindamycin (450 mg PO QID) for a total of 14 days.

G. **Recommended regimens:**
   1. **Levofloxacin** (Levoquin, 500 mg IV Q24h) plus metronidazole (500 mg IV Q8h)
   2. A broad spectrum cephalosporin plus doxycycline with or without metronidazole
   3. Ertapenem (Invanz, 1 g IV Q24h)

H. For patients younger than 18 years of age, the second regimen should be used since levofloxacin is not approved for use in this age group when other effective alternatives are available.

I. Some providers prescribe azithromycin (Zithromax, 1 g PO once) as soon as the patient is tolerating oral intake if the patient is unlikely to comply with doxycycline administration. Parenteral therapy should continue until the pelvic tenderness is absent (two to five days).

J. **Treatment for PID** must be accompanied by a discussion of sexually transmitted infections, partner treatment, and future safe sex practices. Male sex partners of women with PID should be examined and empirically treated if they had sexual contact during the preceding 60 days. Other important components of the evaluation include:
   1. Serology for human immunodeficiency virus (HIV)
   2. Papanicolaou smear
   3. Hepatitis B surface antigen determination and initiation of the vaccine series for patients who are antigen negative and unvaccinated
   4. Hepatitis C virus serology

5. Serologic tests for syphilis
References: See page 372.

Genital Chlamydia Trachomatis Infections

Chlamydia trachomatis is the most common sexually transmitted genital infection. Infants born to mothers through an infected birth canal can develop conjunctivitis and pneumonia. These syndromes are caused by the C. trachomatis serovars B and D through K. The L serovars cause lymphogranuloma venereum (LGV), a genital ulcer syndrome. Chlamydia trachomatis serovars A to C cause endemic trachoma, a common ocular infection in the developing world.

I. **Microbiology and epidemiology**
   A. C. trachomatis is a small gram-negative bacterium and an obligate intracellular parasite.
   B. Chlamydia cannot be cultured on artificial media; tissue culture has been required. Rapid screening tests are now available.
   C. 4,000,000 cases of C. trachomatis infection occur annually. C. trachomatis and Neisseria gonorrhoeae cause similar clinical syndromes, but chlamydia infections tend to have fewer acute symptoms and more significant long-term complications.
   D. **Prevalence.** The rates of chlamydia are highest in adolescent women. Between 18 and 26 years of age, the prevalence of chlamydial infection is 4.2%. The highest rates are in African American women (14%) and are higher in women than men.
   E. **Risk factors for Chlamydia trachomatis infection:**
      1. Adolescents and young adults
      2. Multiple sex partners or a partner with other partners during the last three months or a recent new sex partner
      3. Inconsistent use of barrier contraceptives
      4. Clinical evidence of mucopurulent cervicitis
      5. Cervical ectopy
      6. Unmarried status
      7. History of prior sexually transmitted disease
      8. Lower socioeconomic class or education not beyond high school.

II. **Clinical manifestations**
   A. The majority of women with C. trachomatis infection are asymptomatic; however, cervicitis or pelvic inflammatory disease may occur.
   B. **Cervicitis.** Cervical infection is the most common chlamydial syndrome in women. More than 50% of these women are asymptomatic. Vaginal discharge, poorly differentiated abdominal pain, or lower abdominal pain are the most frequent symptoms.
   C. **Physical examination** is often unremarkable, mucopurulent cervical discharge, cervical friability, cervical edema, and endocervical ulcers may be seen.
   D. **Perihepatitis (Fitzhugh-Curtis syndrome).** Patients with chlamydia infection occasionally develop perihepatitis, an inflammation of the liver capsule and adjacent peritoneal surfaces. Perihepatitis is more commonly seen in PID, occurring in 5% of cases.
   E. **Pelvic inflammatory disease.** 30% of women with chlamydia infection will develop PID if left untreated. While PID caused by N. gonorrhoeae infection may be more acutely symptomatic, PID due to C. trachomatis tends to cause higher rates of infertility.
   F. **Pregnancy.** Untreated chlamydia infection can increase the risk for premature rupture of the membranes and low birth weight. If the mother is untreated, 20 to

50% of newborns will develop conjunctivitis, and 10 to 20% will develop pneumonia.

III. Diagnosis

A. **Nucleic acid amplification (NAAT)** uses polymerase chain reaction (PCR). These sensitive and specific tests have replaced poorly standardized cell culture methods as the "gold standard."

1. Another advantage of NAATs is the ability to perform testing on urine as well as urethral specimens. Since urine collection is noninvasive, it is a preferred method.

2. The PCR assay has a sensitivity and specificity of 83 and 99.5% for urine samples and 86 and 99.6% for cervical samples.

B. **Antigen detection** requires a swab from the cervix or urethra. The sensitivity of this method is 80 to 95% compared to culture.

IV. Chlamydia screening

A. Clinical practice guidelines strongly recommend routine chlamydia screening for sexually-active women below the age of 25.

V. Treatment. Chlamydiae are susceptible to the tetracyclines and the macrolides. Treatment efficacy with recommended regimens is >95%.

A. Azithromycin (Zithromax, 1 g PO as a single dose) or doxycycline (100 mg PO BID for 7 days) are the two recommended regimens.

B. Alternative regimens include seven days of erythromycin base (500 mg PO QID), erythromycin ethylsuccinate (800 mg PO), ofloxacin (300 mg PO BID), or levofloxacin (500 mg PO QD). Erythromycin is associated with significant gastrointestinal side effects; ofloxacin and levofloxacin are expensive alternatives.

Treatment of chlamydia trachomatis infection and related syndromes
Urethritis, cervicitis, conjunctivitis, or proctitis
Azithromycin (Zithromax) 1 g oral once **OR** Doxycycline 100 mg oral twice daily for seven days **Alternatives** Ofloxacin (Floxin) 300 mg oral twice daily for seven days Levofloxacin (Levaquin) 500 mg oral daily for seven days Erythromycin 500 mg oral four times daily for seven days
Infection in pregnancy
Azithromycin (Zithromax) 1 g oral once **OR** Amoxicillin 500 mg oral three times daily for seven days Alternatives Erythromycin 500 mg oral four times daily for seven days
Neonatal ophthalmia or pneumonia
Azithromycin 20 mg/kg oral once daily for three days Alternatives Erythromycin 12.5 mg/kg oral four times daily for 14 days§

Lymphogranuloma venereum

Doxycycline 100 mg oral twice daily for 21 days
Alternatives
Erythromycin 500 mg oral four times daily for 21 days

C. **Adjunctive measures:**
1. Presumptive treatment of partners
2. Evaluation for other STDs (syphilis serology, gonococcal testing)
3. HIV counseling and testing
4. Safer-sex counseling and condom provision
5. Contraception provision or referral
6. Test of cure. Testing for C. trachomatis following treatment with azithromycin or doxycycline is not recommended. Exceptions include:
   a. Patients with persisting symptoms or
   b. Those in whom compliance with the treatment regimen is suspected.
   c. Pregnant females
7. If a test for cure is performed, this should be done more than three weeks after the completion of therapy.
8. Repeat screening should be considered within the first three to four months after therapy is completed or at least when the patient has her next encounter with the healthcare system within the first 12 months because patients who have the disease once are at a higher risk for acquiring it again.

References: See page 372.

Vaginitis

Approximately 8-18% of women report an episode of vaginal symptoms each year. The etiology of vaginal complaints includes infection of the vagina, cervix, and upper genital tract, chemicals or irritants (eg, spermicides or douching), hormone deficiency, and rarely systemic diseases.

I. **Clinical evaluation**
   A. Symptoms of vaginitis include vaginal discharge, pruritus, irritation, soreness, odor, dyspareunia and dysuria. Dyspareunia is a common feature of atrophic vaginitis. Abdominal pain is suggestive of pelvic inflammatory disease and suprapubic pain is suggestive of cystitis.
   B. A new sexual partner increases the risk of acquiring sexually transmitted diseases, such as trichomonas, chlamydia, or Neisseria gonorrheae. Trichomoniasis often occurs during or immediately after the menstrual period; candida vulvovaginitis often occurs during the premenstrual period.
   C. Antibiotics and high-estrogen oral contraceptive pills may predispose to candida vulvovaginitis; increased physiologic discharge can occur with oral contraceptives; pruritus unresponsive to antifungal agents suggests vulvar dermatitis.

II. **Physical examination**
   A. The vulva usually appears normal in bacterial vaginosis. Erythema, edema, or fissure formation suggest candidiasis, trichomoniasis, or dermatitis.
   B. Trichomonas is associated with a purulent discharge; candidiasis is associated with a thick, adherent, "cottage cheese-like" discharge; and bacterial vaginosis is associated with a thin, homogeneous, "fishy smelling" discharge. The cervix in women with cervicitis is usually erythematous and friable, with a mucopurulent discharge.

    C. Abdominal or cervical motion tenderness is suggestive of PID.

III. Diagnostic studies

A. Vaginal pH. The pH of the normal vaginal secretions is 4.0 to 4.5. A pH above 4.5 suggests bacterial vaginosis or trichomoniasis (pH 5 to 6), and helps to exclude candida vulvovaginitis (pH 4 to 4.5).

B. Saline microscopy should look for candidal buds or hyphae, motile trichomonads, epithelial cells studded with adherent coccobacilli (clue cells), and polymorphonuclear cells (PMNs). The addition of 10% potassium hydroxide to the wet mount is helpful in diagnosing candida vaginitis. Culture for candida and trichomonas may be useful if microscopy is negative.

C. Cervical culture. A diagnosis of cervicitis, typically due to Neisseria gonorrhoeae or Chlamydia trachomatis, must always be considered in women with purulent vaginal discharge. The presence of high-risk behavior or any sexually transmitted disease requires screening for HIV, hepatitis B, and other STDs.

Clinical Manifestations of Vaginitis	
Candidal Vaginitis	Nonmalodorous, thick, white, "cottage cheese-like" discharge that adheres to vaginal walls Hyphal forms or budding yeast cells on wet-mount Pruritus Normal pH (<4.5)
Bacterial Vaginosis	Thin, dark or dull grey, homogeneous, malodorous discharge that adheres to the vaginal walls Elevated pH level (>4.5) Positive KOH (whiff test) Clue cells on wet-mount microscopic evaluation
Trichomonas Vaginalis	Copious, yellow-gray or green, homogeneous or frothy, malodorous discharge Elevated pH level (>4.5) Mobile, flagellated organisms and leukocytes on wet-mount microscopic evaluation Vulvovaginal irritation, dysuria
Atrophic Vaginitis	Vaginal dryness or burning

IV. Bacterial vaginosis

A. Incidence. Bacterial vaginosis is the most common cause of vaginitis in women of childbearing age, with prevalence of 5-60%.

B. Microbiology and risk factors. Bacterial vaginosis represents a change in vaginal flora characterized by a reduction of lactobacilli and an increase of Gardnerella vaginalis, Mobiluncus species, Mycoplasma hominis, anaerobic gram-negative rods, and Peptostreptococcus species. Risk factors for bacterial vaginosis include multiple or new sexual partners, early age of first coitus, douching, cigarette smoking, and use of an intrauterine contraceptive device.

C. Clinical features. Symptoms include a "fishy smelling" discharge that is more noticeable after unprotected intercourse. The discharge is off-white, thin, and homogeneous. Pruritus and inflammation are absent.

D. Complications

    1. Pregnant women appear to be at higher risk of preterm delivery.

    2. Bacterial vaginosis may cause plasma-cell endometritis, postpartum fever, post-hysterectomy vaginal-cuff cellulitis, and postabortal infection.

    3. Bacterial vaginosis is a risk factor for HIV acquisition and transmission.

E. Diagnosis. Three of the four criteria listed below are necessary for diagnosis.
  1. Homogeneous, grayish-white discharge
  2. Vaginal pH >4.5
  3. Positive whiff-amine test, defined as the presence of a fishy odor when 10% KOH is added to vaginal discharge samples
  4. Clue cells on saline wet mount (epithelial cells studded with coccobacilli)

F. Therapy. Treatment is indicated in women with symptomatic infection and those with asymptomatic infection prior to abortion or hysterectomy.
  1. Metronidazole or clindamycin administered either orally or intravaginally will result in a high rate of clinical cure (70-80%). Oral medication is more convenient.
  2. The oral regimen is 500 mg twice daily for 7 days. Topical vaginal therapy with 0.75% metronidazole gel (MetroGel, 5 g once daily for 5 days) is as effective as oral metronidazole.
  3. Single-dose therapy with 2 g of metronidazole achieves a similar immediate rate of clinical response.
  4. Side effects of metronidazole include a metallic taste, nausea, a disulfiram-like effect with alcohol, interaction with warfarin, and peripheral neuropathy.

G. Relapse
  1. Approximately 30% of patients have a recurrence within three months. Recurrence usually reflects a failure to eradicate the offending organisms. Management of symptomatic relapse includes prolonged therapy for 10 to 14 days.
  2. Most women with a history of recurrent infection benefit from suppressive therapy with metronidazole gel 0.75% for 10 days, followed by twice-weekly applications for three to six months.

V. Candida vulvovaginitis

A. Incidence. Candida vulvovaginitis accounts for one-third of vaginitis. Up to 75% of women report having had at least one episode of candidiasis. The condition is rare before menarche. It is less common in postmenopausal women, unless they are taking estrogen replacement therapy.

B. Microbiology and risk factors. Candida albicans is responsible for 80-92% of vulvovaginal candidiasis.
  1. **Antibiotics.** A minority of women are prone to vulvovaginal candidiasis while taking antibiotics.
  2. **Intrauterine devices** have been associated with vulvovaginal candidiasis.
  3. **Pregnancy.** Symptomatic infection is more common in pregnancy.

C. Clinical features. Vulvar pruritus is the dominant feature. Women may also complain of dysuria (external rather than urethral), soreness, irritation, and dyspareunia. There is often little or no discharge. Physical examination often reveals erythema of the vulva and vaginal mucosa. The discharge is thick, adherent, and "cottage cheese-like."

D. Diagnosis
  1. The vaginal pH is typically 4 to 4.5, which distinguishes candidiasis from Trichomonas or bacterial vaginosis. The diagnosis is confirmed by finding the organism on a wet mount; adding 10% potassium hydroxide facilitates recognition of budding yeast and hyphae. Microscopy is negative in 50% of patients with vulvovaginal candidiasis.
  2. Empiric therapy is often considered in women with typical clinical features, a normal vaginal pH, and no other pathogens visible on microscopy. Culture should be performed in patients with persistent or recurrent symptoms.

E. Therapy
  1. Women with mild infection usually respond to treatment within a couple of days. More severe infections require a longer course of therapy and may take up to 14 days to fully resolve.

2. **Uncomplicated infection.** Both oral and topical antimycotic drugs achieve comparable clinical cure rates that are in excess of 80%.

3. Oral azole agents are more convenient. Side effects of single-dose fluconazole (150 mg) tend to be mild and infrequent, including gastrointestinal intolerance, headache, and rash.

Treatment regimens for yeast vaginitis*

1-day regimens
Clotrimazole vaginal tablets (Mycelex G), 500 mg hs**
Fluconazole tablets (Diflucan), 150 mg PO
Itraconazole capsules (Sporanox), 200 mg PO bid
Tioconazole 6.5% vaginal ointment (Vagistat-1), 4.6 g hs** [5 g]

3-day regimens
Butoconazole nitrate 2% vaginal cream (Femstat 3), 5 g hs [28 g]
Clotrimazole vaginal inserts (Gyne-Lotrimin 3), 200 mg hs**
Miconazole vaginal suppositories (Monistat 3), 200 mg hs**
Terconazole 0.8% vaginal cream (Terazol 3), 5 g hs
Terconazole vaginal suppositories (Terazol 3), 80 mg hs
Itraconazole capsules (Sporanox), 200 mg PO qd

5-day regimen
Ketoconazole tablets (Nizoral), 400 mg PO bid

7-day regimens
Clotrimazole 1% cream (Gyne-Lotrimin, Mycelex-7, Sweet'n Fresh Clotrimazole-7), 5 g hs**
Clotrimazole vaginal tablets (Gyne-Lotrimin, Mycelex-7, Sweet'n Fresh Clotrimazole-7), 100 mg hs**
Miconazole 2% vaginal cream (Femizol-M, Monistat 7), 5 g hs**
Miconazole vaginal suppositories (Monistat 7), 100 mg hs**
Terconazole 0.4% vaginal cream (Terazol 7), 5 g hs

14-day regimens
Nystatin vaginal tablets (Mycostatin), 100,000 U hs

*Suppositories can be used if inflammation is predominantly vaginal; creams if vulvar; a combination if both. Cream-suppository combination packs available: clotrimazole (Gyne-Lotrimin, Mycelex); miconazole (Monistat, M-Zole). Use 1-day or 3-day regimen if compliance is an issue. Miconazole nitrate may be used during pregnancy.

**Nonprescription formulation. If nonprescription therapies fail, use terconazole 0.4% cream or 80-mg suppositories at bedtime for 7 days.

---

4. **Complicated infections.** Factors that predispose to complicated infection include uncontrolled diabetes, immunosuppression, and a history of recurrent vulvovaginal candidiasis. Women with severe inflammation or complicated infection require seven to 14 days of topical therapy or two doses of oral therapy 72 hours apart.

Management options for complicated or recurrent yeast vaginitis

Extend any 7-day regimen to 10 to 14 days
Eliminate use of nylon or tight-fitting clothing
Consider discontinuing oral contraceptives
Consider eating 8 oz yogurt (with Lactobacillus acidophilus culture) per day
Improve glycemic control in diabetic patients
For long-term suppression of recurrent vaginitis, use ketoconazole, 100 mg (½ of 200-mg tablet) qd for 6 months

---

     5. Partner treatment is not necessary since this is not a primary route of transmission.

     6. Pregnancy. Topical azoles applied for seven days are recommended for treatment during pregnancy.

VI. Trichomoniasis

  A. Trichomoniasis, the third most common cause of vaginitis, is caused by the flagellated protozoan, Trichomonas vaginalis. The disorder is virtually always sexually transmitted.

  B. Clinical features. Trichomoniasis in women ranges from an asymptomatic state to a severe, acute, inflammatory disease. Signs and symptoms include a purulent, malodorous, thin discharge (70%) with associated burning, pruritus, dysuria, and dyspareunia. Physical examination reveals erythema of the vulva and vaginal mucosa; the classic green-yellow frothy discharge is observed in 10-30%. Punctate hemorrhages may be visible on the vagina and cervix in 2%.

  C. Complications. Infection is associated with premature rupture of the membranes and prematurity; however, treatment of asymptomatic infection has not been shown to reduce these complications. Trichomoniasis is a risk factor for development of post-hysterectomy cellulitis. The infection facilitates transmission of the human immunodeficiency virus.

  D. Diagnosis

     1. The presence of motile trichomonads on wet mount is diagnostic of infection, but this occurs in only 50-70% of cases. Other findings include an elevated vaginal pH (>4.5) and an increase in polymorphonuclear leukocytes on saline microscopy.

  E. Culture on Diamond's medium has a high sensitivity (95%) and specificity (>95%) and should be considered in patients with elevated vaginal pH, increased numbers of polymorphonuclear leukocytes and an absence of motile trichomonads and clue cells on wet mount.

  F. The OSOM Trichomonas Rapid Test for Trichomonas antigens has a sensitivity of 88.3% and specificity of 98.8%. Results can be read in 10 minutes. The Affirm VP III Microbial Identification System (Becton Dickinson) test uses a nucleic acid probe and is read in 45 minutes.

  G. Cervical cytology. Trichomonads are sometimes reported on conventional Papanicolaou (Pap) smears. Conventional Pap smears are inadequate for diagnosis of trichomoniasis because this technique has a sensitivity of only 60 to 70% and false positive results are common (at least 8%). Asymptomatic women with trichomonads identified on conventional Pap smear should be evaluated by wet mount and should not be treated until the diagnosis is confirmed.

  H. Treatment of asymptomatic women with trichomonads noted on liquid-based cervical cytology is appropriate.

VII. Treatment of Trichomonas vaginitis

A. Nonpregnant women

1. The 5-nitroimidazole drugs (metronidazole or tinidazole) are the only class of drugs that provide curative therapy of trichomoniasis. Cure rates are 90 to 95%.

2. Treatment consists of a single oral dose of 2 grams (four 500 mg tablets) of either tinidazole (Fasigyn) or metronidazole (Flagyl). Cure rates with tinidazole are comparable to those of metronidazole, but better tolerated.

3. Similar cure rates are obtained with single and multiple dose regimens (82 to 88%). Side effects (eg, nausea, vomiting, headache, metallic taste, dizziness) appear to be dose related and occur less frequently with the lower doses of multiple dose, prolonged therapy (eg, metronidazole 500 mg twice daily for seven days. There is no multiple dose regimen for tinidazole).

4. Oral is preferred to vaginal therapy since systemic administration achieves therapeutic drug levels in the urethra and periurethral glands.

5. Patients should be advised to not consume alcohol for 24 hours after metronidazole treatment and 72 hours after tinidazole treatment because of the possibility of a disulfiram-like (Antabuse effect) reaction.

6. Follow-up is unnecessary for women who become asymptomatic after treatment.

B. Male partners. T vaginalis infection in men is often asymptomatic and transient (spontaneous resolution within 10 days). Symptoms, when present, consist of a clear or mucopurulent urethral discharge and/or dysuria. Complications include prostatitis, balanoposthitis, epididymitis, and infertility. Maximal cure rates are achieved when sexual partners are treated simultaneously with the affected woman. Neither partner should resume intercourse until both partners have completed treatment, otherwise reinfection can occur.

C. Pregnancy

1. Metronidazole is the drug of choice for treatment of symptomatic trichomoniasis in pregnancy. Meta-analysis has not found any relationship between metronidazole exposure during the first trimester of pregnancy and birth defects. The Centers for Disease Control and Prevention no longer discourage the use of metronidazole in the first trimester.

2. In pregnant women, some clinicians prefer metronidazole 500 mg twice daily for five to seven days to the 2 g single dose regimen because of the lower frequency of side effects.

3. Asymptomatic infections during pregnancy should not be treated because treatment does not prevent, and may even increase, the risk of preterm delivery.

Treatment options for trichomoniasis

Initial measures

Tinidazole (Fasigyn) 2 g PO in a single dose. Cure rates with tinidazole are comparable to those of metronidazole, but better tolerated.

Metronidazole (Flagyl, Protostat), 2 g PO in a single dose, or metronidazole, 500 mg PO bid X 7 days, or metronidazole, 375 mg PO bid X 7 days

Treat male sexual partners

Measures for treatment failure

Treatment sexual contacts

Re-treat with tinazole 2 gm PO or metronidazole, 500 mg PO bid X 7 days

If infection persists, confirm with culture and re-treat with metronidazole, 2-4 g PO qd X 3-10 days

VIII. **Other causes of vaginitis and vaginal discharge**
  A. **Atrophic vaginitis**
    1. Reduced endogenous estrogen causes thinning of the vaginal epithelium. Symptoms include vaginal soreness, postcoital burning, dyspareunia, and spotting. The vaginal mucosa is thin with diffuse erythema, occasional petechiae or ecchymoses, and few or no vaginal folds. There may be a serosanguineous or watery discharge with a pH of 5.0-7.0.
    2. Treatment consists of topical vaginal estrogen. **Vaginal ring estradiol (Estring)**, a silastic ring impregnated with estradiol, is the preferred means of delivering estrogen to the vagina. The silastic ring delivers 6 to 9 µg of estradiol to the vagina daily. The rings are changed once every three months. Concomitant progestin therapy is not necessary.
    3. **Conjugated estrogens (Premarin)**, 0.5 gm of cream, or one-eighth of an applicatorful daily into the vagina for three weeks, followed by twice weekly thereafter is also effective. Concomitant progestin therapy is not necessary.
    4. **Estrace cream (estradiol)** can also by given by vaginal applicator at a dose of one-eighth of an applicator or 0.5 g (which contains 50 µg of estradiol) daily into the vagina for three weeks, followed by twice weekly thereafter. Concomitant progestin therapy is not necessary.
    5. **Oral estrogen (Premarin)** 0.3 mg qd should also provide relief.
  B. **Desquamative inflammatory vaginitis**
    1. Chronic purulent vaginitis usually occurs perimenopausally, with diffuse exudative vaginitis, massive vaginal-cell exfoliation, purulent vaginal discharge, and occasional vaginal and cervical spotted rash.
    2. Laboratory findings included an elevated pH, increased numbers of parabasal cells, the absence of gram-positive bacilli and their replacement by gram-positive cocci on Gram staining. Clindamycin 2% cream is usually effective.
  C. **Noninfectious vaginitis and vulvitis**
    1. Noninfectious causes of vaginitis include irritants (eg, minipads, spermicides, povidone-iodine, topical antimycotic drugs, soaps and perfumes) and contact dermatitis (eg, latex condoms and antimycotic creams).
    2. Typical symptoms include pruritus, irritation, burning, soreness, and variable discharge. The diagnosis should be suspected in symptomatic women who do not have an otherwise apparent infectious cause.
    3. Management of noninfectious vaginitis includes identifying and eliminating the offending agent. Sodium bicarbonate sitz baths and topical vegetable oils. Topical corticosteroids are not recommended.

References, see page 372.

Trichomonas Vaginitis

Trichomonas vaginalis is the causative agent of trichomoniasis, accounting for 35% of vaginitis. The prevalence of trichomoniasis in black, white, and Mexican-American women is 13.5, 1.2, and 1.5%, respectively.

I. **Microbiology and risk factors**
  A. Trichomonas is a flagellated protozoan, which may be found in the vagina, urethra, paraurethral glands, and Bartholins and Skene's glands.
  B. Trichomoniasis is virtually always sexually transmitted, although survival on fomites has been reported. It is associated with a high prevalence of coinfection with other sexually transmitted diseases.

II. Clinical features

- **A.** Trichomoniasis in women ranges from an asymptomatic carrier state to a severe, acute, inflammatory disease.
- **B.** **Signs and symptoms** include a purulent, malodorous, thin discharge (70% of cases) with burning, pruritus, dysuria, frequency, and dyspareunia. Postcoital bleeding can occur. The urethra is also infected in the majority of women.
- **C.** **Physical examination** often reveals erythema of the vulva and vaginal mucosa; green-yellow frothy discharge is observed in 10 to 30%. Punctate hemorrhages may be visible on the vagina and cervix ("strawberry cervix") in 2%.

Clinical Features of Vaginitis				
Variable	Normal	Vulvovaginal candidiasis	Bacterial vaginosis	Trichomoniasis
Symptoms	None	Pruritus, soreness, change in discharge, dyspareunia	Malodorous discharge, no dyspareunia	Malodorous, purulent discharge, dyspareunia
Signs	-	Vulvar erythema, edema, fissure	Adherent discharge	Purulent discharge, vulvovaginal erythema
pH	4.0-4.5	4.0-4.5	>4.5	5.0-6.0
Saline microscopy	PMN:EC ratio <1; rods dominate; squames +++	PMN:EC ratio <1; rods dominate; squames +++; pseudohyphae (about 40%)	PMN:EC <1; loss of rods; increased coccobacilli; clue cells (>90%)	PMN ++++; mixed flora; motile trichomonads (60%)
10% potassium hydroxide examination	Negative	Pseudohyphae (about 70%)	Negative	Negative
Miscellaneous	-	Culture if microscopy negative	Culture of no value	Culture if microscopy negative
Differential diagnosis	Physiologic leukorrhea	Contact irritant or allergic vulvitis, chemical irritation, focal vulvitis (vulvodynia)		Purulent vaginitis, desquamative inflammatory vaginitis, atrophic vaginitis plus secondary infection, erosive lichen planus

III. Complications

- **A.** Trichomoniasis is a risk factor for post-hysterectomy cellulitis, tubal infertility, and cervical neoplasia. Infection facilitates transmission of the human immunodeficiency virus (HIV).

  B. **Trichomoniasis in pregnancy** is associated with premature rupture of the membranes and preterm delivery; however, treatment of asymptomatic infection has not been shown to reduce these complications.
IV. **Diagnosis**
  A. **Microscopy and pH.** The presence of motile trichomonads on wet mount is diagnostic of infection, but this occurs in only 50 to 70% of cases. Other findings include an elevated vaginal pH (>4.5) and an increase in polymorphonuclear leukocytes.
  B. **Culture on Diamond's medium** has a high sensitivity (95%) and specificity (>95%) and should be considered in patients with elevated vaginal pH, increased numbers of polymorphonuclear leukocytes and an absence of motile trichomonads and clue cells on wet mount.
  C. **OSOM Trichomonas Rapid Test for Trichomonas antigens** has a sensitivity of 88.3% and specificity of 98.8%. Results can be read in 10 minutes. The Affirm VP III Microbial Identification System (Becton Dickinson) test uses a nucleic acid probe and is read in 45 minutes.
  D. **Cervical cytology.** Trichomonads are sometimes reported on Papanicolaou (Pap) smears. Pap smears are inadequate for diagnosis of trichomoniasis because this technique has a sensitivity of only 60 to 70% and false positive results are common (at least 8%). Asymptomatic women with trichomonads identified on conventional Pap smear should be evaluated by wet mount and should not be treated until the diagnosis is confirmed.
  E. Treatment of asymptomatic women with trichomonads noted on liquid-based cervical cytology is appropriate.
V. **Treatment of Trichomonas vaginitis**
  A. **Nonpregnant women**
    1. The 5-nitroimidazole drugs (metronidazole or tinidazole) are the only class of drugs that provide curative therapy of trichomoniasis. Cure rates are 90 to 95%.
    2. Treatment consists of a single oral dose of 2 grams (four 500 mg tablets) of either tinidazole or metronidazole. Cure rates with tinidazole are comparable to those of metronidazole, but better tolerated.
    3. Similar cure rates are obtained with single and multiple dose regimens (82 to 88%). Side effects (eg, nausea, vomiting, headache, metallic taste, dizziness) appear to be dose related and occur less frequently with the lower doses of multiple dose, prolonged therapy (eg, metronidazole 500 mg twice daily for seven days. There is no multiple dose regimen for tinidazole).
    4. Oral is preferred to vaginal therapy since systemic administration achieves therapeutic drug levels in the urethra and periurethral glands.
    5. Patients should be advised to not consume alcohol for 24 hours after metronidazole treatment and 72 hours after tinidazole treatment because of the possibility of a disulfiram-like (Antabuse effect) reaction.
    6. Follow-up is unnecessary for women who become asymptomatic after treatment.
  B. **Male partners.** T vaginalis infection in men is often asymptomatic and transient. Symptoms, when present, consist of a clear or mucopurulent urethral discharge and/or dysuria. Complications include prostatitis, balanoposthitis, epididymitis, and infertility. Maximal cure rates are achieved when sexual partners are treated simultaneously with the affected woman. Neither partner should resume intercourse until both partners have completed treatment
  C. **Pregnancy**
    1. Metronidazole is the drug of choice for treatment of symptomatic trichomoniasis in pregnancy.

2. In pregnant women, some clinicians prefer metronidazole 500 mg twice daily for five to seven days to the 2 g single dose regimen because of the lower frequency of side effects.
3. Asymptomatic infections during pregnancy should not be treated because treatment does not prevent, and may even increase, the risk of preterm delivery.

References, see page 372.

Breast Cancer Screening and Diagnosis

Breast cancer is the second most commonly diagnosed cancer among women, after skin cancer. Approximately 182,800 new cases of invasive breast cancer are diagnosed in the United States per year. The incidence of breast cancer increases with age. White women are more likely to develop breast cancer than black women. The incidence of breast cancer in white women is about 113 cases per 100,000 women and in black women, 100 cases per 100,000.

I. Risk factors

Risk Factors for Breast Cancer	
Age >50 years	Age >30 at first birth
Prior history of breast cancer	Obesity
Family history	High socioeconomic status
Early menarche, before age 12	Atypical hyperplasia on biopsy
Late menopause, after age 50	Ionizing radiation exposure
Nulliparity	

A. Family history is highly significant in a first-degree relative (ie, mother, sister, daughter), especially if the cancer has been diagnosed premenopausally. Women who have premenopausal first-degree relatives with breast cancer have a three- to fourfold increased risk of breast cancer. Having several second-degree relatives with breast cancer may further increase the risk of breast cancer. Most women with breast cancer have no identifiable risk factors.

B. Approximately 8% of all cases of breast cancer are hereditary. About one-half of these cases are attributed to mutations in the BRCA1 and BRCA2 genes. Hereditary breast cancer commonly occurs in premenopausal women. Screening tests are available that detect BRCA mutations.

II. Diagnosis and evaluation

A. **Clinical evaluation of a breast mass** should assess duration of the lesion, associated pain, relationship to the menstrual cycle or exogenous hormone use, and change in size since discovery. The presence of nipple discharge and its character (bloody or tea-colored, unilateral or bilateral, spontaneous or expressed) should be assessed.

B. **Menstrual history.** The date of last menstrual period, age of menarche, age of menopause or surgical removal of the ovaries, previous pregnancies should be determined.

C. **History of previous breast biopsies**, cyst aspiration, dates and results of previous mammograms should be determined.

D. **Family history** should document breast cancer in relatives and the age at which family members were diagnosed.

III. Physical examination

A. The breasts should be inspected for asymmetry, deformity, skin retraction, erythema, peau d'orange (breast edema), and nipple retraction, discoloration, or inversion.

B. **Palpation**

1. The breasts should be palpated while the patient is sitting and then supine with the ipsilateral arm extended. The entire breast should be palpated systematically. The mass should be evaluated for size, shape, texture, tenderness, fixation to skin or chest wall.

2. mass that is suspicious for breast cancer is usually solitary, discrete and hard. In some instances, it is fixed to the skin or the muscle. A suspicious mass is usually unilateral and nontender. Sometimes, an area of thickening may represent cancer. Breast cancer is rarely bilateral. The nipples should be expressed for discharge.

3. The axillae should be palpated for adenopathy, with an assessment of size of the lymph nodes, number, and fixation.

C. **Mammography.** Screening mammograms are recommended every year for asymptomatic women 40 years and older. Unfortunately, only 60% of cancers are diagnosed at a local stage.

Screening for Breast Cancer in Women	
Age	American Cancer Society guidelines
20 to 39 years	Clinical breast examination every three years Monthly self-examination of breasts
Age 40 years and older	Annual mammogram Annual clinical breast examination Monthly self-examination of breasts

IV. Methods of breast biopsy

A. **Palpable masses. Fine-needle aspiration biopsy (FNAB)** has a sensitivity ranging from 90-98%. Nondiagnostic aspirates require surgical biopsy.

1. The skin is prepped with alcohol and the lesion is immobilized with the nonoperating hand. A 10 mL syringe, with a 14 gauge needle, is introduced in to the central portion of the mass at a 90° angle. When the needle enters the mass, suction is applied by retracting the plunger, and the needle is advanced. The needle is directed into different areas of the mass while maintaining suction on the syringe.

2. Suction is slowly released before the needle is withdrawn from the mass. The contents of the needle are placed onto glass slides for pathologic examination.Excisional biopsy is done when needle biopsies are negative but the mass is clinically suspected of malignancy.

B. **Stereotactic core needle biopsy.** Using a computer-driven stereotactic unit, the lesion is localized in three dimensions, and an automated biopsy needle obtains samples. The sensitivity and specificity of this technique are 95-100% and 94-98%, respectively.

C. **Nonpalpable lesions**

1. **Needle localized biopsy**

a. Under mammographic guidance, a needle and hookwire are placed into the breast parenchyma adjacent to the lesion. The patient is taken to the operating room along with mammograms for an excisional breast biopsy.

b. The skin and underlying tissues are infiltrated with 1% lidocaine with epinephrine. For lesions located within 5 cm of the nipple, a periareolar incision may be used or use a curved incision located over the mass and parallel to the areola. Incise the skin and subcutaneous fat, then palpate the lesion and excise the mass.

c. After removal of the specimen, a specimen x-ray is performed to confirm that the lesion has been removed. The specimen can then be sent fresh for pathologic analysis.

d. Close the subcutaneous tissues with a 4-0 chromic catgut suture, and close the skin with 4-0 subcuticular suture.

2. **Ultrasonography.** Screening is useful to differentiate between solid and cystic breast masses when a palpable mass is not well seen on a mammogram. Ultrasonography is especially helpful in young women with dense breast tissue when a palpable mass is not visualized on a mammogram. Ultrasonography is not used for routine screening because microcalcifications are not visualized and the yield of carcinomas is negligible.

References, see page 372.

Secondary Amenorrhea

Amenorrhea (absence of menses) can be a transient, intermittent, or permanent condition resulting from dysfunction of the hypothalamus, pituitary, ovaries, uterus, or vagina. Amenorrhea is classified as either primary (absence of menarche by age 16 years) or secondary (absence of menses for more than three cycles or six months in women who previously had menses). Pregnancy is the most common cause of secondary amenorrhea.

I. **Diagnosis of secondary amenorrhea**
   A. **Step 1: Rule out pregnancy.** A pregnancy test is the first step in evaluating secondary amenorrhea. Measurement of serum beta subunit of hCG is the most sensitive test.
   B. **Step 2: Assess the history**
      1. Recent stress; change in weight, diet or exercise habits; or illnesses that might result in hypothalamic amenorrhea should be sought.
      2. Drugs associated with amenorrhea, systemic illnesses that can cause hypothalamic amenorrhea, recent initiation or discontinuation of an oral contraceptive, androgenic drugs (danazol) or high-dose progestin, and antipsychotic drugs should be evaluated.
      3. Headaches, visual field defects, fatigue, or polyuria and polydipsia may suggest hypothalamic-pituitary disease.
      4. Symptoms of estrogen deficiency include hot flashes, vaginal dryness, poor sleep, or decreased libido.
      5. Galactorrhea is suggestive of hyperprolactinemia. Hirsutism, acne, and a history of irregular menses are suggestive of hyperandrogenism.
      6. A history of obstetrical catastrophe, severe bleeding, dilatation and curettage, or endometritis or other infection that might have caused scarring of the endometrial lining suggests Asherman's syndrome.
   C. **Step 3: Physical examination.** Measurements of height and weight, signs of other illnesses, and evidence of cachexia should be assessed. The skin, breasts, and genital tissues should be evaluated for estrogen deficiency. The breasts should be palpated, including an attempt to express galactorrhea. The skin should be examined for hirsutism, acne, striae, acanthosis nigricans, vitiligo, thickness or thinness, and easy bruisability.

D. **Step 4: Basic laboratory testing**. In addition to measurement of serum hCG to rule out pregnancy, minimal laboratory testing should include measurements of serum prolactin, thyrotropin, and FSH to rule out hyperprolactinemia, thyroid disease, and ovarian failure (high serum FSH). If there is hirsutism, acne or irregular menses, serum dehydroepiandrosterone sulfate (DHEA-S) and testosterone should be measured.

E. **Step 5: Follow-up laboratory evaluation**
1. **High serum prolactin concentration**. Prolactin secretion can be transiently increased by stress or eating. Therefore, serum prolactin should be measured at least twice before cranial imaging is obtained, particularly in those women with small elevations (<50 ng/mL). These women should be screened for thyroid disease with a TSH and free T4 because hypothyroidism can cause hyperprolactinemia.
2. Women with verified high serum prolactin values should have a cranial MRI unless a very clear explanation is found for the elevation (eg, antipsychotics). Imaging should rule out a hypothalamic or pituitary tumor.
3. **High serum FSH concentration.** A high serum FSH concentration indicates the presence of ovarian failure. This test should be repeated monthly on three occasions to confirm. A karyotype should be considered in most women with secondary amenorrhea age 30 years or younger.

Causes of Primary and Secondary Amenorrhea	
Abnormality	**Causes**
Pregnancy	
Anatomic abnormalities	
Congenital abnormality in Müllerian development	Isolated defect Testicular feminization syndrome 5-Alpha-reductase deficiency Vanishing testes syndrome Defect in testis determining factor
Congenital defect of urogenital sinus development	Agenesis of lower vagina Imperforate hymen
Acquired ablation or scarring of the endometrium	Asherman's syndrome Tuberculosis
Disorders of hypothalamic-pituitary ovarian axis Hypothalamic dysfunction Pituitary dysfunction Ovarian dysfunction	

Causes of Amenorrhea due to Abnormalities in the Hypothalamic-Pituitary-Ovarian Axis	
Abnormality	**Causes**

Hypothalamic dysfunction	Functional hypothalamic amenorrhea
	    Weight loss, eating disorders
	    Exercise
	    Stress
	    Severe or prolonged illness
	Congenital gonadotropin-releasing hormone deficiency
	Inflammatory or infiltrative diseases
	Brain tumors - eg, craniopharyngioma
	Pituitary stalk dissection or compression
	Cranial irradiation
	Brain injury - trauma, hemorrhage, hydrocephalus
	Other syndromes - Prader-Willi, Laurence-Moon-Biedl

Pituitary dysfunction	Hyperprolactinemia Other pituitary tumors- acromegaly, corticotroph adenomas (Cushing's disease) Other tumors - meningioma, germinoma, glioma Empty sella syndrome Pituitary infarct or apoplexy

Ovarian dysfunction	Ovarian failure (menopause)
	    Spontaneous
	    Premature (before age 40 years)
	    Surgical

Other	Hyperthyroidism Hypothyroidism Diabetes mellitus Exogenous androgen use

Drugs Associated with Amenorrhea	
Drugs that Increase Prolactin	Antipsychotics Tricyclic antidepressants Calcium channel blockers
Drugs with Estrogenic Activity	Digoxin, marijuana, oral contraceptives
Drugs with Ovarian Toxicity	Chemotherapeutic agents

4. **High serum androgen concentrations**. A high serum androgen value may suggest the diagnosis of polycystic ovary syndrome or may suggest an androgen-secreting tumor of the ovary or adrenal gland. Further testing for a tumor might include a 24-hour urine collection for cortisol and 17-ketosteroids, determination of serum 17-hydroxyprogesterone after intravenous injection of corticotropin (ACTH), and a dexamethasone suppression test. Elevation of 17-ketosteroids, DHEA-S, or 17-hydroxyprogesterone is more consistent with an adrenal, rather than ovarian, source of excess androgen.

5. **Normal or low serum gonadotropin concentrations and all other tests normal**
   a. This result is one of the most common outcomes of laboratory testing in women with amenorrhea. Women with hypothalamic amenorrhea (caused by excessive exercise or weight loss) have normal to low serum FSH values. Cranial MRI is indicated in all women without an a clear explanation for hypogonadotropic hypogonadism and in most women who have visual field defects or headaches. No further testing is required if the onset of amenorrhea is recent or is easily explained (eg, weight loss, excessive exercise) and there are no symptoms suggestive of other disease.
   b. High serum transferrin saturation may indicate hemochromatosis, high serum angiotensin-converting enzyme values suggest sarcoidosis, and high fasting blood glucose or hemoglobin A1c values indicate diabetes mellitus.

6. **Normal serum prolactin and FSH concentrations with history of uterine instrumentation preceding amenorrhea**
   a. Evaluation for Asherman's syndrome should be completed. A progestin challenge should be performed (medroxyprogesterone acetate 10 mg for 10 days). If withdrawal bleeding occurs, an outflow tract disorder has been ruled out. If bleeding does not occur, estrogen and progestin should be administered.
   b. Oral conjugated estrogens (0.625 to 2.5 mg daily for 35 days) with medroxyprogesterone added (10 mg daily for days 26 to 35); failure to bleed upon cessation of this therapy strongly suggests endometrial scarring. In this situation, a hysterosalpingogram or hysteroscopy can confirm the diagnosis of Asherman syndrome.

II. **Treatment**
   A. **Athletic women** should be counseled on the need for increased caloric intake or reduced exercise. Resumption of menses usually occurs.
   B. **Nonathletic women who are underweight** should receive nutritional counseling and treatment of eating disorders.
   C. **Hyperprolactinemia** is treated with a dopamine agonist. Cabergoline (Dostinex) or bromocriptine (Parlodel) are used for most adenomas. Ovulation, regular menstrual cycles, and pregnancy may usually result.
   D. **Ovarian failure** should be treated with hormone replacement therapy.
   E. **Hyperandrogenism** is treated with measures to reduce hirsutism, resume menses, and fertility and preventing endometrial hyperplasia, obesity, and metabolic defects.
   F. **Asherman's syndrome** is treated with hysteroscopic lysis of adhesions followed by long-term estrogen administration to stimulate regrowth of endometrial tissue.

References, see page 372.

Abnormal Vaginal Bleeding

Menorrhagia (excessive bleeding) is most commonly caused by anovulatory menstrual cycles. Occasionally it is caused by thyroid dysfunction, infections or cancer.

I. **Pathophysiology of normal menstruation**
   A. In response to gonadotropin-releasing hormone from the hypothalamus, the pituitary gland synthesizes follicle-stimulating hormone (FSH) and luteinizing hormone (LH), which induce the ovaries to produce estrogen and progesterone.
   B. During the follicular phase, estrogen stimulation causes an increase in endometrial thickness. After ovulation, progesterone causes endometrial maturation. Menstruation is caused by estrogen and progesterone withdrawal.
   C. **Abnormal bleeding** is defined as bleeding that occurs at intervals of less than 21 days, more than 36 days, lasting longer than 7 days, or blood loss >80 mL.

II. **Clinical evaluation of abnormal vaginal bleeding**
   A. A menstrual and reproductive history should include last menstrual period, regularity, duration, frequency; the number of pads used per day, and intermenstrual bleeding.
   B. Stress, exercise, weight changes and systemic diseases, particularly thyroid, renal or hepatic diseases or coagulopathies, should be sought. The method of birth control should be determined.
   C. Pregnancy complications, such as spontaneous abortion, ectopic pregnancy, placenta previa and abruptio placentae, can cause heavy bleeding. Pregnancy should always be considered as a possible cause of abnormal vaginal bleeding.

III. **Puberty and adolescence – menarche to age 16**
   A. Irregularity is normal during the first few months of menstruation; however, soaking more than 25 pads or 30 tampons during a menstrual period is abnormal.
   B. Absence of premenstrual symptoms (breast tenderness, bloating, cramping) is associated with anovulatory cycles.
   C. Fever, particularly in association with pelvic or abdominal pain may, indicate pelvic inflammatory disease. A history of easy bruising suggests a coagulation defect. Headaches and visual changes suggest a pituitary tumor.
   D. **Physical findings**
      1. Pallor not associated with tachycardia or signs of hypovolemia suggests chronic excessive blood loss secondary to anovulatory bleeding, adenomyosis, uterine myomas, or blood dyscrasia.
      2. Fever, leukocytosis, and pelvic tenderness suggests PID.
      3. Signs of impending shock indicate that the blood loss is related to pregnancy (including ectopic), trauma, sepsis, or neoplasia.
      4. Pelvic masses may represent pregnancy, uterine or ovarian neoplasia, or a pelvic abscess or hematoma.
      5. Fine, thinning hair, and hypoactive reflexes suggest hypothyroidism.
      6. Ecchymoses or multiple bruises may indicate trauma, coagulation defects, medication use, or dietary extremes.
   E. **Laboratory tests**
      1. CBC and platelet count and a urine or serum pregnancy test should be obtained.
      2. Screening for sexually transmitted diseases, thyroid function, and coagulation disorders (partial thromboplastin time, INR, bleeding time) should be completed.

     3. **Endometrial sampling** is rarely necessary for those under age 20.
- **F. Treatment of infrequent bleeding**
    1. Therapy should be directed at the underlying cause when possible. If the CBC and other initial laboratory tests are normal and the history and physical examination are normal, reassurance is usually all that is necessary.
    2. Ferrous gluconate, 325 mg bid-tid, should be prescribed.
- **G. Treatment of frequent or heavy bleeding**
    1. Treatment with nonsteroidal anti-inflammatory drugs (NSAIDs) improves platelet aggregation and increases uterine vasoconstriction. NSAIDs are the first choice in the treatment of menorrhagia because they are well tolerated and do not have the hormonal effects of oral contraceptives.
        - a. **Mefenamic acid (Ponstel)** 500 mg tid during the menstrual period.
        - b. **Naproxen (Anaprox, Naprosyn)** 500 mg loading dose, then 250 mg tid during the menstrual period.
        - c. **Ibuprofen (Motrin, Nuprin)** 400 mg tid during the menstrual period.
        - d. Gastrointestinal distress is common. NSAIDs are contraindicated in renal failure and peptic ulcer disease.
    2. Iron should also be added as ferrous gluconate 325 mg tid.
- **H. Patients with hypovolemia or a hemoglobin level below 7 g/dL** should be hospitalized for hormonal therapy and iron replacement.
    1. Hormonal therapy consists of estrogen (Premarin) 25 mg IV q6h until bleeding stops. Thereafter, oral contraceptive pills should be administered q6h x 7 days, then taper slowly to one pill qd.
    2. If bleeding continues, IV vasopressin (DDAVP) should be administered. Hysteroscopy may be necessary, and dilation and curettage is a last resort. Transfusion may be indicated in severe hemorrhage.
    3. Iron should also be added as ferrous gluconate 325 mg tid.

IV. **Primary childbearing years – ages 16 to early 40s**
- **A.** Contraceptive complications and pregnancy are the most common causes of abnormal bleeding in this age group. Anovulation accounts for 20% of cases.
- **B.** Adenomyosis, endometriosis, and fibroids increase in frequency as a woman ages, as do endometrial hyperplasia and endometrial polyps. Pelvic inflammatory disease and endocrine dysfunction may also occur.
- **C. Laboratory tests**
    1. CBC and platelet count, Pap smear, and pregnancy test.
    2. Screening for sexually transmitted diseases, thyroid-stimulating hormone, and coagulation disorders (partial thromboplastin time, INR, bleeding time).
    3. If a non-pregnant woman has a pelvic mass, ultrasonography or hysterosonography (with uterine saline infusion) is required.
- **D. Endometrial sampling**
    1. Long-term unopposed estrogen stimulation in anovulatory patients can result in endometrial hyperplasia, which can progress to adenocarcinoma; therefore, in perimenopausal patients who have been anovulatory for an extended interval, the endometrium should be biopsied.
    2. Biopsy is also recommended before initiation of hormonal therapy for women over age 30 and for those over age 20 who have had prolonged bleeding.
    3. Hysteroscopy and endometrial biopsy with a Pipelle aspirator should be done on the first day of menstruation (to avoid an unexpected pregnancy) or anytime if bleeding is continuous.
- **E. Treatment**
    1. Medical protocols for anovulatory bleeding (dysfunctional uterine bleeding) are similar to those described above for adolescents.

2. Hormonal therapy

a. In women who do not desire immediate fertility, hormonal therapy may be used to treat menorrhagia.

b. A 21-day package of oral contraceptives is used. The patient should take one pill three times a day for 7 days. During the 7 days of therapy, bleeding should subside, and, following treatment, heavy flow will occur. After 7 days off the hormones, another 21-day package is initiated, taking one pill each day for 21 days, then no pills for 7 days.

c. Alternatively, medroxyprogesterone (Provera), 10-20 mg per day for days 16 through 25 of each month, will result in a reduction of menstrual blood loss. Pregnancy will not be prevented.

d. Patients with severe bleeding may have hypotension and tachycardia. These patients require hospitalization, and estrogen (Premarin) should be administered IV as 25 mg q4-6h until bleeding slows (up to a maximum of four doses). Oral contraceptives should be initiated concurrently as described above.

3. Iron should also be added as ferrous gluconate 325 mg tid.

4. Surgical treatment can be considered if childbearing is completed and medical management fails to provide relief.

V. Premenopausal, perimenopausal, and postmenopausal years--age 40 and over

A. Anovulatory bleeding accounts for about 90% of abnormal vaginal bleeding in this age group. However, bleeding should be considered to be from cancer until proven otherwise.

B. History, physical examination and laboratory testing are indicated as described above. Menopausal symptoms, personal or family history of malignancy and use of estrogen should be sought. A pelvic mass requires an evaluation with ultrasonography.

C. Endometrial carcinoma

1. In a perimenopausal or postmenopausal woman, amenorrhea preceding abnormal bleeding suggests endometrial cancer. Endometrial evaluation is necessary before treatment of abnormal vaginal bleeding.

2. Before endometrial sampling, determination of endometrial thickness by transvaginal ultrasonography is useful because biopsy is often not required when the endometrium is less than 5 mm thick.

D. Treatment

1. Cystic hyperplasia or endometrial hyperplasia without cytologic atypia is treated with depo-medroxyprogesterone, 200 mg IM, then 100 to 200 mg IM every 3 to 4 weeks for 6 to 12 months. Endometrial hyperplasia requires repeat endometrial biopsy every 3 to 6 months.

2. Atypical hyperplasia requires fractional dilation and curettage, followed by progestin therapy or hysterectomy.

3. If the patient's endometrium is normal (or atrophic) and contraception is a concern, a low-dose oral contraceptive may be used. If contraception is not needed, estrogen and progesterone therapy should be prescribed.

4. **Surgical management**

a. **Vaginal or abdominal hysterectomy** is the most absolute curative treatment.

b. **Dilatation and curettage** can be used as a temporizing measure to stop bleeding.

c. **Endometrial ablation and resection** by laser, electrodiathermy "rollerball," or excisional resection are alternatives to hysterectomy.

References, see page 372.

Menopause

Menopause is defined as the cessation of menstrual periods, menopause occurs at a mean age of 51.4 years in normal women.

I. Definitions

  A. **Menopausal transition** begins with variation in menstrual cycle length and an elevated FSH concentration and ends with the final menstrual period (12 months of amenorrhea). Stage -2 (early) is characterized by variable cycle length (>7 days different from normal menstrual cycle length, which is 21 to 35 days). Stage -1 (late) is characterized by ≥2 skipped cycles and an interval of amenorrhea ≥60 days; women at this stage often have hot flashes as well.

  B. **Perimenopause** begins in stage -2 of the menopausal transition and ends 12 months after the last menstrual period.

  C. **Menopause** is defined by 12 months of amenorrhea after the final menstrual period. It results from complete, or near complete, ovarian follicular depletion and absence of ovarian estrogen secretion.

  D. **Postmenopause.** Stage +1 (early) is defined as the first five years after the final menstrual period. It is characterized by further and complete decline in ovarian function and accelerated bone loss; many women in this stage continue to have hot flashes. Stage +2 (late) begins five years after the final menstrual period and ends with death.

II. Epidemiology

  A. The average age at menopause is 51 years; however, for 5% of women it occurs after age 55 (late menopause), and for another 5%, between ages 40 to 45 years (early menopause). Menopause that occurs before age 40 years is premature ovarian failure.

  B. The age of menopause is reduced by about two years in women who smoke. Women who have never had children and who have had regular cycles tend to have an earlier age of menopause.

III. Clinical manifestations

  A. **Bleeding patterns.** Chronic anovulation and progesterone deficiency in this transition period may cause long periods of unopposed estrogen exposure and result in anovulatory bleeding and endometrial hyperplasia.

  B. **Oligomenorrhea** (irregular cycles) for six or more months, or an episode of heavy dysfunctional bleeding is an indication for endometrial surveillance. Endometrial biopsy is the standard to rule out the occurrence of endometrial hyperplasia.

  C. **Irregular or heavy bleeding** during the menopausal transition may be treated with low-dose oral contraceptives or intermittent progestin therapy.

  D. **Hot flashes**

   1. The most common symptom during menopause is the hot flash, occurring in up to 75%. Hot flashes are self-limited, usually resolving without treatment within one to five years, although some women will continue to have hot flashes until after age 70.

   2. Hot flashes begin as the sudden sensation of heat in the upper chest and face that rapidly becomes generalized. The sensation of heat lasts from two to four minutes, is often associated with perspiration and occasionally palpitations, and is often followed by chills and shivering, and sometimes anxiety. Hot flashes usually occur several times per day and are common at night.

  E. **Genitourinary symptoms**

   1. **Vaginal dryness.** The vagina and urethra are very sensitive to estrogen, and estrogen deficiency leads to thinning of the vaginal epithelium. This

results in vaginal atrophy (atrophic vaginitis), causing symptoms of vaginal dryness, itching and often, dyspareunia.

2. The vagina typically appears pale, with lack of the normal rugae and often has visible blood vessels or petechial hemorrhages.

3. **Sexual dysfunction.** Estrogen deficiency causes a decrease in blood flow to the vagina and vulva, decreased vaginal lubrication, and sexual dysfunction.

4. Atrophic urethritis results from low estrogen production after the menopause, predisposing to stress and urge urinary incontinence. The prevalence of incontinence increases with age.

IV. Diagnosis

A. Menopause is defined as 12 months of amenorrhea in a woman over age 45 in the absence of other causes. Further evaluation is not necessary for women in this group.

B. The best approach to diagnosing the menopausal transition is an assessment of menstrual cycle history and menopausal symptoms (vasomotor flushes, mood changes, sleep disturbances). Measuring serum FSH, estradiol, or inhibin levels is usually not necessary. Serum FSH concentrations increase across the menopausal transition, but at times may be suppressed into the normal premenopausal range (after a recent ovulation).

C. **Differential diagnosis.** Hyperthyroidism should be considered in the differential diagnosis because irregular menses, sweats (although different from typical hot flashes), and mood changes are all potential clinical manifestations of hyperthyroidism. Other etiologies for menstrual cycle changes that should be considered include pregnancy, hyperprolactinemia, and thyroid disease. Atypical hot flashes and night sweats may be caused by medications, carcinoid, pheochromocytoma, or underlying malignancy.

V. Treatment of menopausal symptoms in women not taking systemic estrogen

A. Many women cannot or choose not to take estrogen to treat symptoms of estrogen deficiency at menopause because of an increased risk of breast cancer and cardiovascular disease.

B. Therapy prevents bone loss and fracture, but does not confir a protective effect on the heart. Continuous combined therapy with conjugated estrogen (0.625 mg/day) and medroxyprogesterone acetate (2.5 mg/day) is ineffective for either primary or secondary prevention of CHD, and slightly increases risk. Other risks included an increased risk of stroke, venous thromboembolism, and breast cancer.

C. **Patient selection.** Estrogen is a reasonable short-term option for most symptomatic postmenopausal women, with the exception of those with a history of breast cancer, coronary heart disease, a previous venous thromboembolic event or stroke, or those at high risk for these complications. Short-term therapy is six months to five years.

D. **Vasomotor instability.** Hot flashes can result in sleep disturbances, headache, and irritability. Although estrogen is the gold standard for relief of hot flashes, a number of other drugs have been shown to be somewhat better than placebo. Venlafaxine (Effexor, 75 mg daily) reduces hot flashes by 61%. Mouth dryness, anorexia, nausea, and constipation are common. Gabapentin (Neurontin) has been used for hot flashes at a dose of 200mg orally once daily to 400mg orally four times daily.

E. **Urogenital atrophy**

1. Both systemic and vaginal estrogen are effective for genitourinary atrophy; however, vaginal estrogen has lesser systemic levels than estrogen tablets.

2. **Moisturizers and lubricants.** The long-acting vaginal moisturizer, Replens, produces a moist film over the vaginal tissue. A water soluble lubricant, such as Astroglide and K-Y Personal Lubricant, should be used at the time of intercourse.

3. **Low-dose vaginal estrogen**
   a. **Estrogen Cream (Premarin)** 0.5 g of cream, or one-eighth of an applicatorful daily into the vagina for three weeks followed by twice weekly administration thereafter. Estrace, which is crystalline estradiol, can also by given by vaginal applicator at a dose of one-eighth of an applicator or 0.5 g (which contains 50 microgram of estradiol).
   b. **Vaginal ring** is a silastic ring impregnated with estradiol (Estring, Phadia) involves insertion of a silastic ring that delivers 6 to 9 mcg of estradiol to the vagina daily for a period of three months.
   c. With low-dose vaginal estrogen, a progestin is not necessary.

F. **Osteoporosis.** Estrogen is no longer a primary therapy for osteoporosis. Exercise, and daily intake of calcium (1500 mg/day) and vitamin D (400 to 800 IU/day) are recommended for prevention of bone loss in perimenopausal and postmenopausal women.

VI. **Treatment of menopausal symptoms with hormone therapy**

A. Estrogen prevents bone loss and fracture, but is not cardioprotective, and slightly increases risk. Other risks seen with combined therapy included an increased risk of stroke, venous thromboembolism, and breast cancer.

B. **Menopausal symptoms**
   1. **Hot flashes**. Estrogen therapy remains the gold standard for relief of menopausal symptoms, in particular, hot flashes, and therefore is a reasonable option for most postmenopausal women, with the exception of those with a history of breast cancer, CHD, a previous venous thromboembolic event or stroke, or those at high risk for these complications. In otherwise healthy women, the absolute risk of an adverse event is extremely low.
   2. Short-term therapy (with a goal of symptom management) is less than five years.
   3. **Adding a progestin.** Endometrial hyperplasia and cancer can occur after as little as six months of unopposed estrogen therapy; as a result, a progestin should be added in women who have not had a hysterectomy. Women who have undergone hysterectomy should not receive a progestin.
   4. Hormone preparations: Combined, continuous conjugated estrogens (0.625 mg) and medroxyprogesterone acetate (MPA 2.5 mg) is commonly used. However, low dose estrogen is a better option (eg, 0.3 mg conjugated estrogens or 0.5 mg estradiol).
   5. **A low-estrogen oral contraceptive** (20 mcg of ethinyl estradiol) remains an appropriate treatment for perimenopausal women who seek relief of menopausal symptoms, and who also desire contraception, and in some instances need bleeding control (in cases of dysfunctional uterine bleeding). Most of these women are between the ages of 40 and 50 years and are still candidates for oral contraception.
   6. When women taking a low-dose oral contraceptive during menopause reach age 50 or 51 years, options include stopping the pill altogether, or changing to an estrogen replacement regimen if necessary for symptoms. Tapering the oral contraceptive by one pill per week is recommended.

References, see page 372.

Urologic Disorders

Male Sexual Dysfunction

Impotence is defined as the inability to develop or sustain erection 75 percent of the time. It is a common abnormality and may be due to psychological causes, medications, hormonal abnormalities, neurologic, or vascular problems.

I. **Causes of sexual dysfunction in men**
   A. Libido declines with androgen deficiency, depression, and with the use of prescription and recreational drugs. Erectile dysfunction may reflect either inadequate arterial blood flow into (failure to fill) or accelerated venous drainage out of (failure to store) the corpora cavernosae.

II. **Sexual history**
   A. **Rapidity of onset.** Sexually competent men who have sudden onset of impotence invariably have psychogenic impotence. Psychologic counseling is the preferred therapy in this setting. Only radical prostatectomy or other overt genital tract trauma causes a sudden loss of male sexual function. In comparison, men suffering from impotence of any other cause complain that sexual function failed sporadically at first, then more consistently.
   B. **Erectile reserve.** Most men experience spontaneous erections during REM sleep, and often wake up with an erection, attesting to the integrity of neurogenic reflexes and corpora cavernosae blood flow. Complete loss of nocturnal erections is present in men with neurologic or vascular disease.
   C. **Nonsustained erection with detumescence** after penetration is most commonly due to anxiety or the vascular steal syndrome. In the vascular steal syndrome, blood is diverted from the engorged corpora cavernosae to accommodate the oxygen requirements of the thrusting pelvis. Vascular surgery to ensure equitable genital and pelvic arterial inflow is useful.
   D. **Assessment of interpersonal conflict.** Unexpressed interpersonal conflict is one of the more common causes of male sexual dysfunction. Couples counseling can restore harmony and sexual function in 25 percent of cases.

Agents That May Cause Erectile Dysfunction	
Antidepressants	Miscellaneous
Monoamine oxidase inhibitors	Cimetidine (Tagamet)
Selective serotonin reuptake inhibitors	Corticosteroids
Tricyclic antidepressants	Finasteride (Proscar)
Antihypertensives	Gemfibrozil (Lopid)
Beta blockers	Drugs of abuse
Centrally acting alpha agonists	Alcohol
Diuretics	Anabolic steroids
Antipsychotics	Heroin
Anxiolytics	Marijuana

Clinical clues to causes of male sexual dysfunction	
Finding	**Cause**
Rapid onset	Psychogenic Genitourinary trauma (eg, radical prostatectomy)
Nonsustained erection	Anxiety Vascular steal
Depression or use of certain drugs	Depression Drug induced
Complete loss of nocturnal erections	Vascular disease Neurologic disease

III. **Physical examination**
   A. **Weak or absent femoral and peripheral pulses** suggest the presence of vasculogenic impotence. If pulses are normal, the presence of femoral bruits suggests pelvic blood occlusion.
   B. **Visual field defects** in hypogonadal men suggests a pituitary tumor.
   C. **Gynecomastia** suggests Klinefelter's syndrome.
   D. **Penile plaques** suggest Peyronie's disease.
   E. **Testicular atrophy** asymmetry or masses should be sought.
   F. **Cremasteric reflex** is an index of the integrity of the thoracolumbar erection center. This is elicited by stroking the inner thighs and observing ipsilateral contraction of the scrotum.

IV. **Laboratory studies and diagnostic tests**
   A. **Hormonal testing** should include serum testosterone, prolactin and thyroid function tests.
   B. **Nocturnal penile tumescence testing.** The Rigi-Scan monitor provides quantifies the number, tumescence and rigidity of erectile episodes. Impotent men with normal NPT are considered to have psychogenic impotence whereas those with impaired NPT are considered to have "organic" impotence usually due to vascular or neurologic disease.
   C. **Duplex Doppler ultrasonography or angiography** of the penile deep arteries, are indicated in men with impaired NPT to identify areas of arterial obstruction or venous leak.

V. **Treatment of male sexual dysfunction**
   A. **First-line therapy** consists of the **phosphodiesterase inhibitors** because of their efficacy, ease of use. **Sildenafil (Viagra), vardenafil (Levitra), and tadalafil (Cialis)** appear to be equally effective, but tadalafil has a longer duration of action. Phosphodiesterase inhibitors are contraindicated in men taking nitrates.
   B. **Second-line therapy** consists of penile self-injectable drugs, intraurethral alprostadil, and vacuum devices.
   C. **Surgical implantation of a penile prosthesis** is reserved for men who have not responded to first- and second-line therapies.
   D. For men with sexual dysfunction and low serum testosterone levels, testosterone replacement therapy should be the initial treatment.

E. Phosphodiesterase-5 inhibitors

1. **Sildenafil, vardenafil and tadalafil** All act to increase intracavernosal cyclic GMP levels, and each one has been proven to be effective in restoring erectile function.

2. **Sildenafil (Viagra)** is taken one hour before planned sexual intercourse, it is effective for a wide range of disorders causing erectile dysfunction.

   a. Detumescence is associated with catabolism of cyclic GMP by type 5 phosphodiesterase. PDE-5 inhibitors act by blocking the latter enzyme.

   b. **Efficacy.** 69 percent of all attempts at sexual intercourse are successful. Headache, flushing, and dyspepsia occur in 6 to 18 percent of the men.

   c. **Testosterone** therapy with sildenafil therapy may be useful in men with serum total testosterone concentrations <400 ng/dL who do not respond to sildenafil alone.

   d. **Dose.** Sildenafil should be taken orally one hour before a planned sexual encounter. The initial dose should be 50 mg, and it should be reduced to 25 mg if side effects occur. The dose can be increased to 100 mg if necessary. Each sildenafil pill costs about $10.00 retail.

   e. **Cardiovascular effects**

      (1) Sildenafil is a vasodilator that lowers the blood pressure by about 8 mmHg; this change typically produces no symptoms.

      (2) The combination of sildenafil and nitrates can lead to severe hypotension (eg, more than 50/25 mmHg) and syncope. Sildenafil is contraindicated in patients taking nitrates. Nitrates should not be prescribed within 24 hours (or longer in patients with renal or hepatic dysfunction) of takeing sildinafil.

      (3) Sildenafil has been associated with myocardial infarction and sudden death. Case reports of MI in association with sildenafil may have been unrelated to the drug. PDE-5 inhibitors are safe for men with stable coronary artery disease who are not taking nitrates.

      (4) The vasodilator properties of sildenafil may have an adverse effect in some patients with a hypertrophic cardiomyopathy; the decrease in preload and afterload can increase the outflow obstruction.

   f. Sildenafil is clearly contraindicated in men taking nitrates. Other men in whom it is potentially hazardous include those who have:

      (1) Active coronary ischemia (eg, positive exercise test) who are not taking nitrates

      (2) Heart failure and borderline low blood pressure or low volume status

      (3) A complicated, multidrug, antihypertensive drug regimen

   g. Men who are considering sildenafil therapy should be questioned regarding exercise tolerance; resumption of sexual activity after a prolonged period of inactivity is analogous to beginning a new exercise regimen. Sildenafil can be considered in men who are participating in aerobic activities that are roughly equivalent in energy expenditure to sex. If such activity cannot be documented, exercise treadmill testing should be considered.

   h. **Alpha adrenergic antagonists**, used for the treatment of benign prostatic hyperplasia, may cause symptomatic hypotension when taken in combination with PDE-5 inhibitors. Sildenafil doses above 25 mg should not be taken within four hours of an alpha-blocker. Tamsulosin (Flomax) is the only alpha adrenergic antagonist which is approved for use with PDE-5 inhibitors, but only with tadalafil.

   i. Side effects associated with sildenafil include headache, lightheadedness, dizziness, flushing, distorted vision, and, in some cases, syncope. Flushing, headaches, dyspepsia, and visual disturbances occur in 12,11, 5, and 3 percent, respectively. Sildenafil causes blue vision in approximately 3 percent of men. This effect lasts two to three hours.

    j. Interactions. Sildenafil should be avoided in patients taking drugs that can prolong the half-life of sildenafil by blocking CYP3A4 (erythromycin, ketoconazole, protease inhibitors, and grapefruit juice); drugs that induce CYP3A4 (rifampin and phenytoin) reduce the effectiveness of sildenafil.

F. Vardenafil (Levitra) and tadalafil (Cialis) are PDE-5 inhibitors. Vardenafil shares a similar structure, onset and duration of action and side-effect profile with sildenafil, whereas tadalafil (Cialis) differs in chemical structure, has an equally rapid onset but longer duration of action and does not cause blue vision but otherwise shares a similar side-effect profile with the other two phosphodiesterase inhibitors.

G. Vardenafil (Levitra) is available as a 10 and 20 mg dose. Vardenafil appears to be as effective as sildenafil.

    1. High-fat, but not moderate-fat meals, may lower the peak serum concentration of vardenafil by 18 percent, and delay absorption by one hour.

    2. A slight prolongation of the QT interval may occur, but this is not clinically important. However, vardenafil should not be used in men with congenital QT prolongation or in those taking antiarrhythmics drugs, such as quinidine, procainamide, amiodarone, or sotalol.

    3. Side effects are similar to those seen with sildenafil, and include headache, flushing, and rhinitis, in 13, 10, 10 and 5 percent, respectively. Changes in color vision (blue vision) have not been reported.

    4. Vardenafil appears to be as effective as sildenafil with no evidence of a more rapid onset of action. Vardenafil is contraindicated in men taking nitrates.

    5. Patients on alpha-blocker therapy should be stable prior to initiating vardenafil (which should be started at the lowest recommended dose).

H. Tadalafil (Cialis) has a different chemical structure than sildenafil and vardenafil. Tadalafil also appears to be as effective as sildenafil but has a longer duration of action. The recommended starting dose is 10 mg, with 5 and 20 mg options available. Food does not interfere with its absorption.

    1. With tadalafil, 75 percent of intercourse attempts are successful compared with 32 percent with placebo.

    2. Side effects are similar to those seen with sildenafil and vardenafil, with headache, dyspepsia, flushing, and rhinitis occurring in 8 to 14, 5 to 10, 4 to 6, and 5 percent, respectively. Mild back pain occurs in six percent. Visual side effects have not been described.

    3. Drug interactions

        a. Tadalafil is contraindicated in men taking concurrent nitrates. Nitrates should be avoided for at least 48 hours after the last tadalafil dose. Other issues related to sexual activity in men with coronary heart disease are similar to those with sildenafil.

        b. Alpha adrenergic antagonists, used for the treatment of benign prostatic hyperplasia, may cause symptomatic hypotension when taken in combination with PDE-5 inhibitors. Tamulosin is the only alpha adrenergic antagonist which is approved for use with PDE-5 inhibitors, but only with tadalafil.

        c. Excessive alcohol intake (5 or more drinks) in combination with tadalafil may potentiate the hypotensive effect of tadalafil.

        d. Potent CYP3A4 inhibitors (erythromycin, ketoconazole, protease inhibitors, grapefruit juice) should be avoided because these drugs that can prolong the half-life of tadalafil; drugs that induce CYP3A4 (rifampin, phenytoin) reduce the effectiveness of tadalafil. Blue vision has not been reported with this medication.

I. Comparisons

1. All PDE-5 inhibitors allow men to have erections after appropriate sexual stimulation but differ in the onset of action as well as duration of effectiveness. Tadalafil differs in two ways. Its absorption is less affected by high fat meals and alcohol and it has a longer duration of action.

2. With sildenafil and vardenafil men are advised that maximum effectiveness is achieved by taking the tablet on an empty stomach (high fat meals and alcohol delay absorption) and then wait at least an hour before attempting sexual intercourse. Tadalafil can be taken without regard to meals.

3. Duration of action that separates one PDE-5 inhibitor from another. Sildenafil and vardenafil are effective as early as 30 minutes and up to 4 hours after dosing whereas tadalafil is effective as early as 16 minutes after and up to 36 hours after dosing.

4. Concomitant treatment with alpha adrenergic antagonists (used for benign prostatic hyperplasia) is contraindicated (due to potential hypotension with combination therapy), with the exception of tamsulosin, which may be used safely with tadalafil.

5. Sildenafil and vardenafil must be taken on an empty stomach, while tadalafil can be taken without regard to food.

Oral Treatments for Male Sexual Dysfunction

Medication	Mechanism	Pros and cons	Dosing
Vardenafil (Levitra)	Inhibits phosphodiesterase 5, allowing cyclic GMP to accumulate within penis	No visual side effects. Side effects: headaches, dyspepsia, vasodilation, diarrhea. Contraindicated if using nitrates	Taken one hour before sex and effective up to four hours. Stimulation needed for erection. **Dose:** 2.5 to 20 mg
Sildenafil (Viagra)	Same as vardenafil	Similar efficacy/side effects to vardenafil but blue tinge to vision. 100 mg effective in 75 percent of men.	Similar onset and duration as vardenafil **Dose:** 25 to 100 mg
Tadalafil (Cialis)	Same as vardenafil	Similar efficacy/side effects to vardenafil but no visual side effects	Similar onset of action as vardenafil. Duration of action is up to 36 hours. **Dose:** 2.5 to 20 mg
SSRIs	Inhibits serotonin reuptake by neurons	May help patients with premature ejaculation, depression	Sertraline (Zoloft) 50 mg/day. Paroxetine (Paxil) 20 mg as needed 3 hours before intercourse.

Pharmacokinetic Characteristics of PDE-5 Inhibitors			
Parameter	Vardenafil (Levitra)	Sildenafil (Viagra)	Tadalafil (Cialis)
Oral dose	20 mg	100 mg	20 mg
Onset of action	30 min	30 min	16 min
Duration of action	4 hours	4 hours	36 hours
Food interaction	Minimal with low-fat foods; delay in time to peak concentration with high-fat foods	With high-fat foods; possible with low-fat foods	None
Alcohol interaction	None	None	Maybe
Age >65 yr	Increased half-life dose adjustment not needed	Increased half-life, dose adjustment may be needed	Increased half-life dose adjustment may not be needed

VI. **Penile self-injection**
   A. Intrapenile injection therapy with alprostadil (prostaglandin E1, Caverject), papaverine, or alprostadil with papaverine and phentolamine (Tri-Mix) have all been used for purposes of inducing erection.
   B. The technique consists of inserting an insulin syringe with a 26 gauge needle through the shaft of the penis and injecting the vasoactive agent into one corporeal body. A full, firm erection can be expected within a few minutes.
   C. **Alprostadil**
      1. Intrapenile alprostadil injections are satisfactory in 87 percent of the men. There is a very high attrition rate with self-injection, suggesting that it may not be a satisfactory long-term solution.
      2. The major side effect of intrapenile alprostadil therapy is penile pain, occurring in 50 percent.
      3. Priapism, or a prolonged erection lasting more than four to six hours, is a medical emergency. Prolonged erections occur in 6 percent of men who use intrapenile alprostadil and about 11 percent of those who use intrapenile papaverine.

VII. **Intraurethral alprostadil (MUSE)** provides an erection sufficient for intercourse in two-thirds of men. After insertion of the alprostadil into the urethra, the penis should be massaged for up to one minute.
      1. Systemic effects are uncommon, and complications such as priapism and penile fibrosis are less common than after alprostadil given by penile injection.

Suppositories, Injections, and Devices for Sexual Dysfunction			
Treatment	**Effect**	**Pros and cons**	**Usage pattern**
Suppository			
MUSE (alprostadil)	Alprostadil (prosta-glandin E1) in gel form delivered by applicator into meatus of penis	Can be used twice daily. Not recom-mended with preg-nant partners	Inserted 5-10 min-utes before sex. Effects last one hour
Penile injection			
Alprostadil (Caverject and Edex)	Prostaglandin E1 injected into base of penis.	Effective in 50-85 percent of cases. May be painful and not recommended for daily use. Priapism occurs uncommonly	Inject 10-20 min-utes before sex. Erections may last hours
Invicorp (VIP and phentolamine)	VIP and alpha-blocker, phentolamine.	Possibly more ef-fective than alprostadil. Causes less pain. Priapism rare	Inject 10-20 min-utes before sex. Requires stimula-tion to have erec-tion
Device			
Vacuum pump	Creates a vacuum, drawing blood into cavernosae. Elastic tourniquet at base.	Safe if erection not maintained more than one hour. May interfere with ejac-ulation	Inflated just before sexual activity. Erection lasts until elastic ring re-moved

VIII. **Vacuum-assisted erection devices** have been developed to encourage increased arterial inflow and create an erection sufficient for sexual intercourse. Men cannot ejaculate externally because the occlusive rings compress the penile urethra.
  A. Vacuum devices successfully create erections in 67 percent. Satisfaction with vacuum-assisted erections has varied between 25 and 49 percent.
IX. **Penile prostheses** remain a viable option for those men who do not respond to sildenafil and find penile injection or vacuum erection therapy distasteful. There are two general types of prostheses: malleable rods and inflatable prostheses.
X. **Premature ejaculation** is defined as an inability to control ejaculation so that both partners enjoy sexual intercourse. Approximately 20 percent of men complain of premature ejaculation.
  A. The selective serotonin reuptake inhibitor (SSRI) sertraline (Zoloft, 50 mg/day) increases the mean ejaculatory latency time to 3.2 minutes. Other SSRIs also appear to be effective.
  B. Intermittent use of SSRIs may be as effective as continuous use. Paroxetine (Paxil, 20 mg) as needed three to four hours before planned intercourse increases the mean ejaculatory latency time to 3.2 minutes.
  C. Serotonin reuptake inhibitors (SSRIs) are first-line therapy, and clomipramine is second-line therapy for premature ejaculation.

References, see page 372.

Benign Prostatic Hyperplasia

Benign prostatic hyperplasia (BPH) is a common disorder that increases in frequency with age in men older than 50 years. Symptoms or BPH include increased frequency of urination, nocturia, hesitancy, urgency, and weak urinary stream. The correlation between symptoms and the presence of prostatic enlargement on rectal examination or by transrectal ultrasonographic assessment of prostate size is poor.

I. **Clinical evaluation of obstructive urinary symptoms**
   A. History of type 2 diabetes, which can cause nocturia
   B. Symptoms of neurologic disease that would suggest a neurogenic bladder
   C. Sexual dysfunction
   D. Gross hematuria or pain in the bladder region suggestive of a bladder tumor or calculi
   E. History of urethral trauma, urethritis, or urethral instrumentation that could lead to urethral stricture
   F. Family history of BPH and prostate cancer
   G. Treatment with drugs that can impair bladder function (anticholinergic drugs) or increase outflow resistance (sympathomimetic drugs)
   H. A 24-hour voiding chart of frequency and volume should be obtained.
   I. Symptoms are classified as mild (total score 0 to 7), moderate (total score 8 to 19) and severe (total score 20 to 35).
   J. **Other disorders that can cause difficulty urinating:**
      1. Urethral stricture
      2. Bladder neck contracture
      3. Carcinoma of the prostate
      4. Carcinoma of the bladder
      5. Bladder calculi
      6. Urinary tract infection and prostatitis
      7. Neurogenic bladder

Benign Prostatic Hyperplasia Symptom Score

For each question, circle the answer that best describes your situation. Add the circled number together to get your total score. See the key at the bottom of this form to determine the overall rating of your symptoms.

	Not at all	Less than one in five times	Less than half of the time	About half of the time	More than half of the time	Almost always
In the past month, how often have you had a sensation of not emptying your bladder completely after you finished voiding?	0	1	2	3	4	5
In the past month, how often have you had to urinate again less than 2 hours after you finished urinating before?	0	1	2	3	4	5

	Not at all	Less than one in five times	Less than half of the time	About half of the time	More than half of the time	Almost always
In the past month, how often have you found you stopped and started again several times when you urinated?	0	1	2	3	4	5
In the past month, how often have you found it difficult to postpone urination?	0	1	2	3	4	5
In the past month, how often have you had a weak urinary stream?	0	1	2	3	4	5
In the past month, how often have you had to push or strain to begin urination?	0	1	2	3	4	5
In the past month, how many times did you typically get up to urinate from the time you went to bed until you arose in the morning?	0	1	2	3	4	5

K. **Physical examination.** A digital rectal examination should be done to assess prostate size and consistency, nodules, induration, and asymmetry, which raise suspicion for malignancy. Rectal sphincter tone should be determined, and a neurological examination performed.

L. **Urinalysis** should be done to detect urinary infection and blood, which could indicate bladder cancer or calculi.

M. **Optional tests**

1. **Serum prostate specific antigen.** Prostate cancer can cause obstructive symptoms. Measurements of serum PSA may be used as a screening test for prostate cancer in men with BPH, preferably in men between the ages of 50 to 69 years. Blood should not be obtained for PSA assay within 24 hours after vigorous digital rectal examination or ejaculation.

   a. The results should be interpreted according to age- and race-based norms. High values occur in men with prostatic diseases other than cancer, including BPH. Some men with prostatic cancer have serum PSA concentrations of 4.0 ng/mL or less.

   b. A combination of digital rectal examination and serum PSA determination provides the most acceptable means for excluding prostate cancer.

2. **Maximal urinary flow rates** greater than 15 mL/sec are thought to exclude bladder outlet obstruction. Maximal flow rates below 15 mL/sec are compatible with obstruction due to prostatic or urethral disease.

3. **Post-void residual urine volume** can be determined by in-out catheterization, radiographic methods, or ultrasonography. Normal men have less than 12 mL of residual urine. A large residual volume is a possible indicator of BPH.

4. Ultrasonography is useful in men who have a high serum creatinine concentration or a urinary tract infection. Total prostate volume can be measured by ultrasonography to assess disease progression, and it is useful when considering medical treatment with a 5-alpha-reductase inhibitor or when considering surgery.

II. Medical treatment of benign prostatic hyperplasia

A. Indications for therapy

1. Obstructive symptoms only require therapy if they have a significant impact on a patient's quality of life. Benign prostatic hypertrophy may require therapy if obstruction is creating a risk for upper tract injury such as hydronephrosis or renal insufficiency, or lower tract injury such as urinary retention, recurrent infection, or bladder decompensation (eg, low pressure detrusor contractions; >25 percent post-void residuals). Patients who develop these symptoms will require invasive therapy.

B. Alpha-1-adrenergic antagonists are more effective for short-term treatment of BPH; however, only 5-alpha-reductase inhibitors have demonstrated the potential for long-term reduction in prostate volume. The efficacy of these classes are similar with long-term therapy, but 5-alpha-reductase inhibitors have been found to reduce the need for surgery. The use of agents from both classes in combination may be superior to using either class alone.

C. Alpha-1-adrenergic antagonists. Four long-acting alpha-1-antagonists, terazosin, doxazosin, tamsulosin, and alfuzosin have been approved for treatment of the symptoms of BPH.

1. Mechanism. Prostatic tissue contains alpha-1 and alpha-2 adrenergic receptors. Alpha-1-adrenergic antagonists target alpha-1A receptors.

2. The alpha-1-antagonists appear to have similar efficacy.

3. Alfuzosin (Uroxatral), terazosin (Hytrin), doxazosin (Cardura), and tamsulosin (Flomax) decrease symptom scores by 30 to 40 percent, and urinary flow rates increase by 16 to 25 percent.

4. Side effects. The frequency of side effects with alfuzosin (Uroxatral) and tamsulosin (Flomax) is similar to placebo, but terazosin and doxazosin cause significant side effects in 10 percent.

a. Side effects include orthostatic hypotension and dizziness. Terazosin and doxazosin need to be initiated at bedtime (to reduce postural lightheadedness) and the dose should be titrated up over several weeks.

b. The hypotensive action can be useful in older men who have hypertension. Alpha-1-adrenergic antagonists may increase the incidence of heart failure when used for hypertension.

D. Tamsulosin (Flomax) and alfuzosin (Uroxatral) have less effect on blood pressure than either terazosin (Hytrin) or doxazosin (Cardura), and tamsulosin (Flomax) may further have slightly less effect on blood pressure than alfuzosin.

a. The hypotensive effects of terazosin and doxazosin can be potentiated by sildenafil (Viagra), vardenafil (Levitra), or tadalafil (Cialis).

b. Other common side effects of alpha-1-antagonists include asthenia and nasal congestion.

Starting dosages of alpha-blocking agents for managing benign prostatic hypertrophy	
Drug	Starting dosage
Afuzosin (Uroxatral)	10 mg qd
Tamsulosin (Flomax)	0.4 mg qd
Terazosin (Hytrin)	1 mg qd, adjusted up to 5 mg qd
Doxazosin mesylate (Cardura)	1 mg qd, adjusted up to 4 mg qd

E. **5-Alpha-reductase inhibitors** include finasteride and dutasteride. Treatment for 6 to 12 months is required before prostate size is reduced enough to improve symptoms. The type 2 form of 5-alpha-reductase catalyzes the conversion of testosterone to dihydrotestosterone in prostatic tissue.
   1. Efficacy. Finasteride (Proscar) for 12 months reduces obstructive and non-obstructive symptoms by 23-18 percent and increases maximal urinary flow rate by 1.6 mL/sec. The mean prostatic volume is reduced by 19-18 percent.
   2. Dutasteride (Avodart) is an inhibitor of both 5-alpha reductase enzymes, and may be more potent than finasteride.
   3. Dutasteride and finasteride are similar in effectiveness and the side effect profiles of these agents are similar. The side effect on hair growth for men with dutasteride has not yet been established.
   4. Side effects of these drugs are decreased libido and ejaculatory or erectile dysfunction, occurring in 4 to 6 percent of men.
   5. Serum prostate-specific antigen (PSA) concentrations decrease by about 50 percent with finasteride. PSA values should be corrected by a factor of 2 for the first 24 months of finasteride use, and by a factor of 2.5 for longer term use.
   6. **Combination therapy.** Long-term therapy with combined alpha adrenergic antagonist and 5-alpha-reductase inhibitor therapy appears to be superior to either agent alone.
III. **Recommendations**
   A. Men who develop upper tract injury (eg, hydronephrosis, renal dysfunction), or lower tract injury (eg, urinary retention, recurrent infection, bladder decompensation) require invasive therapy.
   B. Alpha-adrenergic antagonists provide immediate therapeutic benefits, while 5-alpha-reductase inhibitors require long-term treatment for efficacy. In most men with mild to moderate symptoms of BPH. Initial treatment consists of an alpha-adrenergic antagonist alone. For severe symptoms (large prostate (>40 g), inadequate response to monotherapy), combination treatment with an alpha-adrenergic antagonist and a 5-alpha-reductase inhibitor is recommended.
   C. The choice of alpha-adrenergic antagonist and 5-alpha-reductase inhibitor may be made on the basis of cost and side-effect profile. Tamsulosin (Flomax) and alfuzosin (Uroxatral) have less effect on blood pressure than either (Hytrin) or doxazosin (Cardura), and tamsulosin may further have slightly less effect on blood pressure than alfuzosin.

References, see page 372.

Acute Epididymoorchitis

I. **Clinical evaluation of testicular pain**
   A. Epididymoorchitis is indicated by a unilateral painful testicle and a history of unprotected intercourse, new sexual partner, urinary tract infection, dysuria, or discharge. Symptoms may occur following acute lifting or straining.
   B. The epididymis and testicle are painful, swollen, and tender. The scrotum may be erythematosus and warm, with associated spermatic cord thickening or penile discharge.
   C. **Differential diagnosis of painful scrotal swelling**
      1. Epididymitis, testicular torsion, testicular tumor, hernia.
      2. Torsion is characterized by sudden onset, age <20, an elevated testicle, and previous episodes of scrotal pain. The epididymis is usually located anteriorly on either side, and there is an absence of evidence of urethritis and UTI.
      3. Epididymitis is characterized by fever, laboratory evidence of urethritis or cystitis, and increased scrotal warmth.

II. **Laboratory evaluation of epididymoorchitis**
   A. Epididymoorchitis is indicated by leukocytosis with a left shift; UA shows pyuria and bacteriuria. Midstream urine culture will reveal gram negative bacilli. Chlamydia and Neisseria cultures should be obtained.
   B. **Common pathogens**
      1. **Younger men.** Epididymoorchitis is usually associated with sexually transmitted organisms such as Chlamydia and gonorrhea.
      2. **Older men.** Epididymoorchitis is usually associated with a concomitant urinary tract infection or prostatitis caused by E. coli, proteus, Klebsiella, Enterobacter, or Pseudomonas.

III. **Treatment of epididymoorchitis**
   A. Bed rest, scrotal elevation with athletic supporter, an ice pack, analgesics, and antipyretics are prescribed. Sexual and physical activity should be avoided.
   B. **Sexually transmitted epididymitis in sexually active males**
      1. Ceftriaxone (Rocephin) 250 mg IM x 1 dose **AND** doxycycline 100 mg PO bid x 10 days **OR**
      2. Ofloxacin (Floxin) 300 mg bid x 10 days.
      3. Treat sexual partners
   C. **Epididymitis secondary to urinary tract infection**
      1. TMP/SMX DS bid for 10 days **OR**
      2. Ofloxacin (Floxin) 300 mg PO bid for 10 days.***References, see page 372.***

Prostatitis and Prostatodynia

Prostatitis is a common condition, with a 5 percent lifetime prevalence to 9 percent. Prostatitis is divided into three subtypes: acute, chronic bacterial prostatitis and chronic nonbacterial prostatitis/chronic pelvic pain syndrome (CNP/CPPS).

I. **Acute Bacterial Prostatitis**
   A. Acute bacterial prostatitis (ABP) should be considered a urinary tract infection. The most common cause is Escherichia coli. Other species frequently found include Klebsiella, Proteus, Enterococci and Pseudomonas. On occasion, cultures grow Staphylococcus aureus, Streptococcus faecalis, Chlamydia or Bacteroides species.
   B. Patients may present with fever, chills, low back pain, perineal or ejaculatory pain, dysuria, urinary frequency, urgency, myalgias and obstruction. The prostate gland is tender and may be warm, swollen, firm and irregular. Vigor-

ous digital examination of the prostate should be avoided because it may induce bacteremia.

C. The infecting organism can often be identified by urine culturing.

D. Treatment consists of trimethoprim-sulfamethoxazole (TMP-SMX [Bactrim, Septra]), a quinolone or tetracycline. Men at increased risk for sexually transmitted disease require antibiotic coverage for Chlamydia.

Common Antibiotic Regimens for Acute Bacterial Prostatitis	
Medication	**Standard dosage**
Trimethoprim-sulfamethoxazole (Bactrim, Septra)	1 DS tablet (160/800 mg) twice a day
Doxycycline (Vibramycin)	100 mg twice a day
Ciprofloxacin (Cipro)	500 mg twice a day
Norfloxacin (Noroxin)	400 mg twice a day
Ofloxacin (Floxin)	400 mg twice a day

E. Antibiotic therapy should be continued for three to four weeks. Extremely ill patients should be hospitalized to receive a parenteral broad-spectrum cephalosporin and an aminoglycoside.

II. Chronic Bacterial Prostatitis

A. Chronic bacterial prostatitis (CBP) is a common cause of recurrent urinary tract infections in men. Men experience irritative voiding symptoms, pain in the back, testes, epididymis or penis, low-grade fever, arthralgias and myalgias. Signs may include urethral discharge, hemospermia and secondary epididymo-orchitis. Often the prostate is normal on rectal examination.

B. CBP presents with negative premassage urine culture results, and greater than 10 to 20 white blood cells per high-power field in the pre- and the postmassage urine specimen. Significant bacteriuria in the postmassage urine specimen suggests chronic bacterial prostatitis.

C. TMP-SMX is the first-line antibiotic for CBP. Norfloxacin (Noroxin) taken twice a day for 28 days achieves a cure rate in 64 percent. Ofloxacin (Floxin) is also highly effective. Some men require long-term antibiotic suppression with TMP-SMX or nitrofurantoin.

III. Chronic Nonbacterial Prostatitis/Chronic Pelvic Pain Syndrome (prostatodynia)

A. Patients with CNP/CPPS have painful ejaculation pain in the penis, testicles or scrotum, low back pain, rectal or perineal pain, and/or inner thigh pain. They often have irritative or obstructive urinary symptoms and decreased libido or impotence. The physical examination is usually unremarkable, but patients may have a tender prostate.

B. No bacteria will grow on culture, but leukocytosis may be found in the prostatic secretions.

C. Treatment begins with 100 mg of doxycycline (Vibramycin) or minocycline (Minocin) twice daily for 14 days. Other therapies may include Allopurinol (Zyloprim), thrice-weekly prostate massage or transurethral microwave thermotherapy.

D. Hot sitz baths and nonsteroidal anti-inflammatory drugs (NSAIDs) may provide some relief. Some men may notice aggravation of symptoms with alcohol or spicy foods and should avoid them. Anticholinergic agents (oxybutynin [Ditropan]) or alpha-blocking agents (doxazosin [Cardura], tamsulosin [Flomax] or terazosin [Hytrin]) may be beneficial.

References, see page 372.

Psychiatric Disorders

Depression

The lifetime prevalence of major depression in the United States is 17 percent. In primary care, depression has a prevalence rate of 4.8 to 8.6 percent.

I. Diagnosis
   A. The Diagnostic and Statistical Manual of Mental Disorders (DSM-IV) includes nine symptoms in the diagnosis of major depression.
   B. These nine symptoms can be divided into two clusters: (1) physical or neurovegetative symptoms and (2) psychologic or psychosocial symptoms. The nine symptoms are: depressed mood plus sleep disturbance; interest/pleasure reduction; guilt feelings or thoughts of worthlessness; energy changes/fatigue; concentration/attention impairment; appetite/weight changes; psychomotor disturbances, and suicidal thoughts.

Diagnostic Criteria for Major Depression, DSM IV

Cluster 1: Physical or neurovegetative symptoms
Sleep disturbance
Appetite/weight changes
Attention/concentration problem
Energy-level change/fatigue
Psychomotor disturbance

Cluster 2: Psychologic or psychosocial symptoms
Depressed mood and/or
Interest/pleasure reduction
Guilt feelings
Suicidal thoughts

Note: Diagnosis of major depression requires at least one of the first two symptoms under cluster 2 and four of the remaining symptoms to be present for at least two weeks. Symptoms should not be accounted for by bereavement.

II. Drug Therapy

Characteristics of Common Antidepressants		
Drug	**Recommended Dosage**	**Comments**
Selective Serotonin Reuptake Inhibitors (SSRIs)		
Escitalopram (Lexapro)	10 mg qd	Minimal sedation, activation, or inhibition of hepatic enzymes, nausea, anorgasmia, headache
Citalopram (Celexa)	Initially 20 mg qd; maximum 40 mg/d	

Drug	Recommended Dosage	Comments
Fluoxetine (Prozac)	10-20 mg qd initially, taken in AM	Anxiety, insomnia, agitation, nausea, anorgasmia, erectile dysfunction, headache, anorexia.
Fluvoxamine (LuVox)	50-100 mg qhs; max 300 mg/d [50, 100 mg]	Headache, nausea, sedation, diarrhea
Paroxetine (Paxil)	20 mg/d initially, given in AM; increase in 10-mg/d increments as needed to max of 50 mg/d. [10, 20, 30, 40 mg]	Headache, nausea, somnolence, dizziness, insomnia, abnormal ejaculation, anxiety, diarrhea, dry mouth.
Sertraline (Zoloft)	50 mg/d, increasing as needed to max of 200 mg/d [50, 100 mg]	Insomnia, agitation, dry mouth, headache, nausea, anorexia, sexual dysfunction.
Secondary Amine Tricyclic Antidepressants		
Desipramine (Norpramin, generics)	100-200 mg/d, gradually increasing to 300 mg/d as tolerated.[10, 25, 50, 75, 100, 150 mg]	No sedation; may have stimulant effect; best taken in morning to avoid insomnia.
Nortriptyline (Pamelor)	25 mg tid-qid, max 150 mg/d. [10, 25, 50, 75 mg]	Sedating
Tertiary Amine Tricyclics		
Amitriptyline (Elavil, generics)	75 mg/d qhs-bid, increasing to 150-200 mg/d. [25, 50, 75, 100, 150 mg]	Sedative effect precedes antidepressant effect. High anticholinergic activity.
Clomipramine (Anafranil)	25 mg/d, increasing gradually to 100 mg/d; max 250 mg/d; may be given once qhs [25, 50, 75 mg].	Relatively high sedation, anticholinergic activity, and seizure risk.
Protriptyline (Vivactil)	5-10 mg PO tid-qid; 15-60 mg/d [5, 10 mg]	Useful in anxious depression; nonsedating
Doxepin (Sinequan, generics)	50-75 mg/d, increasing up to 150-300 mg/d as needed [10, 25, 50, 75, 100, 150 mg]	Sedating. Also indicated for anxiety. Contraindicated in patients with glaucoma or urinary retention.
Imipramine (Tofranil, generics)	75 mg/d in a single dose qhs, increasing to 150 mg/d; 300 mg/d. [10, 25, 50 mg]	High sedation and anticholinergic activity. Use caution in cardiovascular disease.

Drug	Recommended Dosage	Comments
Miscellaneous		
Bupropion (Wellbutrin, Wellbutrin SR)	100 mg bid; increase to 100 mg tid [75, 100 mg] Sustained release: 100-200 mg bid [100, 150 mg]	Agitation, dry mouth, insomnia, headache, nausea, constipation, tremor. Good choice for patients with sexual side effects from other agents; contraindicated in seizure disorders.
Venlafaxine (Effexor)	75 mg/d in 2-3 divided doses with food; increase to 225 mg/d as needed. [25, 37.5, 50, 75, 100 mg]. Extended-release: initially 37.5 mg qAM. The dosage can be increased by 75 mg every four days to a max of 225 mg qd [37.5, 75, 100, 150 mg].	Inhibits norepinephrine and serotonin reuptake. Hypertension, nausea, insomnia, dizziness, abnormal ejaculation, headache, dry mouth, anxiety.
Duloxetine (Cymbalta)	20 mg bid or 60 mg qd or 30 mg bid. Start at a dose of 30 mg and increase the dose to 60 mg daily; up to 120 mg daily [30, 60 mg].	Inhibits norepinephrine and serotonin reuptake. Contraindicated in hepatic or renal insufficiency. Food delays absorption. Nausea, dry mouth, constipation. Diarrhea and vomiting less often. Insomnia, dizziness, somnolence, and sweating also seen. Sexual side effects may be less common than with the SSRIs. Marketed for physical pain associated with depression.
Maprotiline (Ludiomil)	75 to 225 in single or divided doses [25, 50, 75 mg].	Delays cardiac conduction; high anticholinergic activity; contraindicated in seizure disorders.
Mirtazapine (Remeron)	15 to 45 PO qd [15, 30 mg]	High anticholinergic activity; contraindicated in seizure disorders.
Nefazodone (Serzone)	Start at 100 mg PO bid, increase to 150-300 mg PO bid as needed [100, 150, 200, 250 mg].	Headache, somnolence, dry mouth, blurred vision. Postural hypotension, impotence.
Reboxetine (Vestra)	5 mg bid	Selective norepinephrine reuptake inhibitor. Dry mouth, insomnia, constipation, increased sweating
Trazodone (Desyrel, generics)	150 mg/d, increasing by 50 mg/d every 3-4 d 400 mg/d in divided doses [50, 100, 150, 300 mg]	Rarely associated with priapism. Orthostatic hypotension in elderly. Sedating.

A. Psychotherapy
1. The efficacy of cognitive therapy, behavioral therapy, and interpersonal therapy are 46, 55, and 52 percent, respectively, in psychiatric patients with major depression.
2. Cognitive behavioral therapy is as effective as medication use for maintenance therapy (over two years) in patients with major depression.

B. **Selective serotonin reuptake inhibitors**
1. Abnormalities in brain serotonergic activity have been implicated in mood disorders. Medications causing increased serotonergic activity are often effective in ameliorating symptoms of depression, anxiety, and obsessive ruminations.
2. The selective-serotonin reuptake inhibitors (SSRIs) block the action of the presynaptic serotonin reuptake pump, thereby increasing the amount of serotonin available in the synapse and increasing postsynaptic serotonin receptor occupancy.
3. **The SSRIs all share several other characteristics:**
   a. They are all hepatically metabolized.
   b. They have relatively little affinity for histaminic, dopaminergic, alpha-adrenergic, and cholinergic receptors.
   c. They tend to have relatively mild side-effect profiles, although they can be associated with sexual dysfunction.
   d. They are relatively safe in overdose.
   e. They all produce changes in sleep architecture (decreased REM latency and decreased total REM sleep).
4. The SSRIs differ in potency, receptor selectivity, and pharmacokinetic properties. The overall efficacy of the different SSRIs appears to be similar. Coadministration of any SSRI with a monoamine oxidase inhibitor (MAOI) is contraindicated due to the potential for producing a sometimes fatal "serotonin syndrome," characterized by agitation, hyperthermia, diaphoresis, tachycardia, and rigidity.
5. **Fluoxetine (Prozac)** has a relatively mild side-effect profile, and a once-daily-dosing schedule. Fluoxetine is indicated for the treatment of major depressive disorder, obsessive-compulsive disorder, and bulimia.
   a. Fluoxetine is 95 percent protein bound. It undergoes oxidative metabolism in the liver by the cytochrome P-450 (CYP) enzyme system. The principal CYP enzymes responsible for its metabolism are CYP2D6 and CYP3A/34. The half-life (t 1/2) of fluoxetine is four to six days. Its active metabolite, norfluoxetine, is formed through demethylation of fluoxetine, is a potent and selective inhibitor of the serotonin reuptake pump, and has a t 1/2 of 7 to 15 days. Fluoxetine is a potent inhibitor of CYP2D6; norfluoxetine is also a mild inhibitor of CYP 3A/34. Drugs metabolized by CYP2D6 (tricyclic antidepressants, antiarrhythmics, beta-blockers) must be used cautiously when coadministered with fluoxetine.
   b. The clinical antidepressant effect may be delayed three to six weeks from the start of treatment.
   c. The usual effective dose of fluoxetine is 20 mg daily. Patients who do not respond to this dosage after several weeks can have their dose increased by 10 to 20 mg as tolerated up to 80 mg daily.
   d. **Fluoxetine (Prozac Weekly)** can be administered once weekly to patients who have responded to daily fluoxetine. Fluoxetine is given as 90 mg per week. Seven days should elapse after the last 20 mg daily dose of fluoxetine before beginning the once weekly regimen.
   e. The most common initial side effects of fluoxetine are nausea, insomnia, and anxiety. These effects usually present at the start of treatment and tend to resolve over one to two weeks. Fluoxetine, like all of the SSRIs, is relatively safe in overdose.
6. **Sertraline (Zoloft)** is approved for the treatment of depressive illness. Sertraline is 98 percent protein bound. Absorption is increased when taken with food. It is metabolized by the hepatic p450 enzyme system and has an active metabolite that is significantly less potent than the active compound. The t 1/2 of sertraline is 26 hours. As opposed to fluoxetine, which is a

potent inhibitor of CYP2D6, sertraline has only mild inhibition of this enzyme. Sertraline has a low likelihood of interactions with coadministered medications.

a. Sertraline is usually started at 50 mg daily; the effective maintenance dose is typically 50 to 100 mg daily, although doses up to 200 mg daily may be necessary. Clinical effect is usually evident by three to six weeks.

b. Common initial side effects of sertraline include nausea, diarrhea, insomnia, and sexual dysfunction. It may be more likely than the other SSRIs to cause nausea. As with fluoxetine, sexual dysfunction can persist. Addition of bupropion (Wellbutrin, 75 to 150 mg/day in divided doses) or buspirone (BuSpar, 10 to 20 mg twice daily) may alleviate decreased libido, diminished sexual arousal, or impaired orgasm. Sertraline is relatively safe in overdose.

7. Paroxetine (Paxil) is indicated for the treatment of depression, panic disorder, generalized anxiety disorder, and social phobia.

a. Paroxetine is 95 percent protein bound. It inhibits the liver enzyme CYP2D6 and must be used cautiously when coadministered with other drugs metabolized by this enzyme (tricyclic antidepressants, antiarrhythmics, beta-blockers). The t 1/2 is 24 hours. It has a mild affinity for muscarinic receptors and can cause more anticholinergic side effects than the other SSRIs (although much less than the tricyclic antidepressants).

b. The starting and maintenance dose of paroxetine is 20 mg daily but can be raised to 40 mg daily if necessary. In contrast to fluoxetine and sertraline, which can be activating, paroxetine is mildly sedating. Other side effects include nausea, dry mouth, and sexual dysfunction. Sexual dysfunction may be slightly higher with paroxetine than with the other SSRIs.

c. An enteric-coated, controlled-release formulation of paroxetine may cause less nausea than the immediate-release formulation. The recommended starting dose of Paxil CR is 12.5 mg/day for panic disorder and 25 mg/day for depression; the maximum dose is 75 mg/day.

8. Citalopram (Celexa) has mild p450 2D6 inhibition, but it has significantly less p450 interactions than the other SSRIs, making it an appealing choice in patients who are on other medications where drug-drug interactions are a concern. Citalopram is touted as causing less sexual dysfunction than the other SSRIs. Anxiety symptoms are improved with citalopram compared with sertraline or placebo.

a. The usual starting dose of citalopram is 20 mg daily. The therapeutic dose range tends to be 20 to 40 mg daily in a single morning dose.

9. Escitalopram (Lexapro) is a single isomer formulation of citalopram. Escitalopram is reported to be a more potent serotonin reuptake inhibitor, and a daily dose of 10 mg is at least comparable to 40 mg of citalopram. There are no clear advantages of escitalopram compared with other SSRIs in terms of efficacy or adverse effects, although, like citalopram, it has little effect on CYP isoenzymes and therefore may prove to have fewer drug interactions than other SSRIs such as fluoxetine or paroxetine.

C. Heterocyclic antidepressants

1. The cyclic antidepressants are less commonly used as first-line antidepressants with the development of the SSRIs. This is mainly due to the less benign side-effect profile of the cyclic antidepressants. In contrast to the SSRIs, the cyclic antidepressants can be fatal in doses as little as five times the therapeutic dose. The toxicity is usually due to prolongation of the

QT interval, leading to arrhythmias. Overdose of cyclic antidepressants can also cause anticholinergic toxicity and seizures.

2. The cyclic antidepressants tend to have anticholinergic and orthostatic effects, as well as sedation, weight gain, and sexual dysfunction. In addition, tricyclic antidepressant users have a higher risk of myocardial infarction compared with SSRI users.

3. As with all antidepressants, the cyclic antidepressants can take up to three to six weeks before reaching full clinical effect.

4. **Tertiary amines** are not frequently used as primary antidepressant agents because of their tendency to cause significant sedative and anticholinergic side effects.

   a. **Imipramine (Tofranil).** The usual starting dose of imipramine is 25 mg daily. The dose can be increased by 25 to 50 mg every three to four days to a typical therapeutic dose range of 150 to 300 mg daily. Patients with combined blood levels of imipramine and desipramine greater than 225 ng/mL have a superior response. Imipramine is moderately sedating and anticholinergic compared with other cyclic antidepressants.

   b. **Amitriptyline (Elavil).** Amitriptyline is demethylated to nortriptyline, which has antidepressant effects. The usual starting dose of is 25 mg, given at bedtime. Therapeutic doses are generally in the range of 100 to 300 mg daily, but many patients find it difficult to reach these doses due to sedation. Blood levels of amitriptyline plus nortriptyline are 95 to 160 ng/mL.

5. **Secondary amines**

   a. **Desipramine (Norpramin)** is an active metabolite of imipramine. Desipramine differs from the tertiary amines in that it is much more selective in its properties of norepinephrine blockade than in its properties of serotonin reuptake blockade. It tends to have much less sedative and anticholinergic side effects. It does, however, share the side effect of orthostatic hypotension. The usual starting dose of desipramine is 25 mg daily.

   b. **Nortriptyline (Aventyl)** is an active metabolite of amitriptyline. Like desipramine, nortriptyline has significantly more effects on norepinephrine than on serotonin receptors. Although nortriptyline has fewer sedative and anticholinergic side effects than the tertiary amines, it has slightly more than desipramine. It is distinctly different from desipramine in that it has very little orthostatic hypotensive effects. Nortriptyline is twice as potent as the other cyclic antidepressants. The starting dose is 25 mg daily.

6. **Cardiac testing.** Before initiating treatment with any of the cyclic antidepressants, patients must be screened for cardiac conduction system disease, which precludes the use of these medications. Patients over age 40 years should have a baseline electrocardiogram (ECG).

D. **Venlafaxine (Effexor XR)** is a phenylethylamine inhibitor of serotonin reuptake and an inhibitor of norepinephrine reuptake. The t 1/2 of the parent compound plus the active metabolite is 11 hours. There is a slow-release form that allows for once-daily dosing. Venlafaxine is excreted by the kidney, and food does not affect its absorption. Venlafaxine is a weak inhibitor of the p450 2D6 enzyme, but it tends to not interact with most coadministered medications (except MAOIs).

   1. Dosing for the immediate-release form of venlafaxine begins at 37.5 mg twice daily. The medication can be increased by 75 mg every four days to a maximum dose of 375 mg daily in three divided doses. The extended-release form of venlafaxine is given as a single-morning dose of 37.5 mg. If this is well tolerated, the dose is increased to 75 mg in a single daily dose.

The medication can be increased by 75 mg every four days to a recommended maximum of 225 mg daily in a single-daily dose.

2. The most common side effects of venlafaxine are nausea, dizziness, insomnia, sedation, and constipation. It can also induce sweating. Venlafaxine may cause blood pressure increases. Three to 7 percent of patients have mild blood pressure elevations (average 1 to 2 mm Hg).

3. Medications that inhibit CYP2D6 can increase the plasma level of venlafaxine. This is sometimes encountered when switching a patient from an SSRI with CYP2D6 inhibiting properties (eg, fluoxetine, paroxetine) to venlafaxine.

4. Venlafaxine overdose is more serious than overdose with SSRIs. Venlafaxine is more likely to cause seizures than tricyclic antidepressants. Rates of serotonin toxicity are also higher with venlafaxine than with tricyclic antidepressants. Venlafaxine should be avoided in patients who are at high risk for deliberate overdose.

5. Patients who do not respond to other antidepressants may respond better to venlafaxine, and venlafaxine may be less likely to lose efficacy over time. Venlafaxine may be more likely to lead to a remission of depression.

E. **Duloxetine (Cymbalta)** is an inhibitor of both serotonin reuptake and norepinephrine reuptake.

1. Duloxetine is metabolized in the liver and should not be administered with hepatic insufficiency. Metabolites are excreted in the urine, and the use of duloxetine is not recommended in end-stage renal disease. Food delays the absorption of duloxetine, and the t 1/2 is 12 hours. Duloxetine is a moderate inhibitor of CYP2D6.

2. Dosage is 20 mg twice daily or 60 mg daily either as a single dose or as 30 mg twice daily. Start at 30 mg daily and increase to 60 mg daily; there may be added benefit to using up to 120 mg daily.

3. Nausea, dry mouth and constipation are common. Diarrhea and vomiting are seen less often. Insomnia, dizziness, somnolence, and sweating occur. Sexual side effects occur, but may be less common than with the SSRIs. Duloxetine is marketed as a treatment for physical pain associated with depression. Duloxetine has shown efficacy in diabetic neuropathy.

4. Medications that inhibit CYP2D6 (paroxetine and fluoxetine) and medications that inhibit CYP1A2 (fluvoxamine) can increase levels of duloxetine.

F. **Mirtazapine (Remeron)** is a tetracyclic compound (a piperazinoazepine), but it is unrelated to TCAs. It has a unique mechanism of action in that it blocks pre- and postsynaptic alpha-2 receptors, as well as the serotonin receptors 5HT2 and 5HT3.

1. Mirtazapine can be particularly helpful in depressed patients with insomnia because of its sedative properties.

2. Mirtazapine is metabolized in the liver primarily by oxidation and demethylation. It is metabolized by several p450 enzymes including 2D6, 1A2, 3A4, and 2C9. Mirtazapine's t 1/2 is 20 to 40 hours, and it is 85 percent protein bound.

3. Some side effects may be greater at lower doses. Sedation appears more pronounced at doses of 15 mg daily than at 30 mg daily. Dosing is most frequently started at 15 mg daily and can be increased to 30 mg or 45 mg daily as needed in one- to two-week intervals. Dosing may be initiated at 30 mg or more in order to reduce sedation.

4. **Side effects** of mirtazapine are sedation, weight gain, and dry mouth. Many patients report a significant increase in appetite. Mirtazapine may have less propensity to cause sexual dysfunction than the SSRIs, TCAs, and MAOIs. Two out of 2796 patients developed agranulocytosis, and a third developed neutropenia. All recovered after the medication was discontinued. There

are no FDA recommendations to monitor white blood cell counts. Mild transaminase elevations have been noted in some patients.

G. Electroconvulsive therapy. Electroconvulsive therapy (ECT) is highly effective in patients with psychotic depression. Patients who continue to have severe melancholic depression on maximum medical therapy also do well with ETC. The quick response and low side-effect profile make ECT one of the most effective ways to alleviate the symptoms of major depression. The relapse rate after ECT is high, and drug therapy should continue following cessation of ETC.

References, see page 372.

Generalized Anxiety Disorder

Generalized anxiety disorder (GAD) is characterized by excessive worry and anxiety that are difficult to control and cause significant distress and impairment. Commonly patients develop symptoms of GAD secondary to other DSM-IV diagnoses such as panic disorder, major depression, alcohol abuse, or an axis II personality disorder.

I. **Epidemiology.** GAD is a common anxiety disorder. The prevalence is estimated to be 5 percent in the primary care setting. Twice as many women as men have the disorder. GAD may also be associated with substance abuse, post-traumatic stress disorder, and obsessive compulsive disorder. Between 35 and 50 percent of individuals with major depression meet criteria for GAD.

II. **Clinical manifestations and diagnosis**

A. **The diagnostic criteria for GAD** suggest that patients experience excessive anxiety and worry about a number of events or activities, occurring more days than not for at least six months, that are out of proportion to the likelihood or impact of feared events. Affected patients also present with somatic symptoms, including fatigue, muscle tension, memory loss, and insomnia, and other psychiatric disorders.

DSM-IV-PC Diagnostic Criteria for Generalized Anxiety Disorder

1. Excessive anxiety and worry about a number of events or activities, occurring more days than not for at least six months, that are out of proportion to the likelihood or impact of feared events.
2. The worry is pervasive and difficult to control.
3. The anxiety and worry are associated with three (or more) of the following six symptoms (with at least some symptoms present for more days than not for the past six months):
   Restlessness or feeling keyed up or on edge
   Being easily fatigued
   Difficulty concentrating or mind going blank
   Irritability
   Muscle tension
   Sleep disturbance (difficulty falling or staying asleep, or restless unsatisfying sleep)
4. The anxiety, worry, or physical symptoms cause clinically significant distress or impairment in social, occupational, or other important areas of functioning.

B. **Comorbid psychiatric disorders** and an organic etiology for anxiety must be excluded by careful history taking, a complete physical examination, and appropriate laboratory studies. The medical history should focus upon current medical disorders, medication side effects, or substance abuse to anxiety (or panic) symptoms.

    C. Psychosocial history should screen for major depression and agoraphobia, stressful life events, family psychiatric history, current social history, substance abuse history (including caffeine, nicotine, and alcohol), and past sexual, physical and emotional abuse, or emotional neglect.

    D. Laboratory studies include a complete blood count, chemistry panel, serum thyrotropin (TSH) and urinalysis. Urine or serum toxicology measurements or drug levels can be obtained for drugs or medications suspected in the etiology of anxiety.

III. Treatment

    A. Drug therapy. While benzodiazepines have been the most traditionally used drug treatments for GAD, selective serotonin reuptake inhibitors (SSRIs), selective serotonin and norepinephrine reuptake inhibitors (SNRIs, eg venlafaxine), and buspirone are also effective, and because of their lower side effect profiles and lower risk for tolerance are becoming first-line treatment.

    B. Antidepressants

        1. Venlafaxine SR (Effexor) may be a particularly good choice for patients with coexisting psychiatric illness, such as panic disorder, major depression, or social phobia, or when it is not clear if the patient has GAD, depression, or both. Venlafaxine can be started as venlafaxine XR 37.5 mg daily, with dose increases in increments of 37.5 mg every one to two weeks until a dose of 150 mg to 300 mg is attained.

    C. Tricyclic antidepressants, SSRIs, or SNRIs may be associated with side effects such as restlessness and insomnia. These adverse effects can be minimized by starting at lower doses and gradually titrating to full doses as tolerated.

        1. Selective serotonin reuptake inhibitors

            a. Paroxetine (Paxil) 5 to 10 mg qd, increasing to 20 to 40 mg.

            b. Sertraline (Zoloft) 12.5 to 25 mg qd, increasing to 50 to 200 mg.

            c. Fluvoxamine (Luvox) 25 mg qd, increasing to 100 to 300 mg.

            d. Fluoxetine (Prozac) 5 mg qd, increasing to 20 to 40 mg.

            e. Citalopram (Celexa) 10 mg qd, increasing to 20 to 40 mg.

            f. Side effects of SSRIs include agitation, headache, gastrointestinal symptoms (diarrhea and nausea), and insomnia. About 20 to 35 percent of patients develop sexual side effects after several weeks or months of SSRI therapy, especially a decreased ability to have an orgasm. Addition of bupropion (75 to 150 mg/day in divided doses) or buspirone (10 to 20 mg twice daily) may alleviate decreased libido, diminished sexual arousal, or impaired orgasm.

        2. Imipramine (Tofranil), a starting dose of 10 to 20 mg po at night can be gradually titrated up to 75 to 300 mg each night. Imipramine has anticholinergic and antiadrenergic side effects. Desipramine (Norpramin), 25-200 mg qhs, and nortriptyline (Pamelor), 25 mg tid-qid, can be used as alternatives.

        3. Trazodone (Desyrel) is a serotonergic agent, but because of its side effects (sedation and priapism), it is not an ideal first-line agent. Daily dosages of 200 to 400 mg are helpful in patients who have not responded to other agents.

        4. Nefazodone (Serzone) has a similar pharmacologic profile to trazodone, but it is better tolerated and is a good alternative; 100 mg bid; increase to 200-300 mg bid.

Physical Causes of Anxiety-Like Symptoms

Cardiovascular
Angina pectoris, arrhythmias, congestive heart failure, hypertension, hypovolemia, myocardial infarction, syncope (multiple causes), valvular disease, vascular collapse (shock)
Dietary
Caffeine, monosodium glutamate (Chinese restaurant syndrome), vitamin-deficiency diseases
Drug-related
Akathesia (secondary to antipsychotic drugs), anticholinergic toxicity, digitalis toxicity, hallucinogens, hypotensive agents, stimulants (amphetamines, cocaine, related drugs), withdrawal syndromes (alcohol, sedative-hypnotics), bronchodilators (theophylline, sympathomimetics)
Hematologic
Anemias
Immunologic
Anaphylaxis, systemic lupus erythematosus
Metabolic
Hyperadrenalism (Cushing's disease), hyperkalemia, hyperthermia, hyperthyroidism, hypocalcemia, hypoglycemia, hyponatremia, hypothyroidism, menopause, porphyria (acute intermittent)
Neurologic
Encephalopathies (infectious, metabolic, toxic), essential tremor, intracranial mass lesions, postconcussive syndrome, seizure disorders (especially of the temporal lobe), vertigo
Respiratory
Asthma, chronic obstructive pulmonary disease, pneumonia, pneumothorax, pulmonary edema, pulmonary embolism
Secreting tumors
Carcinoid, insulinoma, pheochromocytoma

D. **Buspirone (BuSpar)** appears to be as effective as the benzodiazepines for the treatment of GAD. However, the onset of action can be several weeks, and there are occasional gastrointestinal side effects. Advantages of using buspirone instead of benzodiazepines include the lack of abuse potential, physical dependence, or withdrawal, and lack of potentiation of alcohol or other sedative-hypnotics. Most patients need to be titrated to doses of 30 to 60 mg per day given in two or three divided doses.

E. **Benzodiazepines.** Several controlled studies have demonstrated the efficacy of benzodiazepines (eg, chlordiazepoxide, diazepam, alprazolam) in the treatment of GAD.

1. Many anxious patients who start on benzodiazepines have difficulty stopping them, particularly since rebound anxiety and withdrawal symptoms can be moderate to severe. Methods of facilitating withdrawal and decreasing rebound symptoms include tapering the medication slowly, converting short-acting benzodiazepines to a long-acting preparation (eg, clonazepam) prior to tapering, and treating the patient with an antidepressant before attempting to taper.

2. Symptoms of anxiety can be alleviated in most cases of GAD with clonazepam (Klonopin) 0.25 to 0.5 mg po bid titrated up to 1 mg bid or tid, or lorazepam (Ativan) 0.5 to 1.0 mg po tid titrated up to 1 mg po tid or qid. Often an antidepressant is prescribed concomitantly. After six to eight weeks, when the antidepressant begins to have its optimal effects, the benzodiazepine usually should be tapered over months, achieving roughly a 10 percent dose reduction per week.

Benzodiazepines Commonly Prescribed for Anxiety Disorders			
Name	Half-life (hours)	Dosage range (per day)	Initial dosage
Alprazolam (Xanax)	14	1 to 4 mg	0.25 to 0.5 mg four times daily
Chlordiazepoxide (Librium)	20	15 to 40 mg	5 to 10 mg three times daily
Clonazepam (Klonopin)	50	0.5 to 4.0 mg	0.5 to 1.0 mg twice daily
Clorazepate (Tranxene)	60	15 to 60 mg	7.5 to 15.0 mg twice daily
Diazepam (Valium)	40	6 to 40 mg	2 to 5 mg three times daily
Lorazepam (Ativan)	14	1 to 6 mg	0.5 to 1.0 mg three times daily
Oxazepam (Serax)	9	30 to 90 mg	15 to 30 mg three times daily

F. Agents with short half-lives, such as oxazepam (Serax), do not cause excessive sedation. These agents should be used in the elderly and in patients with liver disease. They are also suitable for use on an "as-needed" basis. Agents with long half-lives, such as clonazepam (Klonopin), should be used in younger patients who do not have concomitant medical problems. The longer-acting agents can be taken less frequently during the day, patients are less likely to experience anxiety between doses and withdrawal symptoms are less severe.

References, see page 372.

Panic Disorder

Panic disorder is characterized by the occurrence of panic attacks--sudden, unexpected periods of intense fear or discomfort. About 15% of the general population experiences panic attacks; 1.6-3.2% of women and 0.4%-1.7% of men have panic disorder.

I. Clinical evaluation
   A. Panic attacks are manifested by the sudden onset of an overwhelming fear, accompanied by feelings of impending doom, for no apparent reason.

DSM-IV Criteria for panic attack

A discrete period of intense fear or discomfort in which four or more of the following symptoms developed abruptly and reached a peak within 10 minutes.

- Chest pain or discomfort
- Choking
- Depersonalization or derealization
- Dizziness, faintness, or unsteadiness
- Fear of "going crazy" or being out of control
- Fear of dying
- Flushes or chills
- Nausea or gastrointestinal distress
- Palpitations or tachycardia
- Paresthesias
- Shortness of breath (or feelings of smothering)
- Sweating
- Trembling or shaking

B. The essential criterion for panic attack is the presence of 4 of 13 cardiac, neurologic, gastrointestinal, or respiratory symptoms that develop abruptly and reach a peak within 10 minutes. The physical symptoms include shortness of breath, dizziness or faintness, palpitations, accelerated heart rate, and sweating. Trembling, choking, nausea, numbness, flushes, chills, or chest discomfort are also common, as are cognitive symptoms such as fear of dying or losing control.

C. One third of patients develop agoraphobia, or a fear of places where escape may be difficult, such as bridges, trains, buses, or crowded areas. Medications, substance abuse, and general medical conditions such as hyperthyroidism must be ruled out as a cause of the patient's symptoms.

D. The history should include details of the panic attack, its onset and course, history of panic, and any treatment. Questioning about a family history of panic disorder, agoraphobia, hypochondriasis, or depression is important. Because panic disorder may be triggered by marijuana or stimulants such as cocaine, a history of substance abuse must be identified. A medication history, including prescription, over-the-counter, and herbal preparations, is essential.

E. The patient should be asked about stressful life events or problems in daily life that may have preceded onset of the disorder. The extent of any avoidance behavior that has developed or suicidal ideation, self-medication, or exacerbation of an existing medical disorder should be assessed.

Diagnostic criteria for panic disorder without agoraphobia

Recurrent, unexpected panic attacks
And
At least one attack has been followed by at least 1 month of one (or more) of the following:
Persistent concern about experiencing more attacks
Worry about the meaning of the attack or its consequences (fear of losing control, having a heart attack, or "going crazy")
A significant behavioral change related to the attacks
And
Absence of agoraphobia
And
Direct physiological effects of a substance (drug abuse or medication) or general medical condition has been ruled out as a cause of the attacks
And
The panic attacks cannot be better accounted for by another mental disorder

II. Management

A. Patients should reduce or eliminate caffeine consumption, including coffee and tea, cold medications, analgesics, and beverages with added caffeine. Alcohol use is a particularly insidious problem because patients may use drinking to alleviate the panic.

Pharmacologic treatment of panic disorder

Drug	Initial dosage (mg/d)	Therapeutic dosage (mg/d)
SSRIs		
Fluoxetine (Prozac)	5-10	10-60
Fluvoxamine (LuVox)	25-50	25-300
Paroxetine (Paxil)	10-20	20-50
Sertraline (Zoloft)	25-50	50-200
Citalopram (Celexa)	10-20 mg qd	20-40
Benzodiazepines		
Alprazolam (Xanax)	0.5 in divided doses, tid-qid	1-4 in divided doses, tid-qid
Alprazolam XR (Xanax XR)	0.5 to 1 mg/day given once in the morning.	3-6 mg qAM
Clonazepam (Klonopin)	0.5 in divided doses, bid-tid	1-4 in divided doses, bid-tid
Diazepam (Valium)	2.0 in divided doses, bid-tid	2-20 in divided doses, bid
Lorazepam (Ativan)	0.5 in divided doses, bid-tid	1-4 in divided doses, bid-tid
TCAs		
Amitriptyline (Elavil)	10	10-300
Clomipramine (Anafranil)	25	25-300
Desipramine (Norpramin)	10	10-300
Imipramine (Tofranil)	10	10-300
Nortriptyline (Pamelor)	10	10-300
MAOIs		
Phenelzine (Nardil)	1510	15-90
Tranylcypromine (Parnate)		10-30

B. **Selective serotonin reuptake inhibitors (SSRIs)** are an effective, well-tolerated alternative to benzodiazepines and TCAs. SSRIs are superior to either imipramine or alprazolam. They lack the cardiac toxicity and anticholinergic effects of TCAs. Fluoxetine (Prozac), fluvoxamine (LuVox), paroxetine (Paxil), sertraline (Zoloft), and citalopram (Celexa) have shown efficacy for the treatment of panic disorder.

C. **Tricyclic antidepressants (TCAs)** have demonstrated efficacy in treating panic. They are, however, associated with a delayed onset of action and side effects--particularly orthostatic hypotension, anticholinergic effects, weight gain, and cardiac toxicity.

D. **Benzodiazepines**
1. Clonazepam (Klonopin), alprazolam (Xanax), and lorazepam (Ativan), are effective in blocking panic attacks. Advantages include a rapid onset of therapeutic effect and a safe, favorable, side-effect profile. Among the drawbacks are the potential for abuse and dependency, worsening of depressive symptoms, withdrawal symptoms on abrupt discontinuation, anterograde amnesia, early relapse on discontinuation, and inter-dose rebound anxiety.
2. Benzodiazepines are an appropriate first-line treatment only when rapid symptom relief is needed. The most common use for benzodiazepines is to stabilize severe initial symptoms until another treatment (eg, an SSRI or cognitive behavioral therapy) becomes effective.
3. The starting dose of alprazolam is 0.5 mg bid. Approximately 70% of patients will experience a discontinuance reaction characterized by increased anxiety, agitation, and insomnia when alprazolam is tapered. Clonazepam's long duration of effect diminishes the need for multiple daily dosing. Initial symptoms of sedation and ataxia are usually transient.

E. **Monoamine oxidase inhibitors (MAOIs).** MAOIs such phenelzine sulfate (Nardil) may be the most effective agents for blocking panic attacks and for relieving the depression and concomitant social anxiety of panic disorder. Recommended doses range from 45-90 mg/d. MAOI use is limited by adverse effects such as orthostatic hypotension, weight gain, insomnia, risk of hypertensive crisis, and the need for dietary monitoring. MAOIs are often reserved for patients who do not respond to safer drugs.

F. **Beta-blockers** are useful in moderating heart rate and decreasing dry mouth and tremor; they are less effective in relieving subjective anxiety.

References, see page 372.

Insomnia

Insomnia is the perception by patients that their sleep is inadequate or abnormal. Insomnia may affect as many as 69% of adult primary care patients. The incidence of sleep problems increases with age. Younger persons are apt to have trouble falling asleep, whereas older persons tend to have prolonged awakenings during the night.

I. **Causes of insomnia**
A. **Situational stress** concerning job loss or problems often disrupt sleep. Patients under stress may experience interference with sleep onset and early morning awakening. Attempting to sleep in a new place, changes in time zones, or changing bedtimes due to shift work may interfere with sleep.
B. **Drugs associated with insomnia** include antihypertensives, caffeine, diuretics, oral contraceptives, phenytoin, selective serotonin reuptake inhibitors, protriptyline, corticosteroids, stimulants, theophylline, and thyroid hormone.
C. **Psychiatric disorders.** Depression is a common cause of poor sleep, often characterized by early morning awakening. Associated findings include hopelessness, sadness, loss of appetite, and reduced enjoyment of formerly pleasurable activities. Anxiety disorders and substance abuse may cause insomnia.

    D. Medical disorders. Prostatism, peptic ulcer, congestive heart failure, and chronic obstructive pulmonary disease may cause insomnia. Pain, nausea, dyspnea, cough, and gastroesophageal reflux may interfere with sleep.

    E. Obstructive sleep apnea syndrome

        1. This sleep disorder occurs in 5-15% of adults. It is characterized by recurrent discontinuation of breathing during sleep for at least 10 seconds. Abnormal oxygen saturation and sleep patterns result in excessive daytime fatigue and drowsiness. Loud snoring is typical. Overweight, middle-aged men are particularly predisposed. Weight loss can be helpful in obese patients.

        2. Diagnosis is by polysomnography. Use of hypnotic agents is contraindicated since they increase the frequency and the severity of apneic episodes.

II. Clinical evaluation of insomnia

    A. Evaluation should include a review of sleep habits, drug and alcohol consumption, medical, psychiatric, and neurologic illnesses, pain, sleep environment, and family history. The physical examination should exclude asthma or congestive heart failure, which may contribute to the patient's sleep problem.

    B. Sleep history. The onset, frequency, duration, and severity of sleep complaints should be assessed. The progression of symptoms, fluctuations over time, and any possible precipitating events should be evaluated.

        1. A sudden onset suggests that a change in sleep environment or a stressful life event may be responsible. Persistent insomnia is usually a consequence of medical, neurologic, or psychiatric disease; persistent insomnia can also result from primary sleep disorders, including restless leg syndrome.

        2. The evaluation should determine if sleep difficulties involve initiation or maintenance of sleep.

        3. Specific symptoms that occur around sleep onset should be sought, including paresthesia or other unpleasant sensations and uncontrollable limb movements of restless leg syndrome; eg, repeated awakenings, snoring, or cessation of breathing in sleep apnea syndromes should be sought; daytime fatigue, irritability, or lack of concentration should be evaluated.

        4. Frequent awakenings may be seen when insomnia occurs secondary to drugs or underlying medical conditions; early morning awakenings frequently occur secondary to anxiety or depression.

        5. The patient's functional status and mood during the daytime should be assessed. Episodes of unintentional sleep are suggestive of sleep apnea syndrome or narcolepsy.

    C. Alcohol and drug history. The patient should be questioned about the use of drugs that can directly cause insomnia (eg, central nervous system stimulants, beta blockers, bronchodilators, corticosteroids), and about withdrawal of central nervous system depressant drugs (eg, sedatives, hypnotics, corticosteroids). Alcohol, caffeine, and tobacco consumption should also be documented, since they can adversely affect sleep.

    D. Psychiatric history. Symptoms or history of depression, anxiety, psychosis, or unusually stressful life events. Sleep disorders that occur secondary to psychiatric illness respond in most cases to psychotherapeutic modalities; an additional cause of disturbed sleep or a primary sleep disorder should be suspected if insomnia complaints.

    E. Medical, neurologic, and family history. A thorough history of medical and neurologic complaints and past illnesses should be obtained to detect potential causes of secondary insomnia. A family history of insomnia may suggest certain primary sleep disorders. A positive family history is found in about one-third of patients with idiopathic restless leg syndrome.

    F. Physical examination. A careful physical examination may direct attention to medical disorders involving the respiratory, cardiovascular, gastrointestinal, endocrine, or neurologic systems. A wide variety of medical conditions or their treatment may result in insomnia.

Medical causes of insomnia

Congestive cardiac failure
Ischemic heart disease
Nocturnal angina
Chronic obstructive pulmonary disease (COPD)
Bronchial asthma including nocturnal asthma
Peptic ulcer disease
Reflux esophagitis
Rheumatic disorders
Lyme disease
Acquired immunodeficiency syndrome (AIDS)
Chronic fatigue syndrome

III. **Laboratory evaluation** may suggest an underlying medical diagnosis in patients with other suggestive historical or physical findings.
   A. **Polysomnography (PSG).** Formal sleep studies are rarely indicated in the initial evaluation of insomnia. PSG may be useful in the following situations:
   1. A sleep-related breathing disorder is suspected.
   2. Insomnia has been present for more than six months, and medical, neurologic, and psychiatric causes have been excluded.
   3. Insomnia has not responded to behavioral or pharmacologic treatment.
IV. **Pharmacologic management**
   A. Hypnotics are the primary drugs used in the management of insomnia. These drugs include the benzodiazepines and the benzodiazepine receptor agonists in the imidazopyridine or pyrazolopyrimidine classes.

Recommended dosages of hypnotic medications (elderly dosages are in parentheses)

Benzodiazepine hypnotics	Recommended dose, mg	T_{max}	Elimination half-life	Receptor selectivity
Benzodiazepine receptor agonists				
Zolpidem (Ambien)	5-10 (5)	1.6	2.6	Yes
Zaleplon (Sonata)	5-10 (5)	1	1	Yes
Eszopiclone (Lunesta)	2-3 (1-2)	1	6	Yes
Hypnotic Medications				
Estazolam (ProSom)	1-2 (0.5-1)	2.7	17.1	No
Flurazepam (Dalmane)	15-30 (15)	1	47.0-100	No
Triazolam (Halcion)	0.250 (0.125)	1.2	2.6	No
Temazepam (Restoril)	7.5-60 (7.5-20)	0.8	8.4	No

Benzodiazepine hypnotics	Recommended dose, mg	T_{max}	Elimination half-life	Receptor selectivity
Quazepam (Doral)	7.5-15.0 (7.5)	2	73	No

B. Zolpidem (Ambien) and zaleplon (Sonata) have the advantage of achieving hypnotic effects with less tolerance and fewer adverse effects.

C. The safety profile of these benzodiazepines and benzodiazepine receptor agonists is good; lethal overdose is rare, except when benzodiazepines are taken with alcohol. Sedative effects may be enhanced when benzodiazepines are used in conjunction with other central nervous system depressants.

D. Zolpidem (Ambien) is a benzodiazepine agonist with a short elimination half-life that is effective in inducing sleep onset and promoting sleep maintenance. Zolpidem may be associated with greater residual impairment in memory and psychomotor performance than zaleplon.

E. Zaleplon (Sonata) is a benzodiazepine receptor agonist that is rapidly absorbed (T_{MAX} = 1 hour) and has a short elimination half-life of 1 hour. Zaleplon does not impair memory or psychomotor functioning at as early as 2 hours after administration, or on morning awakening. Zaleplon does not cause residual impairment when the drug is given in the middle of the night. Zaleplon can be used at bedtime or after the patient has tried to fall asleep naturally.

F. Eszopiclone (Lunesta) is a benzodiazepine receptor agonist with a half-life of 6 hours. It is approved for prolonged use; the use of the other agents is restricted to 35 days.

G. Benzodiazepines with long half-lives, such as flurazepam (Dalmane), may be effective in promoting sleep onset and sustaining sleep. These drugs may have effects that extend beyond the desired sleep period, however, resulting in daytime sedation or functional impairment. Patients with daytime anxiety may benefit from the residual anxiolytic effect of a long-acting benzodiazepine administered at bedtime. Benzodiazepines with intermediate half-lives, such as temazepam (Restoril), facilitate sleep onset and maintenance with less risk of daytime residual effects.

H. Benzodiazepines with short half-lives, such as triazolam (Halcion), are effective in promoting the initiation of sleep but may not contribute to sleep maintenance.

I. Sedating antidepressants are sometimes used as an alternative to benzodiazepines or benzodiazepine receptor agonists. Amitriptyline (Elavil), 25-50 mg at bedtime, or trazodone (Desyrel), 50-100 mg, are common choices.

References, see page 372.

Nicotine Dependence

Smoking causes approximately 430,000 smoking deaths each year, accounting for 19.5% of all deaths. Daily use of nicotine for several weeks results in physical dependence. Abrupt discontinuation of smoking leads to nicotine withdrawal within 24 hours. The symptoms include craving for nicotine, irritability, frustration, anger, anxiety, restlessness, difficulty in concentrating, and mood swings. Symptoms usually last about 4 weeks.

I. Drugs for treatment of nicotine dependance

A. Treatment with nicotine is the only method that produces significant withdrawal rates. Nicotine replacement comes in three forms: nicotine polacrilex gum (Nicorette), nicotine transdermal patches (Habitrol, Nicoderm, Nicotrol), and nicotine nasal spray (Nicotrol NS) and inhaler (Nicotrol). Nicotine patches provide steady-state nicotine levels, but do not provide a bolus of nicotine on demand as do sprays and gum.

B. Bupropion (Zyban) is an antidepressant shown to be effective in treating the craving for nicotine. The symptoms of nicotine craving and withdrawal are reduced with the use of bupropion, making it a useful adjunct to nicotine replacement systems.

Treatments for nicotine dependence

Drug	Dosage	Comments
Nicotine gum (Nicorette)	2- or 4-mg piece/30 min	Available OTC; poor compliance
Nicotine patch (Habitrol, Nicoderm CQ)	1 patch/d for 6-12 wk, then taper for 4 wk	Available OTC; local skin reactions
Nicotine nasal spray (Nicotrol NS)	1-2 doses/h for 6-8 wk	Rapid nicotine delivery; nasal irritation initially
Nicotine inhaler (Nicotrol Inhaler)	6-16 cartridges/d for 12 wk	Mimics smoking behavior; provides low doses of nicotine
Bupropion (Zyban)	150 mg/day for 3 d, then titrate to 300 mg	Treatment initiated 1 wk before quit day; contraindicated with seizures, anorexia, heavy alcohol use

C. Nicotine polacrilex (Nicorette) is available OTC. The patient should use 1-2 pieces per hour. A 2-mg dose is recommended for those who smoke fewer than 25 cigarettes per day, and 4 mg for heavier smokers. It is used for 6 weeks, followed by 6 weeks of tapering. Nicotine gum improves smoking cessation rates by about 40%-60%. Drawbacks include poor compliance and unpleasant taste.

D. Transdermal nicotine (Habitrol, Nicoderm, Nicotrol) doubles abstinence rates compared with placebo, The patch is available OTC and is easier to use than the gum. It provides a plateau level of nicotine at about half that of what a pack-a-day smoker would normally obtain. The higher dose should be used for 6-12 weeks followed by 4 weeks of tapering.

E. Nicotine nasal spray (Nicotrol NS) is available by prescription and is a good choice for patients who have not been able to quit with the gum or patch or for heavy smokers. It delivers a high level of nicotine, similar to smoking. Nicotine nasal spray doubles the rates of sustained abstinence. The spray is used 6-8 weeks, at 1-2 doses per hour (one puff in each nostril). Tapering over about 6 weeks. Side effects include nasal and throat irritation, headache, and eye watering.

F. Nicotine inhaler (Nicotrol Inhaler) delivers nicotine orally via inhalation from a plastic tube. It is available by prescription and has a success rate of 28%, similar to nicotine gum. The inhaler has the advantage of avoiding some of the adverse effects of nicotine gum, and its mode of delivery more closely resembles the act of smoking.

G. Bupropion (Zyban)

1. Bupropion is appropriate for patients who have been unsuccessful using nicotine replacement. Bupropion reduces withdrawal symptoms and can be used in conjunction with nicotine replacement therapy. The treatment is associated with reduced weight gain. Bupropion is contraindicated with a history of seizures, anorexia, heavy alcohol use, or head trauma.

2. Bupropion is started at a dose of 150 mg daily for 3 days and then increased to 300 mg daily for 2 weeks before the patient stops smoking. Bupropion is then continued for 3 months. When a nicotine patch is added to this regimen, the abstinence rates increase to 50% compared with 32% when only the patch is used.

References

References are available at www.ccspublishing.com.

Index

Order Form

Current Clinical Strategies books can also be purchased at all medical bookstores

Title	Book	CD
Treatment Guidelines in Medicine, 2008 Edition	$19.95	$36.95
Psychiatry History Taking, Third Edition	$12.95	$28.95
Psychiatry, 2008 Edition	$12.95	$28.95
Pediatric Drug Reference, 2004 Edition	$9.95	$28.95
Anesthesiology, 2008 Edition	$16.95	$28.95
Medicine, 2007 Edition	$16.95	$28.95
Pediatric Treatment Guidelines, 2007 Edition	$19.95	$29.95
Physician's Drug Manual	$9.95	$28.95
Surgery, Sixth Edition	$12.95	$28.95
Gynecology and Obstetrics, 2008 Edition	$16.95	$30.95
Pediatrics, 2007 Edition	$12.95	$28.95
Family Medicine, 2008 Edition	$26.95	$46.95
History and Physical Examination in Medicine, Tenth Edition	$14.95	$28.95
Outpatient and Primary Care Medicine, 2008 Edition	$16.95	$28.95
Critical Care Medicine, 2007 Edition	$16.95	$32.95
Handbook of Psychiatric Drugs, 2008 Edition	$14.95	$28.95
Pediatric History and Physical Examination, Fourth Edition	$12.95	$28.95
Current Clinical Strategies CD-ROM Collection for Palm, Pocket PC, Windows, and Macintosh		$59.95

CD-ROMs are compatible with Palm, Pocket PC, Windows and Macintosh.

Quantity	Title	Amount

Order by Phone: 800-331-8227 or 949-348-8404
Fax: 800-965-9420 or 949-348-8405
Internet Orders: http://www.ccspublishing.com/ccs
Mail Orders:

> Current Clinical Strategies Publishing
> PO Box 1753
> Blue Jay, CA 92317

Credit Card Number: _____

Exp: ____/____

A shipping charge of $5.00 will be added to each order

Signature: _____

Phone Number: (_____)_____

Name and Address (please print):

_____

_____

_____

_____